Quality and Performance Improvement in Healthcare

Theory, Practice, and Management

Eighth Edition

Patricia Shaw, EdD, RHIA, FAHIMA,
and Darcy Carter, DHSc, MHA, RHIA

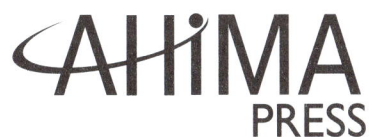

Copyright ©2025 by the American Health Information Management Association. All rights reserved. Except as permitted under the Copyright Act of 1976, no part of this publication may be reproduced, stored in a retrieval system, or transmitted, in any form or by any means, electronic, photocopying, recording, or otherwise, without the prior written permission of AHIMA, 35 West Wacker Ste. 1600, Chicago, Illinois, 60601-5809 (https://www.ahima.org/reprint).

ISBN: **978-1-58426-966-3**
eISBN: **978-1-58426-967-0**
AHIMA Product No.: AB102723

AHIMA Staff:
Jasmine T. Agnew, DHPE, MHIIM, RHIA, CPHIMS, Senior Vice President of Academic Affairs and Professional Credentials
Christine Scheid, Content Development Manager
Rachel Schratz, MA, Associate Digital Content Developer

Cover image: © natrot: iStock

Limit of Liability/Disclaimer of Warranty: This book is sold, as is, without warranty of any kind, either express or implied. While every precaution has been taken in the preparation of this book, the publisher and author assume no responsibility for errors or omissions. Neither is any liability assumed for damages resulting from the use of the information or instructions contained herein. It is further stated that the publisher and author are not responsible for any damage or loss to your data or your equipment that results directly or indirectly from your use of this book.

The websites listed in this book were current and valid as of the date of publication. However, webpage addresses and the information on them may change at any time. Users are encouraged to perform their own general web searches to locate any site addresses listed here that are no longer valid.

CPT® is a registered trademark of the American Medical Association. All other copyrights and trademarks mentioned in this book are the possession of their respective owners. AHIMA makes no claim of ownership by mentioning products that contain such marks.

For more information, including updates, about AHIMA Press publications, visit **https://www.ahima.org/education-events/education-by-product/books/**.

American Health Information Management Association
35 West Wacker Ste. 1600
Chicago, Illinois 60601-5809
ahima.org

Contents

Detailed Table of Contents	v
About the Authors	xvii
Preface	xix
Acknowledgments	xxiii

Part I A Performance Improvement Model — 1

Chapter 1	Introduction and History of Performance Improvement	3
Chapter 2	Defining a Performance Improvement Model	23
Chapter 3	Identifying Improvement Opportunities Based on Performance Measurement	41
Chapter 4	Using Teamwork in Performance Improvement	53
Chapter 5	Aggregating and Analyzing Performance Improvement Data	69
Chapter 6	Communicating Performance Improvement Activities and Recommendations	95

Part II Continuous Monitoring and Improvement Functions — 105

Chapter 7	Measuring Customer Satisfaction	107
Chapter 8	Refining the Continuum of Care	125
Chapter 9	Improving the Provision of Care, Treatment, and Services	147
Chapter 10	Preventing and Controlling Infectious Disease	163
Chapter 11	Managing Risk Exposure	181
Chapter 12	Building a Safe Medication Management System	205
Chapter 13	Managing the Environment of Care	219
Chapter 14	Developing Staff and Human Resources	261

Part III	Management of Performance Improvement Programs	291
Chapter 15	Organizing and Evaluating Performance Improvement	293
Chapter 16	Navigating the Accreditation, Certification, and Licensure Process	319
Chapter 17	Implementing Effective Information Management Tools for Performance Improvement	343
Chapter 18	Managing Healthcare Performance Improvement Projects	361
Chapter 19	Managing the Human Side of Change	377
Chapter 20	Understanding the Legal Implications of Performance Improvement	387

Glossary 397
Check Your Understanding Answer Key 407
Index 423

On the Website:
Student Review Quizzes

Detailed Contents

QI Toolbox Techniques Table of Contents	xv
About the Authors	xvii
Preface for Students	xix
Preface for Educators and Practitioners	xxi
Acknowledgments	xxiii

Part I   A Performance Improvement Model   1

Chapter 1   Introduction and History of Performance Improvement   3

Early Quality and Performance Improvements in Healthcare	4
Healthcare Institutions	4
Medical Practice	6
Nursing Practice	7
Other Health Professions	8
Historically Significant Contributions of Individual Healthcare Professionals	8
Hospital Standardization and Accreditation	9
Check Your Understanding 1.1	10
Quality, PI, and Modern Healthcare	11
Medicare and Medicaid Programs	11
Managed Care	13
Paying for Value	13
Accountable Care Organizations	13
Increased Transparency	13
Check Your Understanding 1.2	14
Evolution of Quality in Healthcare	14
Check Your Understanding 1.3	18
Why Care About Quality and PI?	18
Case Study	19
Review Questions	19
References	19
Resources	21

Chapter 2   Defining a Performance Improvement Model   23

Performance Improvement as a Cyclical Process	24
Monitoring Performance through Data Collection	27
Team-Based PI Processes	30

	Check Your Understanding 2.1	31
	Systems Thinking	31
	Systems Analysis Tools	32
	Systems Control Tools	32
	Check Your Understanding 2.2	33
	Performance Improvement Frameworks	33
	Six Sigma	33
	Lean	34
	Lean Six Sigma	35
	High Reliability Organizations	35
	Check Your Understanding 2.3	36
	Real-Life Example	36
	Case Study	37
	Review Questions	38
	References	38
	Resources	39
Chapter 3	**Identifying Improvement Opportunities Based on Performance Measurement**	**41**
	Continuous Improvement Builds on Continuous Monitoring: Steps to Success	43
	Step 1: Identify Performance Measures	43
	Step 2: Identify the Customers for Each Monitored Process	45
	Step 3: Identify Customers' Actual Requirements with Respect to the Outcomes	45
	Step 4: Determine if the Outcomes of Current Processes Meet Customers' Requirements	46
	Check Your Understanding 3.1	46
	QI Toolbox Techniques	47
	Brainstorming	47
	Affinity Diagrams	47
	Nominal Group Technique	47
	Check Your Understanding 3.2	48
	Real-Life Example #1	48
	Real-Life Example #2	49
	Case Study	50
	Review Questions	51
	References	51
	Resources	52
Chapter 4	**Using Teamwork in Performance Improvement**	**53**
	Effective Teams and Team Composition	54
	Team Roles	55
	Team Charters	57
	Check Your Understanding 4.1	57
	Mission, Vision, and Values Statements	59
	Ground Rules for Meetings	61
	Problem-Solving Techniques, Listening, and Questioning	62
	People Issues	63
	Check Your Understanding 4.2	64
	QI Toolbox Technique	64
	Agenda	64
	Team Charter	65
	Real-Life Example #1	65

	Real-Life Example #2	66
	Real-Life Example #3	66
	Case Study	67
	Review Questions	68
	Reference	68
	Resources	68

Chapter 5   Aggregating and Analyzing Performance Improvement Data — 69

- Data Collection Tools — 72
  - *Check Sheets* — 72
  - *Types of Data* — 73
- Check Your Understanding 5.1 — 76
- Management of Data Sets — 77
- Analysis of Data — 78
  - *Data Quality* — 78
  - *Statistical Analysis* — 79
  - *Artificial Intelligence* — 82
  - *Predictive Analytics* — 83
- Check Your Understanding 5.2 — 83
- QI Toolbox Techniques — 84
  - *Bar Graphs* — 84
  - *Histograms* — 84
  - *Pareto Charts* — 85
  - *Pie Charts* — 86
  - *Pivot Tables* — 86
  - *Line Charts* — 87
  - *Control Charts* — 87
  - *Scatter Diagram* — 88
- Real-Life Example — 89
- Check Your Understanding 5.3 — 91
- Case Study — 91
- Review Questions — 93
- References — 93
- Resources — 94

Chapter 6   Communicating Performance Improvement Activities and Recommendations — 95

- Minutes — 96
- Quarterly Report — 98
- Check Your Understanding 6.1 — 99
- Storytelling — 99
  - *Methods of Storytelling* — 99
  - *Benefits of Storytelling* — 100
- QI Toolbox Technique: Report Cards — 101
- Check Your Understanding 6.2 — 101
- Real-Life Example — 101
- Case Study — 102
- Review Questions — 103
- References — 103
- Resources — 103

Part II Continuous Monitoring and Improvement Functions — 105

Chapter 7 Measuring Customer Satisfaction — 107

Types of Customers — 108
Check Your Understanding 7.1 — 111
Monitoring and Improving Customer Satisfaction: Steps to Success — 111
   Step 1: Identify Internal and External Customers — 112
   Step 2: Identify Products and Services Important to Customers — 112
   Step 3: Identify Quality Measures and Satisfaction Scales for Each Product and Service — 113
   Step 4: Collect and Aggregate Data on Each Performance Measure — 114
   Step 5: Analyze and Compare Collected Data — 114
   Step 6: Identify Opportunities for Improvement — 115
Check Your Understanding 7.2 — 115
QI Toolbox Techniques — 115
   Survey Design — 115
   Interview Design — 118
Check Your Understanding 7.3 — 118
Real-Life Example — 119
Case Study — 121
Review Questions — 122
References — 122
Resources — 123

Chapter 8 Refining the Continuum of Care — 125

Healthcare in the US — 127
Shift to Paying for Value — 131
   Medicare's Hospital Value-Based Purchasing Program — 131
   Hospital Outpatient Quality Reporting Program — 133
   Physician Practice Program — 133
   Ambulatory Surgical Center Quality Reporting Program — 134
   Other Medicare Value-Based Programs — 134
   Hospital Readmission Reduction Program — 135
Check Your Understanding 8.1 — 135
Refining the Continuum of Care: Steps to Success — 135
   Step 1: Perform Preadmission Care Planning — 136
   Step 2: Perform Care Planning at the Time of Admission — 136
   Step 3: Review the Progress of Care — 137
   Step 4: Conduct Discharge Planning — 138
   Step 5: Conclude Postdischarge Planning — 138
Check Your Understanding 8.2 — 138
QI Toolbox Techniques — 139
   Indicators — 139
   Gantt Charts — 142
Check Your Understanding 8.3 — 142
Real-Life Example — 142
Case Study — 144
Review Questions — 144
References — 145
Resources — 145

Chapter 9 Improving the Provision of Care, Treatment, and Services — 147

The Patient Care Process Cycle — 148

Core Process 1: Assessing the Patient's Needs	149
Core Process 2: Planning Care, Treatment, and Services	150
Core Process 3: Providing Care, Treatment, and Services	151
Core Process 4: Coordinating Care, Treatment, and Services	151
Check Your Understanding 9.1	153
Optimizing Patient Care: Steps to Success	153
Step 1: Conduct Patient Care Outcomes Review	153
Step 2: Conduct Evaluations of the Organization's Use of Seclusion, Restraints, and Protective Devices	154
Step 3: Conduct Evaluations of Laboratory Services and the Use of Blood Products	155
Step 4: Conduct Evaluations of the Organization's Medication Systems and Processes	155
Step 5: Conduct Policy, Procedure, and Documentation Review	156
Step 6: Evaluate the Organization's Standards of Care and Care Pathways	156
Check Your Understanding 9.2	156
Ongoing Developments	157
Focus on Patient Safety: National Patient Safety Goals	157
National Standardization of Care Processes	158
Patient-Centered Care Initiatives	158
Long-Term Care and Home Healthcare Monitoring	159
Check Your Understanding 9.3	160
Real-Life Example	160
Case Study	161
Review Questions	161
References	162
Resources	162

Chapter 10 Preventing and Controlling Infectious Disease — 163

Managing Infectious Disease: Steps to Success	165
Step 1: Control Infection through the Use of Standard Precautions	167
Step 2: Conduct Ongoing Infection Surveillance and Epidemiologic Investigations	167
Step 3: Conduct Educational and Screening Programs	169
Check Your Understanding 10.1	170
QI Toolbox Technique: Flow Chart	170
Real-Life Example #1	171
Real-Life Example #2	177
Case Study	177
Review Questions	179
References	179
Resources	180

Chapter 11 Managing Risk Exposure — 181

Patient Rights	182
Risk	185
Check Your Understanding 11.1	186
Managing Risk Exposure: Steps to Success	186
Step 1: The Healthcare Organization Develops a Risk Management Plan, Policies, and Procedures	188
Step 2: The Risk Management Team Teaches Risk Management Concepts and Principles to All Employees	188
Step 3: The Team Evaluates Occurrence Reports	188
Step 4: The Risk Management Team Examines Structure, Process, and Knowledge Issues	195

Step 5: The Team Identifies Practice Patterns, Trends in Risk Occurrences, and Sentinel Events	195
Step 6: The Team Provides Direction in the Patient Advocacy Function	197
Step 7: The Team Communicates All Relevant Data and Information to Legal Support When PCEs Occur	197
Step 8: The Risk Team and Legal Counsel Lead the Development of an Appropriate Insurance Strategy for the Organization	198
Check Your Understanding 11.2	198
QI Toolbox Techniques	198
Cause-and-Effect Diagram	199
Root-Cause Analysis	200
Check Your Understanding 11.3	201
Case Study	202
Review Questions	202
References	203
Resources	203

Chapter 12 Building a Safe Medication Management System — 205

Building a Safe and Effective Medication Management System: Steps to Success	207
Step 1: Select and Procure Medications	209
Step 2: Properly and Safely Store Medications	209
Step 3: Order (Prescribe) and Transcribe Medications	210
Step 4: Prepare and Dispense Medications	211
Step 5: Administer Medications	212
Step 6: Monitor the Effects of Medications on Patients	213
Step 7: Evaluate the Medication Management System	214
Check Your Understanding 12.1	215
QI Toolbox Technique: Failure Mode and Effects Analysis	215
Real-Life Example	216
Case Study	217
Review Questions	217
References	218
Resources	218

Chapter 13 Managing the Environment of Care — 219

Improving the Environment of Care: Steps to Success	220
Step 1: Monitor and Improve the Safety Management Program	221
Step 2: Monitor and Improve the Security Management Program	221
Step 3: Monitor and Improve the Hazardous Materials and Waste Management Program	227
Step 4: Monitor and Improve the Emergency Operations Plan	233
Step 5: Monitor and Improve the Life (Fire Prevention) Safety Management Plan	245
Step 6: Monitor and Improve the Medical Equipment Management Program	247
Step 7: Monitor and Improve the Utilities Management Program	248
Check Your Understanding 13.1	253
Criteria for an Annual Evaluation	253
Information Collection and Evaluation System	255
QI Toolbox Technique: Postprogram Assessment	256
Check Your Understanding 13.2	257
Real-Life Example	257
Case Study	257

	Review Questions	258
	References	258
	Resources	259

Chapter 14 Developing Staff and Human Resources — 261

- Steps to Success: Developing Staff and Human Resources — 263
  - *Step 1: Manage the Recruitment Process* — 263
  - *Step 2: Onboarding of New Employees* — 267
  - *Step 3: Manage the Performance Appraisal Process* — 268
  - *Step 4: Manage the Retention Process* — 268
  - *Step 5: Credential and Extend Privileges to Providers* — 269
- QI Toolbox Technique: Provider Profile Summary — 271
- Check Your Understanding 14.1 — 271
- Real-Life Example — 272
- Case Study — 273
- Review Questions — 289
- Resources — 289

Part III Management of Performance Improvement Programs — 291

Chapter 15 Organizing and Evaluating Performance Improvement — 293

- Leading PI Activities — 294
- Strategic Planning — 296
- Check Your Understanding 15.1 — 297
- PI Plan Design — 297
- Decision Matrix — 305
- Implementing the PI Plan — 306
- Check Your Understanding 15.2 — 307
- Evaluating the Performance Improvement Program — 307
  - *Components of Program Review* — 308
- Check Your Understanding 15.3 — 311
- Managing the Board of Directors' PI Activities — 311
- Other Resources for PI Programs — 314
  - *Standing Committees of the Medical Staff* — 314
  - *PI Education* — 314
  - *Formal Quality Management Structures* — 315
- Check Your Understanding 15.4 — 315
- QI Toolbox Techniques — 315
  - *Dashboard* — 315
  - *Decision Matrix* — 316
  - *SWOT Analysis* — 316
- Case Study — 316
- Review Questions — 317
- References — 318
- Resources — 318

Chapter 16 Navigating the Accreditation, Certification, and Licensure Process — 319

- Healthcare Accreditation, Certification, and Licensure Standards — 320
  - *The Joint Commission and Its Accreditation Activities* — 320
  - *DNV Accreditation* — 321

CARF Accreditation ... 321
National Committee for Quality Assurance ... 322
Accreditation Association for Ambulatory Health Care ... 322
CMS Conditions of Participation ... 322
State Licensure ... 322
Check Your Understanding 16.1 ... 323
Development of Policies and Procedures to Meet Multiple Standards and Regulations ... 323
Surviving the Survey Process ... 323
Accreditation of Acute Care and Other Facilities: The Joint Commission ... 324
Survey Team ... 324
Survey Process ... 325
Public Disclosure ... 329
Check Your Understanding 16.2 ... 330
Certification and Licensure of Long-Term Care Facilities: State Departments of Health ... 330
Accreditation of Psychiatric and Rehabilitative Care Facilities: CARF ... 331
Certification: Compliance with the CMS *Conditions of Participation* ... 332
Check Your Understanding 16.3 ... 333
Real-Life Example ... 333
Case Study ... 340
Review Questions ... 340
References ... 341
Resource ... 341

Chapter 17 Implementing Effective Information Management Tools for Performance Improvement ... 343

Data Governance ... 344
Business Intelligence ... 345
Data Repositories ... 346
Information Warehouses ... 352
Web-Based PI Team Collaboration Technologies ... 352
Check Your Understanding 17.1 ... 352
Comparative Performance Data ... 352
Check Your Understanding 17.2 ... 355
Information Resources Management Professionals ... 355
Joint Commission Information Management Standards ... 355
Check Your Understanding 17.3 ... 357
Case Study ... 357
Review Questions ... 359
References ... 359
Resources ... 359

Chapter 18 Managing Healthcare Performance Improvement Projects ... 361

Project Management and Organizational Structure ... 362
Project Life Cycle ... 362
Initiating Processes ... 362
Planning Processes ... 366
Executing Processes ... 368
Monitoring and Controlling Processes ... 369
Closing Processes ... 369
Why Projects Fail ... 370

	Check Your Understanding 18.1	371
	QI Toolbox Techniques	371
	Gantt chart	371
	PERT chart	371
	Real-Life Example	371
	Case Study	373
	Review Questions	374
	References	374
	Resources	375
Chapter 19	**Managing the Human Side of Change**	**377**
	The Three Phases of Change	378
	Phase 1: Unfreezing/Ending	379
	Phase 2: Moving/Transition	379
	Phase 3: Freezing/Beginning	379
	Change Management	380
	Create a Sense of Urgency	380
	Build a Guiding Coalition	380
	Form a Strategic Vision and Initiatives	381
	Enlist a Volunteer Army	381
	Enable Action by Removing Barriers	381
	Generate Short-Term Wins	381
	Sustain Acceleration	382
	Institute Change	382
	Real-Life Example	382
	Check Your Understanding 19.1	383
	Case Study	384
	Review Questions	384
	References	385
	Resources	385
Chapter 20	**Understanding the Legal Implications of Performance Improvement**	**387**
	Tort Law	388
	Four Basic Elements of Negligence or Malpractice	388
	Avoidance of Risk from a Malpractice Perspective	389
	The Organized Medical Staff	390
	Peer Review Protection	390
	Immunity from Liability	391
	Occurrence Reports and Sentinel Events	392
	Responsibility for Disclosing Adverse Events to the Patient or Patient's Family	392
	Distinguishing Quality Improvement from Research	393
	Public Health Activities	394
	Check Your Understanding 20.1	394
	Case Study	394
	Review Questions	395
	References	395

Glossary	397
Check Your Understanding Answer Key	407
Index	423

QI Toolbox Techniques
Table of Contents

Affinity diagrams	47
Agenda	64
Bar graphs	84
Brainstorming	47
Cause-and-effect diagram	199
Control charts	87
Dashboard	315
Decision matrix	316
Failure mode and effects analysis	215
Flow chart	170
Gantt charts	142
Histograms	84
Indicators	139
Interview design	118
Line charts	87
Nominal group technique	47
Pareto charts	85
PERT chart	371
Pie charts	86
Pivot tables	86
Postprogram assessment	256
Provider profile summary	271
Report cards	101
Root-cause analysis	200
Scatter diagram	88
Survey design	115
SWOT analysis	316
Team charter	65

About the Authors

Patricia Shaw, EdD, RHIA, FAHIMA, holds a doctorate and master's degree in education. She is currently professor emeritus at Weber State University. Prior to her position at Weber State, Dr. Shaw managed hospital health information management services departments and was a nosologist for 3M Health Information Systems. Dr. Shaw is also coeditor of *Registered Health Information Administrator (RHIA) Exam Preparation* and *Registered Health Information Technician (RHIT) Exam Preparation* published by AHIMA.

Darcy Carter, DHSc, MHA, RHIA, earned her doctorate degree in health science with an emphasis in leadership and organizational behavior and her master's degree in healthcare administration. Dr. Carter is currently department chair, associate professor, and MHA program director at Weber State University, where she teaches courses in reimbursement, quality management, and healthcare management. Dr. Carter is also coeditor of *Registered Health Information Administrator (RHIA) Exam Preparation* and *Registered Health Information Technician (RHIT) Exam Preparation* published by AHIMA.

Preface for Students

You will soon be entering your chosen profession in the healthcare field. The issues involved in the management of quality in healthcare span the various clinical and administrative disciplines and must be approached from a variety of perspectives. Many improvements for healthcare services are developed through team-based activities. Employers also will expect you to be able to apply performance improvement (PI) data analysis and presentation tools. Prepare now for the possibility that at some point in the future you will be asked to facilitate a PI team meeting.

The authors of this text hope that this tool for programmed, incremental learning of the PI process will prepare you well for the challenges you will face in your new career. If you use this text carefully, you will probably find yourself miles ahead of your fellow students in preparation for today's healthcare environment.

Preface for Educators and Practitioners

This textbook from AHIMA presents a comprehensive introduction to the theory, practice, and management of performance and quality improvement processes for quality of patient care in healthcare organizations. Parts I and II provide a basic background in performance improvement (PI) philosophy and methodology for healthcare practice today. Each chapter has real-life examples and case studies from healthcare settings that bring home the importance of quality in healthcare services. QI toolbox techniques are presented both in theory and in practice so that your students can see how the techniques can actually be used in PI activities. Healthcare information management students will find the textbook's unique step-by-step and case study–based approach to the subject easy to use and understand. Students also will gain hands-on practice applying the analytical and graphic tools used in performance and quality improvement. Integrated into the chapter discussions are student projects that range from designing specific improvement projects to ongoing quality monitoring and managing quality improvement programs and staff.

Part III focuses on the issues inherent in the management of quality and PI programs in healthcare. Each chapter presents the issues and their backgrounds and most conclude with a case study to reinforce student learning and encourage critical thinking about the issues.

Acknowledgments

AHIMA Press would like to thank Angela Campbell, MSHI, RHIA, FAHIMA, AHIMA-Approved ICD-10-CM/PCS Trainer, and Lynn Ward, EdD, RHIA, CPHIMS, for their technical review of this textbook.

Online Resources

For Students

Resources for students include online quizzes to review each section of the book.

For Instructors

Instructor materials for this book are provided only to approved educators. Materials include instructor manual, PowerPoint slides, course plans, test bank, curriculum map, and other useful instructional tools, tips, reminders, and resources. Please visit http://www.ahima.org/publications/educators.aspx for further instruction. If you have any questions regarding the instructor materials, please contact AHIMA Customer Relations at (800) 335-5535 or submit a customer support request at https://my.ahima.org/.

PART I
A Performance Improvement Model

Introduction and History of Performance Improvement

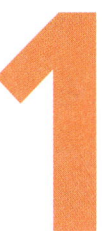

Learning Objectives

- Summarize the historical events that have contributed to modern performance improvement programs
- Relate how key legislation has influenced healthcare quality initiatives
- Illustrate how key individuals and organizations have shaped the theory and developed models for use in performance improvement activities

Key Terms

Accountable care organization (ACO)
Affordable Care Act (ACA)
Cost
Increased transparency
Outcome
Performance improvement (PI)
Process
Prospective payment system

Quality
Quality assurance (QA)
Retrospective payment system
Social determinants of health (SDOH)
Structure
Total quality management (TQM)
Value-based purchasing

People naturally expect their world to improve over time. This expectation affects everything people come into contact with, including food, housing, cars, education, and healthcare, and stimulates general social progress. Progress may take considerable time to develop, and the desire for progress sometimes takes a counterproductive path, as during times of war and political upheaval. Still, the objective of making the human situation better is a constant in human endeavors.

Progress is commonly accomplished in one of two ways. First, progress can be achieved through an understanding of the scientific basis of the natural world and its constituent parts. For example, understanding the way the human body functions through biochemistry facilitated the development of the pharmaceuticals in use today. Second, progress can be achieved through improvements in the ways that people perform their work. For example, understanding the procedures that healthcare professionals must perform to help people get well facilitated the development of one of the best healthcare delivery systems in the world. This textbook examines the second approach to progress.

The focus of this textbook is how US healthcare organizations use **quality** and **performance improvement (PI)** methods to improve healthcare delivery. Quality is defined as the degree or grade of excellence of goods or services. In healthcare, this means meeting expectations for outcomes of care. Performance improvement is the continuous adaptation of a healthcare organization's functions and processes to increase the likelihood of achieving the desired outcomes. For healthcare organizations to improve the quality of care delivered they must be engaged in performance improvement activities. Every healthcare professional needs to understand the issues surrounding quality and PI in healthcare because society expects that healthcare entities will produce progressively better healthcare products and services.

Early Quality and Performance Improvements in Healthcare

There is a long tradition of quality and performance improvement in healthcare, a representation of which is shown in figure 1.1. From colonial times to the present, healthcare in the US has undergone a series of developments and reforms, from the creation of hospitals in the 18th century and the scientific discoveries of the 19th century, to the professionalization of medical and nursing practices in the early 20th century and the technological advances of the late 20th and early 21st centuries. Healthcare institutions, professional associations, individual leaders, and political visionaries all laid the foundations of modern healthcare.

Healthcare Institutions

During the mid-1700s, before the American colonies became a nation, the citizens of Philadelphia, PA, recognized the need for a place to house the mentally ill and to provide relief to the sick and injured. They also recognized the need to sequester newly arrived immigrants, who often contracted diseases during their long voyages as a means of infection control. Thousands of people immigrated to the Pennsylvania colony in an attempt to improve their lives. Although most healthcare was provided in people's homes, established inhabitants, particularly the poor, were sometimes in need of a place to rest and recover during times of illness and injury. Recognizing these needs, Dr. Thomas Bond, with the help of Benjamin Franklin, persuaded the Pennsylvania legislature to undertake the organization and development of a hospital for the community. The famous Pennsylvania Hospital was the first in the growing nation (Morton and Woodbury 1973, 5–7).

Over the next 150 years, the Pennsylvania Hospital became a model for the development of hospitals in other communities. The hospital even standardized its care processes by publishing rules and regulations for its physicians and staff (Morton and Woodbury 1973, 549–552). These regulations represent early attempts at healthcare improvement.

The annals of Massachusetts General Hospital provide an early example of an action taken by a hospital board of trustees to ensure the quality of care provided in the institution. In 1837, the trustees became aware that the son of a resident surgeon (a surgeon who had not attained appointment to the hospital) had practiced in the hospital during his father's absence. The trustees reiterated to all of the medical staff the need for allowing only those accorded privileges at the institution to practice there:

The Trustees have recently seen with great pain, that a violation of the rules of the institution by one of its officers has become the subject of newspaper animadversion. In an institution like this, to which it is so difficult to attract, and in which it is so important to command, public confidence, the strictest and most scrupulous adherence to rules, of which the propriety is unquestioned, is required by a just regard as well to its usefulness to the public, as to the character of those who have any agency in its direction and control. Where many persons are connected in different departments, the reputation of all is more or less affected by the conduct of each; and all are therefore bound, by respect for others as well as themselves to conduct in such a manner as to give no reasonable ground of complaint. (Bowditch 1972, 135)

Figure 1.1. Historical perspectives on quality and PI in healthcare.

1700s and 1800s	1900s	2000s	2010+
Mid-1700s Pennsylvania Hospital becomes the model for the organization and development of hospitals. **1760** New York State begins the practice of medical licensure. **1771** New Jersey begins the practice of medical licensure. **1837** Massachusetts General Hospital sets limitations on clinical practice in the first granting of clinical privileges. **1853** Massachusetts General Hospital establishes the first disease/procedure index by classifying patient disposition. **Mid-1800s** Medical licensure is deemed undemocratic and is stopped. **1872** New England Hospital for Women and Children organizes a general training school for nurses. **1874** American Medical Association (AMA) encourages the creation of independent state licensing boards.	**1903** North Carolina passes the first nurse registration bill in the United States. **1910** Flexner Report indicates unacceptable variation in medical school curricula. **1917** American College of Surgeons (ACS) establishes the Hospital Standardization Program. **1920** Most medical colleges meet rigorous academic by the Association of American Medical Colleges. **1946** Hill-Burton Act establishes funding to build new hospitals. **1952** Joint Commission on Accreditation of Hospitals (JCAH) was formed by the AMA, the American College of Physicians (ACP), the American Hospital Association (AHA), and the Canadian Medical Association (CMA). **1965** Public Law 89–97 establishes Medicare and Medicaid. **1972** Local peer review organizations are formed. **1980s** Prospective payment system is established. State and regional peer review organizations contract with Health Care Financing Administration (HCFA). **1990s** JCAH becomes JCAHO (Joint Commission on Accreditation of Healthcare Organizations). Deming's total quality management (TQM) philosophy begins to spread in US healthcare. JCAHO integrates quality improvement into the accreditation process.	**2001** Ambulatory payment classification system is initiated. **2002** HCFA becomes the Centers for Medicare and Medicaid Services (CMS). **2003** JCAHO implements the National Patient Safety Goals. **2005** JCAHO begins unannounced and tracer methodology surveys. **2007** JCAHO renames itself the Joint Commission. **2008** Medicare Severity diagnosis-related groups (MS-DRGs) are implemented **2009** Health Information Technology for Economic and Clinical Health (HITECH) legislation is passed.	**2010** Patient Protection and Affordable Care Act (ACA) is passed **2015** ICD-10-CM and ICD-10- PCS scheduled for implementation. **2020** Hospital Compare is consolidated with the other CMS "Compare" sites on Care Compare. **2021** Hospital Price Transparency Rule is in effect. **2022** CMS released the CMS Framework for Health Equity

It is also interesting to note that the trustees believed that the expectations of the members of their community—their customers—should be considered.

The annals of Massachusetts General Hospital include other examples of the hospital's concern about service quality. In 1851, the hospital hired a watchman to guard against the danger of fire during the night (Bowditch 1972, 367). In 1853, the hospital commended one of its surgical staff members for compiling an analytical index for the surgical records of the institution and reflecting on the quality of the surgical services provided (Bowditch 1972, 483). In 1872, the trustees decided to regulate the use of restraints at the institution, and they identified each by type and set the conditions under which the restraint could be used (Bowditch 1972, 679–680). Throughout the history of the institution, the trustees received regular reports on the number of patients treated as well as the classification of each patient's outcome at discharge: "well," "relieved," "not relieved," or "dead" (Bowditch 1972, 447).

Medical Practice

Human anatomy and physiology were not well understood before the 20th century. At one time, it was believed that four basic fluids, called *humors,* determined a person's temperament and health and that imbalances in the proportion of humors in the body caused disease. The therapeutic bleeding of patients was practiced into the early 20th century. Early physicians also treated patients by administering a variety of substances with no scientific basis for their effectiveness. The science of medicine began to evolve in the late 19th century but was not fully realized until the second and third decades of the 20th century.

Early on, the medical profession recognized that some of its members achieved better results than others and attempted to regulate the practice of medicine. At first, the regulation took the form of licensure, beginning in New York in 1760 and New Jersey in 1771. The New Jersey law stated that "no person whatsoever shall practice as a physician or surgeon, within this colony of New Jersey, before he shall have first been examined in physic and surgery, approved of, and admitted by any two of the judges of the Supreme Court" (Wickes 1879, 103). The examination was to be performed before a board of "medical men" appointed by the state medical society (Trent 1977, 91). Various states developed similar legislation over the following decades.

However, by the middle of the 19th century, medical licensure had been repudiated as undemocratic, and the penalties for practicing medicine without a license were removed in most states. "Buyer beware" was the rule of thumb because the title of "doctor" could be used by anyone who wanted to sell medical services (Haller 1981, 200–201). During this period, medical education consisted primarily of an apprenticeship with an already established practitioner of some kind. After the apprenticeship, the new doctor could hang out a shingle and begin to treat patients. Some trainees did attend schools that claimed to teach them how to become physicians, but there was no established medical curriculum. Many people received diplomas just by paying a fee. Many others with no education, apprenticeship, or license just hung out a sign and began collecting fees. Effectively, doctoring had become a commercial enterprise. Any man with sufficient entrepreneurial talents could enter the practice of medicine. The emphasis was on making a living rather than joining a true profession. The result was an overabundance of "medical men" who provided medical care based on all kinds of traditions and, at times, no tradition at all.

The American Medical Association (AMA) was established in 1840 to represent the interests of physicians across the US. The organization was dominated by members who had strong ties to medical schools and the status quo. The organization's ability to lead reform was limited until it broke its ties with the medical colleges in 1874. At that time, the association encouraged the creation of independent state licensing boards (Haller 1981, 214).

In 1876, the Association of American Medical Colleges (AAMC) was established. The AAMC was dedicated to standardizing the curriculum of US medical schools and developing the public's appreciation of the need for medical licensure.

Together, the AMA and the AAMC pushed for medical licensing. By the 1890s, 35 states had established or reestablished a system of licensure for physicians. Fourteen states granted medical licenses only to graduates of reputable medical schools. The state licensing boards discouraged the worst medical schools, but the criteria for licensing continued to vary by state and were not fully enforced (Haller 1981, 223).

By the early 20th century, it had become apparent that promoting quality in medical practice required regulation through curriculum reform as well as licensure, but the AMA membership was divided on this issue. Conservative members continued to believe that the organization should stay out of the regulatory arena. Progressive members advocated the continuing development of state licensure systems and the development of a model medical curriculum.

The situation attracted the attention of the Carnegie Foundation for the Advancement of Teaching and its president, Henry S. Pritchett. Pritchett offered to sponsor and fund an independent review of the medical curricula and the medical colleges of the US. The review was undertaken in 1906 by Abraham Flexner, an educator from Louisville, KY (Flexner 1910).

Over the next four years, Flexner visited every medical college in the country and carefully documented his findings. In his 1910 report to the Carnegie Foundation, the AMA, and the AAMC, he documented the unacceptable variation in curricula that existed across the schools. He also noted that applicants to medical schools frequently lacked knowledge of the basic sciences. Flexner reported how the absence of appropriate hospital-based training limited the clinical skills of medical school graduates. Perhaps most importantly, he documented the huge number of graduates produced by the colleges each year, most with unacceptable levels of medical expertise.

Several reform initiatives grew out of Flexner's report and the recommendations made by the AMA's Committee on Medical Education. One reform required medical college applicants to hold a baccalaureate degree. Another required that the medical curriculum be founded in the basic sciences. Reforms also required that medical students receive practical, hospital-based training. Flexner recommended the closing of most medical schools in the country. Most of these recommendations were instituted over the decade after the release of Flexner's report, but only about half of the medical colleges actually closed. By 1920, most of the colleges met rigorous academic standards and were approved by the AAMC.

Nursing Practice

During the 19th century and throughout the first part of the 20th century, more than half of the hospitals in the US were sponsored by religious organizations. Nursing care at that time was usually provided by members of religious orders. As the US population grew and more towns and cities were established, hospitals were built to accommodate the healthcare needs of new communities. Older cities were also growing, and city hospitals became more and more crowded.

In the late 19th century, nurses received no formal education or training. Nursing staffs for the hospitals were often recruited from the surrounding communities, and many poor women who had no other skills became nurses. The nature of nursing care at that time was unsophisticated, and ignorance of basic hygiene often promoted disease rather than wellness. For example, in 1871 at Bellevue Hospital in New York City, 15 percent of patients died while hospitalized, and hospital-acquired infections were common (Kalisch and Kalisch 1995, 71). Even simple surgical procedures and maternity care often resulted in death due to infection.

In 1868, the AMA president, Dr. Samuel Gross, called the medical profession's attention to the need for trained nurses. During the years that followed, the public began to call for better nursing care in hospitals.

A small group of women physicians working in the northeast area of the country created the first formal program for training nurses. Dr. Susan Dimock, working with Dr. Marie Zakrzewska at the New England Hospital for Women and Children, organized a general training school for nurses in 1872 (Kalisch and Kalisch 1995, 67–70). The school became a model for other institutions throughout the US. As hospital after hospital struggled to find competent nursing staff, many institutions developed their own nurse training programs to meet staffing needs.

The responsibilities of nurses in the late 19th and early 20th centuries included housekeeping duties such as cleaning furniture and floors, making beds, changing linens, and controlling temperature, humidity, and ventilation. Nurses also cooked meals for patients in kitchens attached to each ward. Direct patient care duties included giving baths, changing dressings, monitoring vital signs, administering medication, and assisting at surgical procedures (Kalisch and Kalisch 1995, 76–79). Nurses generally worked 12-hour shifts, 7 days per week.

During this time, nurses were not required to hold a license to practice. Because licensure was not required, and because it was difficult to attract women to nursing staff positions, many women who had no training at all continued to work as nurses in the nation's hospitals and as private-duty nurses.

In the years immediately following the turn of the 20th century, nurses began to organize state nursing associations to advocate for the registration of nurses. Their goal was to increase the level of competence among nurses nationwide. Despite opposition from many physicians who believed that nurses did not need formal education or licensure, North Carolina passed the first nurse registration bill in the US in 1903. Many other states initiated similar legislation in subsequent years. Today, all states have carefully developed boards of nursing registration that maintain basic standards for nursing practice, promulgate advanced standards for clinical and managerial nurse specialists, license the professional membership, and require ongoing education for maintenance of nursing skills.

Other Health Professions

In the US other healthcare professions developed as specialized areas of practice during the 20th century. These health professions include radiologic technology, respiratory therapy, occupational therapy, physical therapy, and others. Each specialized area underwent periods of formalization in similar ways. Each became regulated either by the states or by national professional associations as membership and professional responsibilities grew and the public demanded that they document their professional competence. For example, health information professionals are certified and registered by the American Health Information Management Association (AHIMA). These developments made important contributions to the quality of healthcare delivered in the US.

Historically Significant Contributions of Individual Healthcare Professionals

Many individual healthcare professionals have made significant contributions to the early improvement of healthcare delivery in the US, including the development and implementation of a variety of improvement strategies. A small sample of these individuals and their contributions is included here. It is important to recognize the progress that can be made when healthcare professionals care about the quality of their work.

Maude E. Callen, an African American public health nurse-midwife, undertook the training of midwives in coastal South Carolina in 1926. A registered nurse, Callen recognized that the midwives' lack of training contributed to high infant and maternal mortality rates in the region, and she traveled extensively throughout the region to assist at deliveries and improve the expertise of midwives (Hill 1997, 49–54).

Robert Latou Dickinson, an obstetrician and gynecologist practicing in New England around the turn of the 20th century, developed a standardized patient questionnaire. He used the patients' answers on the questionnaire to structure his examinations. His questionnaire represents one of the first uses of a structured health assessment tool in the US (Bullough 1997, 75–78).

Lavinia Lloyd Dock, a nurse and early nurse educator, developed important approaches to disaster nursing at the end of the 19th century. After graduating from a nurse training program, Dock worked to institute appropriate nursing practices during the yellow fever epidemic in Jacksonville, FL, in 1888, and during the aftermath of the Johnstown, PA, flood in 1889 (Leighow 1997, 79–85).

Roswell Park, a physician and surgeon during the late 19th century, helped disseminate the principles of antisepsis during surgical procedures in the US. Park used the findings of English scientist Joseph Lister to advocate for the use of antiseptic techniques and appropriate wound care in the treatment of surgical cases, well before such approaches were common in the US (Gage 1997, 204–208).

Nicholas J. Pisacano, a physician who practiced during the mid- to late 20th century, recognized the need to upgrade the general practitioner's skills as new technologies and treatments were developed. He worked tirelessly to develop and promote the specialty of family practice in the US (Adams and Moore 1997, 222–226).

Ernst P. Boas, a physician who practiced in New York City during the first half of the 20th century, was among the first to call for the coordinated, interdisciplinary care of the chronically ill. Prior to his advocacy, the chronically ill often were considered incurable. He believed that the development of new therapeutics and restorative technologies could return people with chronic illnesses to better health and productivity. His work led to the establishment of the Goldwater Memorial Hospital for Chronic Diseases on Welfare Island in New York City (Brickman 1997, 21).

Mary Steichen Calderone, medical director of the Planned Parenthood Federation of America during the 1950s, launched a clinical investigation program to scientifically identify effective contraceptive methods. Hers was one of the first efforts to identify appropriate clinical practice through the use of scientific evidence in a controversial area (Meldrum 1997, 43–48).

Hospital Standardization and Accreditation

In 1910, Dr. Edward Martin suggested that the surgical area of medical practice become more concerned with patient outcomes. He had been introduced to this concept through discussions with Dr. Ernest Codman, a physician who believed that hospital practitioners should track their patients for a significant time after treatment to determine whether the end result was positive or negative. Dr. Codman also advocated the use of outcome information to identify practices that led to the best results.

Dr. Martin and others had been concerned about the conditions in US hospitals for some time. Many observers felt that part of the problem was related to the absence of organized medical staffs in hospitals and to lax professional standards. In the early 20th century, hospitals were used primarily by surgeons who required their facilities to treat patients with surgical modalities. Therapies based on medical regimens were not developed until later in the century. It was natural, therefore, for the impetus for improvement in hospital care to come from the surgical community.

In November 1912, the Third Clinical Congress of Surgeons of North America was held. At this meeting, Dr. Franklin Martin made a proposal that eventually led to the formation of the American College of Surgeons (ACS). Dr. Edward Martin made the following resolution:

> Be it resolved by the Clinical Congress of Surgeons of North America here assembled, that some system of standardization of hospital equipment and hospital work should be developed to the end that those institutions having the highest ideals may have proper recognition before the profession, and that those of inferior equipment and standards should be stimulated to raise the quality of their work. In this way, patients will receive the best type of treatment, and the public will have some means of recognizing those institutions devoted to the highest levels of medicine. (Roberts et al. 1987, 936)

Through the proposal and the resolution, the ACS and the hospital improvement movement became intimately tied. Immediately upon formation, officers of the college realized how important their work would be. They were forced to reject 60 percent of the fellowship applications during the college's first three years because applicants were unable to provide documentation to support their clinical competence (Roberts et al. 1987, 937). Medical records from many hospitals were so inadequate that they could not supply information about the applicants' practices in the institutions. Because of this situation and many others of which they became aware, in 1917 college officers petitioned the Carnegie Foundation for funding to plan and develop a hospital standardization program.

That same year, the ACS formed a committee on standards and met to consider the development of a minimum set of standards that US hospitals would have to meet if they wanted ACS approval. On December 20, 1917, the ACS formally established the Hospital Standardization Program and published a formal set of hospital standards called *The Minimum Standard.*

During 1918 and part of 1919, the ACS undertook a review of hospitals across the US and Canada as a field trial to see whether *The Minimum Standard* would be effective as a measurement tool. In total, 692 hospitals were surveyed, of which only 89 met the standard entirely. Some of the most prestigious institutions in the US failed to meet the standard. Brief and clear in its delineation of what was believed to promote good hospital-based patient care in 1918, *The Minimum Standard* stated

1. That physicians and surgeons privileged to practice in the hospital be organized as a definite group or staff. Such organization has nothing to do with the question as to whether the hospital is "open" or "closed," nor need it affect the various existing types of staff organization. The word staff is here defined as the group of doctors who practice in the hospital inclusive of all groups such as the "regular staff," the "visiting staff," and the "associate staff."

2. That membership upon the staff be restricted to physicians and surgeons who are (a) full graduates of medicine in good standing and legally licensed to practice in their respective states or provinces; (b) competent in their respective fields; and (c) worthy in character and in matters of professional ethics; that in this latter connection the practice of the division of fees, under any guise whatever, be prohibited.

3. That the staff initiate and, with the approval of the governing board of the hospital, adopt rules, regulations, and policies governing the professional work of the hospital; that these rules, regulations, and policies specifically provide: (a) that staff meetings be held at least once each month (In large hospitals, the departments may choose to meet separately); and (b) that the staff review and analyze at regular intervals their clinical experience in the various departments of the hospital, such as medicine, surgery, obstetrics, and the other specialties; the clinical records of patients, free and pay, to be the basis of such review and analysis.

4. That accurate and complete records be written for all patients and filed in an accessible manner in the hospital—a complete case record being one which includes identification data; complaint; personal and family history; history of present illness; physical examination; special examinations, such as consultations, clinical laboratory, x-ray, and other examinations; provisional or working diagnosis; medical or surgical treatment; gross and microscopic pathological findings; progress notes; final diagnosis; condition on discharge; follow-up; and, in case of death, autopsy findings.

5. That diagnostic and therapeutic facilities under competent supervision be available for the study, diagnosis, and treatment of patients, these to include, at least (a) a clinical laboratory providing chemical, bacteriological, serological, and pathological services; and (b) an x-ray department providing radiographic and fluoroscopic services. (ACS 1930, 3)

The adoption of *The Minimum Standard* marked the beginning of the accreditation process for healthcare organizations. A similar process is still followed today. The process is based on the development of reasonable quality standards and a survey of the organization's performance in relation to the standards. The accreditation program is voluntary, and healthcare organizations request participation to improve patient care (Roberts et al. 1987, 938).

The ACS continued to examine and approve hospitals for three decades. However, by 1950 the number of hospitals being surveyed every year had grown to be unmanageable, and the ACS could no longer afford to administer the program alone. After considerable discussion and organizing activity, four professional associations from the US and Canada—the AMA, the American College of Physicians (ACP), the American Hospital Association (AHA), and the Canadian Medical Association (CMA)—decided to join the ACS to develop the Joint Commission on Accreditation of Hospitals. The new accrediting agency was formally incorporated in 1952 and began accreditation activities in 1953. It continued its activities almost 50 years later as the Joint Commission on Accreditation of Healthcare Organizations (JCAHO) before renaming itself the Joint Commission in 2007.

Check Your Understanding 1.1

1. Describe how the American College of Surgeons' *Minimum Standard* laid the ground work for quality standards in healthcare?

2. After early attempts at licensure for physicians were challenged and efforts to standardize the curriculum of US medical schools were tested, the Carnegie Foundation volunteered to sponsor and fund the first review of medical college curriculum and education processes, leading to more rigorous academic standards for medical schools. The end-product of this review was the Flexner Report. What were the major findings of the Flexner Report?

Quality, PI, and Modern Healthcare

Until World War II, most healthcare was still provided in the home. Quality in healthcare services was considered a byproduct of physicians' appropriate medical practice and oversight. The positive and negative effects of other factors and the contributions of other healthcare workers were not given much consideration.

In the 1950s, the number of hospitals grew to support developments in diagnostic, therapeutic, and surgical technology and pharmacology. Fueled by an expanding economy, the Hill-Burton Act of 1946 funded extensive hospital construction. A renewed insurance industry helped pay for the new healthcare services provided to groups of individual beneficiaries.

During this period, the Hospital Standardization Program was replaced by the Joint Commission on Accreditation of Hospitals (JCAH) (JCAH 1952). A whole new set of standards covered every aspect of hospital care. The intent was to ensure that the care provided to patients in accredited hospitals would be of the highest quality.

The construction of new facilities and the growth of the medical insurance industry did not guarantee access to services. As new treatments and "miracle" drugs such as antibiotics were developed, healthcare services became more and more costly. Many Americans, particularly the poor and older adults, could not afford to buy health insurance or pay for the services themselves.

Medicare and Medicaid Programs

The idea of federal funding for healthcare services goes back to the 1930s, the Great Depression, and Franklin Roosevelt's New Deal. Harry Truman also supported a universal healthcare program in the late 1940s. But it was not until the 1960s and the presidency of Lyndon Johnson that the federal government developed a program to pay for healthcare services provided to low-income individuals and families and the older population (AHA 1999, 52–53).

In 1965, the US Congress passed Public Law 89-97, an amendment to the Social Security Act of 1935 (Social Security Amendments 1965). Title XVIII of Public Law 89-97 established health insurance for adults age 65 and older and individuals with disabilities. This program soon became known as Medicare. Title XIX of Public Law 89-97 provided grants to states for establishing medical assistance programs for low-income individuals and families. The Title XIX program became known as Medicaid. The objective of the programs was to ensure access to healthcare for people who could not afford to pay for it themselves. The Great Society, as the geopolitics of the US was called in the 1960s, marshaled billions of federal tax dollars to fund care for millions of Americans.

The changes that most significantly improved patient outcomes in the 1970s involved the development and use of sophisticated medical technology and pharmaceuticals. The overall benefits of modern healthcare were evident in increased life spans and better medical outcomes. Also during the 1970s, attempts were made to further standardize and improve the clinical services provided by physicians and hospitals. Under the authority of Medicare officials, hospital audits of health records were mandated to identify physicians with substandard practice patterns or excessive patient care costs. Local peer review organizations (PROs), usually sponsored by local medical societies, reviewed the findings at each local institution and developed recommendations for physician continuing education. These audit activities were designed to measure the quality of services, products, or processes, followed by remedial action to improve care delivery. These activities were referred to as **quality assurance (QA)**. Such retrospective QA efforts were only partially successful and had little effect on the mounting cost to the government of the Medicare and Medicaid programs. As a result, utilization review (UR) programs were mandated to justify hospital admissions. The concept and practice of UR survives today. To be reimbursed, institutions must still provide payers a rationale for the level of services provided.

By 1980 it was obvious that healthcare spending in the US would consume even more economic resources if left unchecked. The Medicare and Medicaid programs were on their way to becoming the most expensive government programs in US history. At the same time, healthcare experts also began to understand that increased spending and technological advances did not automatically guarantee quality healthcare.

In the early 1980s, a new nationwide system was developed to standardize reimbursement for hospital services provided to Medicare and Medicaid beneficiaries. Until 1983, Medicare and Medicaid reimbursement was based on a **retrospective payment system**. In a retrospective payment system, a type of fee-for-service payment, providers are paid for the services they provided to a patient in the past. The patient goes to the doctor, the doctor cares for the patient, the doctor assigns charges and submits a bill to a payer, and the doctor is reimbursed. The problem with this system is that there is no incentive for the doctor to hold down costs. A doctor who provides more services and bills more consequently gets paid more. So, this type of arrangement did not help rein in ever-increasing healthcare costs.

To slow the growth in cost of federal healthcare programs, a **prospective payment system** was developed. In a prospective payment system, providers receive a fixed, predetermined payment for the services they provide. The reimbursement amounts are determined annually by the Centers for Medicare and Medicaid Services (CMS), and billing of insurance carriers and patients cannot exceed these assigned amounts. Because the amount of reimbursement is fixed and often lower than the provider would otherwise charge, healthcare professionals are theoretically motivated to provide only those services that are absolutely necessary for the patient's care. In this way, costs could supposedly be controlled and unnecessary services avoided. However, by the first decade of the 21st century, this system became less and less capable of controlling costs due to a variety of factors, none of which are completely understood. Healthcare costs continue to be one of the fastest-growing segments of the gross domestic product as well as one of the most contentious subjects in the US political arena.

In the Medicare and Medicaid prospective payment system, reimbursement for hospital inpatient services has long been based on a classification known as the diagnosis-related group (DRG). This system assumes that similar diseases and treatments consume similar amounts of resources and therefore have similar total costs, at least on a regional, if not national, basis. Since 1984, hospital inpatients have been assigned to an appropriate DRG based on their diagnosis. Reimbursement levels for each DRG are updated annually and adjusted for the geographic location of the healthcare facility. For federal fiscal year 2009, CMS undertook a major revision of the DRG structure to create groups that reflect the medical severity of the patient's condition (Medicare severity DRGs [MS-DRGs]). MS-DRGs identify conditions that significantly inflate the use of resources and the overall costs of care when they occur concurrently with the reason for admission.

The Healthcare Common Procedure Coding System (HCPCS) was developed in the early 1980s. HCPCS codes are used to report the healthcare services provided to Medicare and Medicaid beneficiaries treated in ambulatory settings. HCPCS initially included three separate levels of codes: Level I, Current Procedural Terminology (CPT) codes; Level II, national codes; and Level III, local codes. The Level III local codes were eliminated by CMS in 2003 (CMS 2024a).

A prospective payment system for hospital outpatient and ambulatory surgery services provided to Medicare and Medicaid beneficiaries was implemented in 2001. This system, known as the Outpatient Prospective Payment System (OPPS), is based on ambulatory payment classification (APC) groups. The APCs are generated on the basis of the HCPCS CPT codes assigned for services such as outpatient diagnostic procedures and outpatient radiology procedures. A similar system was implemented for the reimbursement of professional fees. This resource-based relative value scale (RBRVS) system takes into consideration the level of services provided in terms of time spent with the patient, complexity of physical examination and information gathering, the diagnostic and procedural actions performed to arrive at the reimbursement amount, and the geographic location of the service.

Hospitals and healthcare providers in the US provide billions of dollars' worth of care to Medicare and Medicaid patients every year. The implementation of prospective payment systems made it necessary for healthcare organizations to devise ways to control costs without endangering safe and effective patient care. It is necessary to recognize, however, that there are limits to the amount of money that can be saved by these methods.

Managed Care

The growth of managed care in the US has had a tremendous impact on healthcare providers. *Managed care* is a broad term used to describe several types of health insurance plans. Health maintenance organizations

(HMOs) are one of the most familiar types of managed care plans. Members of an HMO (or their employers) pay a set premium and are entitled to a specific range of healthcare services. HMOs control costs by requiring members to seek services from a preapproved list of providers, by limiting access to specialists and expensive diagnostic and treatment procedures, and by requiring preauthorization for inpatient hospitalization and surgery.

Other types of managed care plans include preferred provider organizations (PPOs) and point-of-service (POS) plans. These types of plans negotiate discounted rates with specific hospitals, physicians, and other healthcare providers. Many also restrict access to specialists and require preauthorization for surgery and other hospital services. In PPOs, enrollees are required to seek care from a limited list of providers who have agreed in advance to accept a discounted payment for their services. Enrollees in POS plans pay for a greater portion of their healthcare expenses when they choose to seek treatment from providers who do not participate in their plan.

Together, the Medicare and Medicaid programs and the managed care insurance industry have virtually eliminated fee-for-service reimbursement arrangements. At the same time, healthcare consumers are demanding more services and greater quality. Hospitals and providers now find that they have no choice but to become more efficient and effective if they are to stay in business. Programs that promote efficiency and effectiveness have become the only way for providers to add value to the services they provide and ensure their financial viability.

Paying for Value

Linking payment for services to quality and performance continued to evolve and led to the development of value-based purchasing, or pay-for-performance initiatives. **Value-based purchasing (VBP)** is defined as a payment model that holds healthcare providers accountable for both the cost and quality of care they provide (Healthcare.gov 2023). In the private sector, pay-for-performance programs base provider payments on performance and incentives.

At the end of the first decade of the 21st century, US politicians tackled the issues of payment and insurance discrimination with the passage of the **Affordable Care Act (ACA)** of 2010. The major focus of the act is providing or improving access to healthcare services for millions of US citizens, including restrictions on the ability of payers to limit coverage on the basis of pre-existing conditions, an end to lifetime limits on coverage, and a requirement for payers to spend the majority of premium dollars on healthcare costs and not administrative costs. Recognizing that access is a financial issue and a quality issue, the act also has requirements directly related to the issue of quality. For example, it included the establishment of a quality measures program for Medicaid; requires long-term care, rehabilitation, and hospice facilities to submit quality data to CMS; and expands the quality reporting in the prospective payment system that can have a negative impact on reimbursement rates when the patient encounters adverse events or complications resulting from inadequate treatment by providers.

Accountable Care Organizations

Established as a key component of the Patient Protection and Affordable Care Act of 2010, an **accountable care organization (ACO)** is a voluntary network of doctors, hospitals, and other healthcare providers that share responsibility for providing care to patients. An ACO agrees to manage all of the healthcare needs for their Medicare beneficiaries for a period of time. ACOs provide coordinated care that helps ensure patient receive the care they need at the right time, reducing unnecessary services and preventing medical errors. When an ACO succeeds in delivering high-quality care, healthcare spending is reduced and the savings are shared between both parties (CMS n.d.).

Increased Transparency

An increased focus on transparency in healthcare has occurred in the 21st century. The large volume of healthcare data and emphasis on quality also led to demands for more transparency within the healthcare system. With the integration of electronic health records (EHRs), healthcare organizations and facilities had the capability to access, analyze and share data more efficiently. As organizations were increasingly tasked with tracking and reporting their performance on quality metrics, this information began to be available to consumers, resulting in increased transparency. Healthcare consumers now have many more options to find information about providers, facilities, insurance options, and even price of services. For example, the website medicare.gov/care-compare/ and many other sources of information are now readily available online. Historically, it was often difficult for consumers to determine how much a service would cost at a hospital. Unlike purchasing an item at a store for which the price is visible, hospital prices for services were not easily assessable or shared. Due to government regulation, the price of hospital services must be shared with consumers in a transparent and convenient manner in an effort to facilitate patient-driven care (CMS, 2023).

Check Your Understanding 1.2

1. In 1965, the US Congress passed Public Law 89-97, an amendment to the Social Security Act of 1935. This law established the Medicare and Medicaid programs. Describe the impact of this legislation and how it changed the healthcare industry.

2. What is the primary purpose of promoting transparency in healthcare?
   a. To limit access to health records
   b. To enhance healthcare provider profits
   c. To foster trust and accountability
   d. To expedite administrative processes

Evolution of Quality in Healthcare

In the 1980s, leaders in the healthcare industry began to take notice of a business theory called **total quality management (TQM)**. The concept of TQM was developed by W. Edwards Deming in the early 1950s as an alternative to authoritarian, top-down management philosophies. Philip Crosby and J. M. Juran each further adapted TQM and developed similar approaches. TQM mobilizes individuals directly involved in a work process to examine and improve the process with the goal of achieving a better product or outcome. It does not matter what the product or outcome might be. TQM is firmly based in the statistical analysis of objective data gathered from observation of the process being examined. The data are then carefully analyzed to identify the steps in the process that lead to a less-than-ideal product or outcome. Once the problematic steps in the process have been identified, individuals or teams can make recommendations for changing the process to produce a better product or outcome. Key to Deming's philosophy is the concept that problematic processes, not people, cause inferior products and outcomes.

TQM revolutionized industrial production in Japan during the post–World War II period. When Japanese automobiles took over much of the US car market in the late 20th century, American manufacturers began to take notice of TQM. They recognized that Deming's management philosophy might help them create more efficient and effective manufacturing processes.

Avedis Donabedian was one of the first theorists to recognize that the TQM philosophy could be applied to healthcare services (Donabedian 1966). Beginning in 1966, Donabedian advocated the assessment of healthcare from four perspectives:

- **Structure**: The foundation of caregiving, which includes buildings, equipment, technology, professional staff, and appropriate policies
- **Process**: The interrelated activities of healthcare organizations—including governance, managerial support, and clinical services—that affect patient outcomes across departments and disciplines within an integrated environment

- **Outcome**: The results of care, treatment, and services in terms of the patient's expectations, needs, and quality of life, which may be positive and appropriate or negative and diminishing
- **Cost**: The amount of financial resources consumed in the provision of healthcare services

It took until the 1990s for his approaches to be widely adopted. The concept of TQM became known as continuous quality improvement (CQI) in the US healthcare system and was integrated into the quest for healthcare improvement. The industry began using Donabedian's four perspectives to identify processes of providing care that could be improved. Using the team approach from Deming and his emphasis on objective data gathering to describe a process clearly, members of the healthcare industry began a self-examination that focused very specifically on the processes of care rather than on the individuals who provided it. Many improvements were made across all types of healthcare organizations using this variant of TQM.

However, by the end of the 1990s some individuals involved in the improvement of quality in healthcare had made a significant realization: quality in healthcare was tied very closely to the performance of individuals in the healthcare organization. Unlike manufacturing firms that utilized machinery to shape raw materials into physical products, the "products" of healthcare organizations were the services provided to patients by healthcare professionals who defined processes of practice. The performance of the professionals often determined the quality of the services. Quality improvement initiatives in healthcare organizations were renamed *performance improvement* initiatives, at least in those organizations affected by the Joint Commission's PI standards. Quality improvement was refocused to examine the performance of the people in the organization, rewarding those who obtained good outcomes or costs, and requiring those working in the healthcare industry to become more accountable for their patient or client outcomes.

The Institute of Medicine (IOM) published a landmark report, *To Err is Human* (IOM 1999), which was instrumental in raising awareness about the status of healthcare quality and patient safety in the US. This report famously estimated that 44,000 to 98,000 deaths occurred every year due to medical errors in hospitals; it is viewed as a catalyst for moving quality and patient safety to the forefront of healthcare organizations. This study was considered such an eye-opening event for US healthcare that all stakeholders, including consumers, took note and expected change.

Early in the 21st century, federal agencies began to emphasize quality improvement in the programs they sponsored. The approach by federal Medicare and Medicaid programs retained the quality improvement terminology but focused largely on the same kinds of process issues. Today, contracted healthcare examiners—once called PROs and now called quality improvement organizations (QIOs)—retrospectively examine the care provided to beneficiaries and compare it with similar providers' performance in different regions of the country.

This comparison of providers' performance was facilitated by the collection and submission of mandated data sets by the Joint Commission and CMS, called core measures, on the most common diagnoses, such as pneumonia, congestive heart failure, or myocardial infarction. The core measures defined the practices used in managing a health condition that achieve the best outcomes, often on the basis of research identifying the best practices and methodologies used across the country. Analysis of the core measure data allowed providers to examine where their performance on various characteristics of care does not measure up to the performance of the general community, allowing them to identify aspects of their services that can be improved. The core measure data collection process has evolved into many other manual and electronic data collection processes, such as abstracting measures or direct feeds from the electronic health record into federal value-based purchasing programs. Much of this data is now available to consumers through websites for this public reporting purpose.

In the first decade of the 21st century, the Joint Commission evolved its philosophy to emphasize patient safety. This was in response to the IOM's analysis in *To Err is Human*, which revealed that tens of thousands of patients die in hospitals every year from mistakes or miscommunication involving the care they are receiving. In particular, the analysis highlighted mistakes occurring in medication administration and provision of surgical procedures. In response to these revelations, the Joint Commission developed a set of National Patient Safety Goals (NPSGs) (Joint Commission 2024). All institutions participating in accreditation must promote and train their staff members who provide care to adhere to the NPSGs. The Joint Commission has continued to revise and fine-tune the original set of NPSGs that went into effect in 2003, moving some of them into the formal accreditation standards. Finally, the Joint Commission undertook radical restructuring of the survey processes used to examine hospitals for accreditation, emphasizing foremost the processes by which nurses and allied health professionals provide care at the bedside, rather than emphasizing the development of policy and procedure and retrospective review of records. This process began with the Joint Commission's move to unannounced surveys in 2006.

In parallel with these changes in the philosophy of the Joint Commission, the federal government has sponsored more and more research into the issues inherent in the US healthcare delivery system through its Agency for Healthcare Research and Quality. In the private sector, organizations such as the National Quality Forum have brought together a variety of stakeholders, including researchers, providers, consumer advocates, payers, and accreditors, to develop quality measures for use across most healthcare organizations. The IOM has used funding from a variety of sources to examine the areas in which the system is failing US healthcare consumers and to make recommendations on systematic improvement. Since its inception, the IOM has published hundreds of reports on different healthcare topics, such the previously discussed *To Err is Human* and *Crossing the Quality Chasm: A New Health System for the 21st Century* (IOM 2001).

Students of healthcare quality improvement might want to read *Crossing the Quality Chasm*. After acknowledging that the current system is overly complex and inequitable with respect to various socioeconomic groups, the IOM cites six core dimensions of quality that are necessary to focus US healthcare delivery in the 21st century: care should be *"safe, effective, patient-centered, timely, efficient, and equitable."* At the same time, the IOM proposed a set of 10 rules or general principles to inform efforts in redesigning the healthcare system:

- Care is based on continuous healing relationships. Patients should receive care whenever they need it and in many forms... [for example,] over the Internet, by telephone, and by other means in addition to in-person visits.
- Care is customized according to patient needs and values....
- The patient is the source of control, [and should be given] the necessary information and opportunity to exercise the degree of control they choose over healthcare decisions that affect them....
- Knowledge is shared and information flows freely. Patients should have unfettered access to their own medical information and to clinical knowledge. Clinicians and patients should communicate effectively and share information.
- Decision-making is evidence-based. Patients should receive care based on the best available scientific knowledge. Care should not vary from clinician to clinician or from place to place.
- Safety is a system [priority].... Reducing risk and ensuring safety require greater attention to systems that help prevent and mitigate errors.
- Transparency is necessary.... Information describing the system's performance on safety, evidence-based practice, and patient satisfaction [should be readily available].
- [Patient] needs are anticipated.
- Waste is continuously decreased.
- Cooperation among clinicians is a priority (IOM 2001, 3–4).

Following publication of *Crossing the Quality Chasm* and heightened discussion between accrediting and licensing agencies regarding some of the report's recommendations, healthcare entities renewed their emphasis on the issues the report raised regarding safety of care, patient centricity of care, the scientific basis for care, and the transparency of the outcomes of care. In 2008, the IOM published *Knowing What Works in Health Care: A Roadmap for the Nation*. This report further reveals how the science on which healthcare is based could be promulgated to US providers and consumers. The report makes recommendations for a national clinical effectiveness assessment program "with authority, overarching responsibility, sustained resources, and adequate capacity to ensure production of credible, unbiased information about what is known and not known about clinical effectiveness." It goes on to make specific recommendations regarding how the assessment should be undertaken:

- Set priorities for, fund, and manage systematic reviews of clinical effectiveness and related topics.
- Develop a common language and standards for conducting systematic reviews of the evidence and for generating clinical guidelines and recommendations.
- Provide a forum for addressing conflicting guidelines and recommendations.
- Prepare an annual [summary] report to Congress. (IOM 2008, 9–10)

Many of these dialogues have taken place alongside political discussions, debates, and demonstration projects about healthcare reform in the face of burgeoning healthcare costs in the first decade of the 21st century and the projected financial inadequacies of the Medicare and Medicaid programs as the century progresses. Many political figures of this period assumed that they had an adequate understanding of the complexities of US healthcare delivery to formulate plans to solve the issues. Few undertook a solid attempt at doing so at the federal level until 2009 and 2010. Prior to that, those charged with administration of the Medicare and Medicaid programs put forward little in the way of reform, except to require the development of more specific data sets: MS-DRGs; the *International Classification of Diseases, Tenth Revision, Clinical Modification* (ICD-10-CM); and the *International Classification of Diseases, Tenth Revision, Procedure Coding System* (ICD-10-PCS).

After many years of debate, the US Congress passed three sets of legislation in an effort to positively impact the quality of care in the healthcare system as a whole. The American Recovery and Reinvestment Act of 2009 (ARRA), the Health Information Technology for Economic and Clinical Health Act (HITECH), and the ACA all have provisions designed to improve the quality of a patient's healthcare: the ARRA by focusing funding on the expansion of the healthcare workforce; HITECH by stimulating investment in the information systems infrastructure of professional practices, clinics, and hospitals; and the ACA by mandating increased quality measure reporting by payers and providers at all levels of care, by implementing penalties for poor care in terms of reimbursement, and by improving access for the millions of Americans who, prior to the act's implementation, had nowhere to turn but the nation's emergency departments.

In 2014, Congress passed the Improving Medicare Post-Acute Care Transformation Act of 2014 (IMPACT Act) that established a quality reporting program for skilled nursing care. This program requires long-term care hospitals, skilled nursing facilities, home health agencies, and inpatient rehabilitation facilities to submit standardized data pertaining to resource use, hospitalization, and discharge to the community. These types of facilities were subject to Medicare payment reductions beginning in fiscal year 2018 for noncompliance with the data reporting and submission requirements.

Each of these actions taken by Congress is part of the National Quality Strategy for better care that is patient-centered, reliable, accessible, and safe; to improve the health of the US population; and to reduce the cost of quality healthcare (CMS 2024b). This National Quality Strategy includes the Medicare Access and CHIP Reauthorization Act of 2015 (MACRA). MACRA created the Quality Payment Program that changed how Medicare reimburses providers and made significant changes to data collection efforts to assess quality of care (CMS 2018b). All of these initiatives have provided the foundation and set the stage for a climate of paying for quality care. Most public and private payers have this premise of paying for value at the core of their reimbursement models. Healthcare providers will no longer be paid for medical errors, complications, and readmissions that resulted from lack of quality care.

Social determinants of health (SDOH) moved to the forefront of healthcare due to an increased interest and focus on improving the overall health of populations. Research showed that the health of individuals was more complex than just providing services and was often directly correlated to their social determinants. These determinants include education, neighborhood, economic stability, healthcare access, and social and community context. Providing quality care to patients includes addressing the SDOH that impact the community served. It also encompasses work to provide equitable care, as SDOH are tied to healthcare outcomes. Healthcare inequities exist with the US healthcare system. Many healthcare organizations are focused on initiatives to remove barriers to equitable care for their communities and are working with community partners to improve the local environment. Some of this work includes housing, transportation, access to food, and education (HHS n.d.). Quality managers in healthcare organizations must consider SDOH issues as part of their performance improvement activities, as this focus helps to ensure quality of care to all patients in the communities served. For example, if a hospital creates a new program to help patients with diabetes better manage their condition but does not provide outreach within areas where patients do not have access to public transportation, the new program will not meet the needs of this population.

Check Your Understanding 1.3

1. A local community has limited access to nutritious food, inadequate educational resources, and a scarcity of job opportunities. Residents in this community often face SDOH challenges related to health disparities. Which of the following is most prominently at play in this scenario?
   a. Genetic factors
   b. Healthcare system efficiency
   c. Physical environment
   d. Lifestyle choices

2. Which of the following entities is responsible for retrospectively examining the care provided to Medicare and Medicaid beneficiaries and comparing it to similar providers' performance in different regions of the US?
   a. Agency for Healthcare Research and Quality
   b. American Medical Association
   c. Quality improvement organizations
   d. The Joint Commission

Why Care About Quality and PI?

An individual working in the US healthcare industry today hears many terms that reflect the long-term development of quality improvement philosophy, including *quality assurance*, *quality improvement*, *quality management*, and *performance improvement*. The differences in meaning are subtle, reflecting the time and place of their origins as well as the individuals and philosophies that generated them. However, they are all, in reality, focused on one thing: helping people with health challenges return to healthier, more productive lives and doing so by the most efficient and effective means possible. This balance is an ongoing challenge to address cost, access, and quality, often referred to as the iron triangle. Each aspect (cost, access, and quality) is represented by a side of the triangle. The challenge of this model is that when the focus is on two of the three sides of the triangle the remaining side often suffers. All three sides of the triangle have to be considered when making changes or improvements. This is an evolving mission and one that is always seeking a better way and has led to further iterations of the iron triangle (Van der Goes et al. 2019).

There is a long tradition of seeking improvement in the healthcare industry, and healthcare professionals must continue to be concerned with PI. Today, PI is the key to ensuring high-quality care, and a PI philosophy pervades leading healthcare organizations. To contribute to personal and organizational success, one must commit to participate in PI. Today's patients are increasingly able to choose their professional and institutional providers on the basis of quality due to increased transparency and public reporting of outcomes. Furthermore, most payers prefer to negotiate with organizations that provide high-quality, cost-effective services.

Today's healthcare organizations must be able to back up their espousal of quality with reliable, objective data. Government-sponsored and commercial health plans, employers, and consumers are all now asking for more information on the quality of the healthcare services they receive and pay for. In addition, a focus on quality is the key to meeting regulatory, licensure, and accreditation requirements. Demonstrating quality and improving performance are the definitive keys to success in the healthcare industry's mission to provide high-quality care.

Case Study

This chapter addresses the historical background of quality and performance improvement in healthcare. One item addressed is the iron triangle, which depicts the balance between cost, access, and quality in healthcare. Many believed that addressing each of these items in an effective manner was a somewhat impossible task as gains in one area may create a deficit in another. Over time this model has evolved into the triple aim, quadruple aim, and most recently, the quintuple aim.

Research each of these models (triple aim, quadruple aim, quintuple aim) and answer the following questions:

1. Are there any issues with the models in which balance is not possible, similar to what was true for the iron triangle? Provide reasoning for your answer.
2. Is one model more effective for healthcare organizations to use to improve their quality of patient care? Why or why not?
3. Why is it important to include patient satisfaction in a model to improve quality of patient care?

Review Questions

1. Select a significant historical event described in the chapter and demonstrate how this event has shaped current performance improvement or quality initiatives in the modern era.
2. Describe some of the ways in which the Patient Protection and Affordable Care Act (ACA) of 2010 changed healthcare delivery in the US.
3. During the mid-1700s, the citizens of Philadelphia, PA, recognized the need to sequester newly arrived immigrants, who often contracted diseases during their long voyages to America. This procedure is an example of early _____.
   a. Infection control
   b. Utilization management
   c. Performance improvement
   d. Standardization
4. Compare and contrast the activities taken by Massachusetts General Hospital in the 1800s with modern day quality and performance improvement activities.
5. Explain why improving the health of a patient within the healthcare organization is not enough based on what is known about the role social determinants of health play in regard to the overall health of the patient.

References

Adams, D. P. and A. L. Moore. 1997. Nicholas J. Pisacano. In *Doctors, Nurses, and Medical Practitioners: A Bio-Bibliographical Sourcebook,* edited by L. N. Magner. Westport, CT: Greenwood Press.

ACS (American College of Surgeons). 1930. Manual of Hospital Standardization and Hospital Standardization Report. Chicago: American College of Surgeons.

AHA (American Hospital Association. 1999. *100 Faces of Health Care*. Chicago: Health Forum.

Bowditch, N. I. 1972. *History of the Massachusetts General Hospital*. Boston: Arno Press and New York Times.

Brickman, J. P. 1997. Ernst P. Boas. In *Doctors, Nurses, and Medical Practitioners: A Bio-Bibliographical Sourcebook,* edited by L. N. Magner. Westport, CT: Greenwood Press.

Bullough, V. L. 1997. Robert Latou Dickinson. In *Doctors, Nurses, and Medical Practitioners: A Bio-Bibliographical Sourcebook,* edited by L. N. Magner. Westport, CT: Greenwood Press.

References

CMS (Centers for Medicare and Medicaid Services. 2024a. "Healthcare Common Procedure Coding Systems (HCPCS)." https://www.cms.gov/medicare/coding-billing/healthcare-common-procedure-system.

CMS (Centers for Medicare and Medicaid Services. 2024b. "CMS National Quality Strategy." https://www.cms.gov/medicare/quality/meaningful-measures-initiative/cms-quality-strategy

CMS (Centers for Medicare and Medicaid Services). 2023. "Hospital Price Transparency Fact Sheet." https://www.cms.gov/newsroom/fact-sheets/hospital-price-transparency-fact-sheet.

CMS (Centers for Medicare and Medicaid Services). 2018b. "What's MACRA?" https://www.cms.gov/Medicare/Quality-Initiatives-Patient-Assessment-Instruments/Value-Based-Programs/MACRA-MIPS-and-APMs/MACRA-MIPS-and-APMs.html.

CMS (Centers for Medicare and Medicaid Services). n.d. "Accountable Care Organizations (ACOs): General Information." https://www.cms.gov/priorities/innovation/innovation-models/aco.

Donabedian, A. 1966. Evaluating the quality of medical care. *Milbank Quarterly* 44:166–203.

Flexner, A. 1910. *Medical Education in the United States and Canada, Bulletin Number Four*. New York: The Carnegie Foundation for the Advancement of Teaching. http://archive.carnegiefoundation.org/publications/pdfs/elibrary/Carnegie_Flexner_Report.pdf

Gage, A. 1997. Roswell Park. In *Doctors, Nurses, and Medical Practitioners: A Bio-Bibliographical Sourcebook*, edited by L. N. Magner. Westport, CT: Greenwood Press.

Haller, J. S. 1981. *American Medicine in Transition 1840–1910*. Chicago: University of Illinois Press.

Healthcare.gov. 2023. "Glossary." https://www.healthcare.gov/glossary/.

Hill, P. E. 1997. Maude E. Callen. In *Doctors, Nurses, and Medical Practitioners: A Bio-Bibliographical Sourcebook*, edited by L. N. Magner. Westport, CT: Greenwood Press.

IOM (Institute of Medicine. 2008. *Knowing What Works in Health Care: A Roadmap for the Nation*. Washington, DC: National Academies Press.

IOM (Institute of Medicine). 2001. *Crossing the Quality Chasm: A New Health System for the 21st Century*. Washington, DC: National Academies Press.

IOM (Institute of Medicine). 1999. *To Err is Human: Building A Safer Health System*. Washington, DC: National Academies Press.

Joint Commission. 2024. "National Patient Safety Goals Fact Sheet." https://www.jointcommission.org/resources/news-and-multimedia/fact-sheets/facts-about-national-patient-safety-goals

JCAH (Joint Commission on Accreditation of Hospitals). 1952. *Standards of Hospital Accreditation*. Oakbrook Terrace, IL: JCAH.

Kalisch, P. A. and B. J. Kalisch. 1995. *The Advance of American Nursing*. Philadelphia: J. B. Lippincott.

Leighow, S. R. 1997. Lavinia Lloyd Dock. In *Doctors, Nurses, and Medical Practitioners: A Bio-Bibliographical Sourcebook*, edited by L. N. Magner. Westport, CT: Greenwood Press.

Meldrum, M. 1997. Mary Steichen Calderone. In *Doctors, Nurses, and Medical Practitioners: A Bio-Bibliographical Sourcebook*, edited by L. N. Magner. Westport, CT: Greenwood Press.

Morton, T. G. and F. Woodbury. 1973. *The History of the Pennsylvania Hospital*. New York: Arno Press.

Roberts, J. S., J. G. Coate, and R. Redman. 1987. A history of the Joint Commission on Accreditation of Hospitals. *JAMA* 256(7):936–940.

Social Security Amendments of 1965. Public Law 89-97.

Trent, J. C. 1977. An early New Jersey medical license. Chapter X in *Legacies in Law and Medicine*, edited by C. R. Burns. New York: Science History Publications.

HHS (US Department of Health and Human Services). n.d. "Healthy People 2030: Social Determinants of Health." Accessed December 20, 2023. https://health.gov/healthypeople/priority-areas/social-determinants-health.

Van der Goes DN, N. Edwardson, V. Rayamajhee, C. Hollis, D. Hunter. 2019. An iron triangle ROI model for health care. Clinicoecon Outcomes Research 11:335–348.

Wickes, S. 1879. *History of Medicine in New Jersey: And of its Medical Men, From the Settlement of the Province to A.D. 1800*. Newark, N.J.: L. J. Hardham.

Resources

AHRQ (Agency for Healthcare Research and Quality). 2023. http://www.ahrq.gov.

Crosby, P. B. 1984. *Quality without Tears*. New York: Plume Books.

Crosby, P. B. 1980. *Quality Is Free*. New York: Mentor Books.

Deming, W. E. 1986. *Out of the Crisis*. Cambridge, MA: MIT Press. First published in 1982 as *Quality, Productivity, and Competitive Position*.

Donabedian, A. 1988. The quality of care: How can it be assessed? *JAMA* 260(12):1743–1748.

Donabedian, A. 1980. *The Definition of Quality and Approaches to Its Management*. Volume 1. *Explorations in Quality Assessment and Monitoring*. Ann Arbor, MI: Health Administration Press.

Hill-Burton Act of 1946. 42 USC 6.

Juran, J. M. 1988. *Juran on Planning for Quality*. New York: Free Press.

Juran, J. M. 1980. *Upper Management and Quality*. New York: Joseph M. Juran.

Juran, J. M. 1970. *Quality Planning and Analysis*. New York: McGraw-Hill.

Juran, J. M. 1967. *Management of Quality Control*. New York: Joseph M. Juran.

Juran, J. M. 1964. *Managerial Breakthrough*. New York: McGraw-Hill.

Juran, J. M. 1951. *Quality Control Handbook*. New York: McGraw-Hill.

Juran, J. M. 1945. *Management of Inspection and Quality Control*. New York: Harper & Brothers.

Silin, C. I. 1977. A state medical board examination in 1816. In *Legacies in Law and Medicine*, edited by C. R. Burns. New York: Science History Publications. 93–106.

Walton, M. 1990. *Deming Management at Work*. New York: G. P. Putnam's Sons.

Walton, M. 1986. *The Deming Management Method*. New York: Perigee Books.

Defining a Performance Improvement Model

Learning Objectives

- Recognize the cyclical nature of performance improvement activities
- Demonstrate mastery of terminology associated with performance improvement (PI) activities
- Describe standards that are commonly applied to PI activities
- Distinguish between organization-wide PI activities and team-based PI activities
- Differentiate the organization-wide and team-based PI cycles

Key Terms

Benchmark
Continuous monitoring
High reliability organizations (HROs)
Leadership group
Lean
Lean Six Sigma
Plan, do, check, act (PDCA)
Plan, do, study, act (PDSA)

Opportunity for improvement
Performance improvement (PI) team
Performance measure
Process redesign
QI toolbox techniques
Six Sigma
Systems thinking

Various efforts to ensure the quality of healthcare services provided in the US have been in place for years. These efforts have had many different names: quality assurance (QA), total quality management (TQM), quality improvement (QI), continuous quality improvement (CQI), quality management (QM), and performance improvement (PI). Each of these terms represents a quality and PI model or methodology that healthcare organizations have used with varying degrees of success. Many books and articles have been written on the subject, and new models and terminology will likely be developed in the future.

A professional entering the healthcare field will probably work for many organizations over the course of their career and participate in many quality and PI projects. They will learn to use specific quality and PI models and techniques as needed. With experience, healthcare professionals will develop the skills necessary to customize the models to specific organizations and healthcare services.

The goal of this chapter is to provide a general overview of quality and PI as it is applied in healthcare organizations. The chapter describes a generic PI model, defines commonly used PI terms, and explains the philosophy of continuous performance improvement. This chapter also discusses various PI techniques and methodologies used in healthcare today.

Performance Improvement as a Cyclical Process

Various healthcare organizations, including accreditation bodies, groups of clinical professionals, QM professionals, healthcare providers, and government regulatory and policy-making entities have unique perspectives on quality in healthcare. Many have developed their own methodologies for quality and PI. Most PI models applied in healthcare today share one structural characteristic: they are cyclical in nature.

W. Edwards Deming developed the **plan, do, check, act (PDCA)** cycle (see figure 2.1):

- P = Plan the change
- D = Do or test the change
- C = Check or analyze the test
- A = Act on the results of the test (ASQ 2023a)

Figure 2.1. Deming's plan, do, check, act cycle

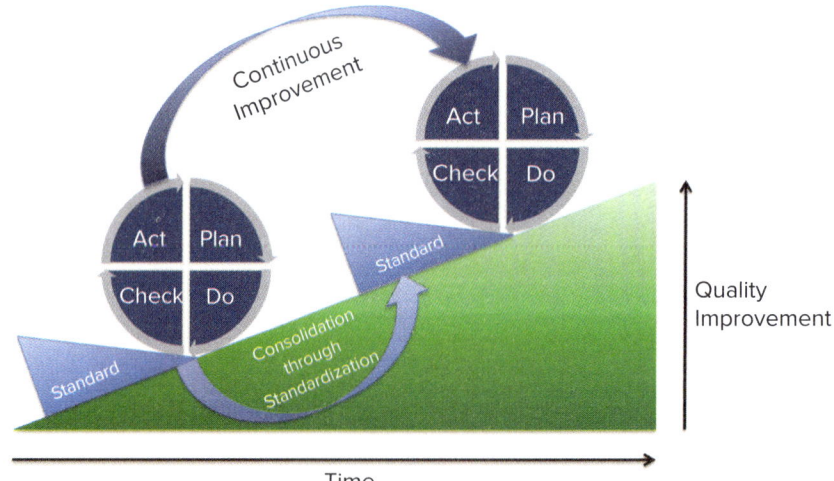

Source: Vietze 2013.

This cycle, sometimes called the Deming cycle or Shewhart cycle, has been modified over the years to become the **plan, do, study, act (PDSA)** cycle. "Check" has been replaced with "study," which refers to observing and learning from the consequences. The PDSA model is a foundation for quality and PI activities in healthcare today (AHRQ 2020; IHI 2023) and the basis for most PI models currently in use.

For example, a manager is reviewing the results from a recent employee satisfaction survey. Based on the survey results, the employees in the department responded that they do not feel adequate recognition for their work. The manager identified the following tasks using the PDSA model to investigate this issue further:

Plan:

- **Objective:** Improve employee satisfaction of recognition for work in the department by 15%.
- **Identify Issues:** Conduct a thorough analysis of the current employee recognition program and create focus groups of employees to discuss meaningful ways to enhance the recognition program.
- **Set Targets:** Establish a specific and measurable goal for improvement.

Do:

- **Implement Changes:** Introduce changes based on the analysis and focus group findings. Some examples would be to develop a multi-tiered recognition program with various levels of "rewards" for employees.
- **Educate Staff:** Ensure that all staff members are educated on the new program and are aware of the opportunities and expectation to earn recognition.

Study:

- **Collect Data:** Track employee performance and response to the new recognition program.
- **Assess Results:** Continue to measure employee satisfaction rates against the entry level results prior to the program change.
- **Gather Feedback:** Obtain feedback from employees and other stakeholders to identify any unforeseen issues or areas for further improvement.

Act:

- **Adjust:** If the results indicate that the employee satisfaction scores regarding employee recognition have not met the target, analyze the data to identify areas that need further improvement.
- **Modify Strategies:** Adjust the recognition program and introduce new strategies based on the feedback and analysis.
- **Standardize:** Once an effective program is identified, standardize the improved process and update protocols to ensure sustainability.

The cyclical model is based on the assumptions that PI activities will take place continually and that services, processes, and outcomes can always be improved. Quality should not be treated as a goal that is accomplished and then forgotten. Rather, it should be an ongoing mission that guides everyday operations.

Accreditation and licensing agencies expect hospitals and other healthcare facilities to strive for the highest possible quality of care at all times. Each organization's healthcare leaders and board of directors are responsible for the quality of the services provided. Many large healthcare organizations employ QM experts who are responsible for organizing PI activities and reporting results to the leadership and boards of directors. In addition, all employees are expected to have a basic understanding of PI principles and to participate in PI activities.

The general PI model presented in this textbook includes two interrelated cycles. The cycle illustrated in figure 2.2 represents the organization's ongoing performance monitoring function.

Figure 2.2. Organization-wide PI process

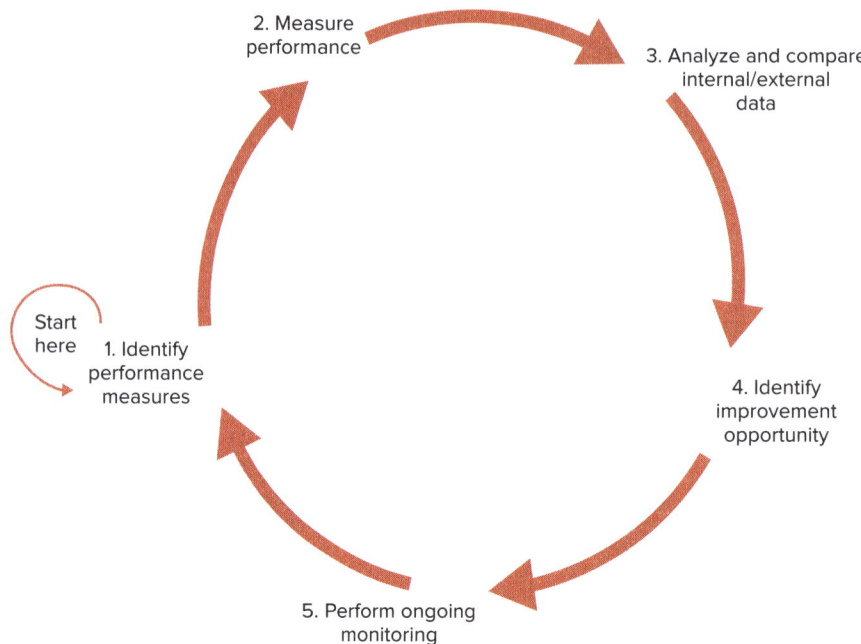

The cycle illustrated in figure 2.3 represents the activities of individual PI teams working on specific PI projects.

Figure 2.3. Team-based PI process

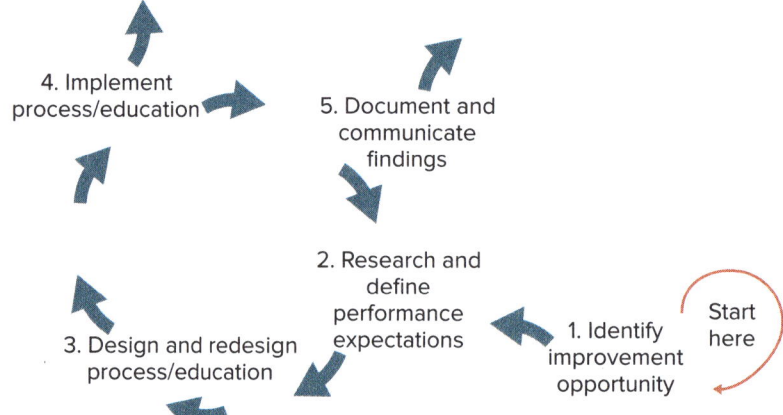

Together, the organization-wide and team-based cycles make up the healthcare PI model shown in figure 2.4.

Figure 2.4. PI model

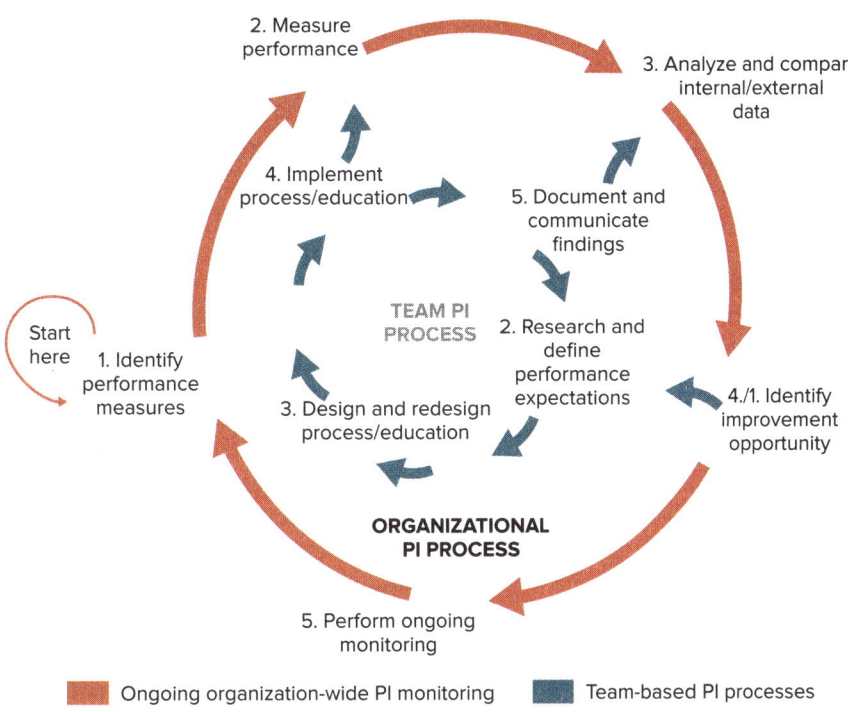

Monitoring Performance through Data Collection

Monitoring performance based on internal and external data is the foundation of all PI activities. Each healthcare organization must identify and prioritize which processes and outcomes (i.e., which types of data) are important to monitor based on its mission and the scope of care and services it provides. Logical areas in which to begin monitoring performance include those that perform important organizational functions, particularly functions that are high risk, high volume, or problem prone, such as a patient's unplanned return to the operating room, medication administration, or transfusions. Outcomes of care, customer feedback, and the requirements of regulatory agencies are additional areas that organizations consider when prioritizing performance monitors. Once the scope and focus of performance monitoring are determined, the organization's leaders define the data collection requirements for each performance measure.

As shown in figure 2.2, monitoring performance depends on the identification of performance measures for each service, process, or outcome deemed important to track. A **performance measure** is "a gauge used to assess the performance of a process or function of any organization" (CMS 2023). Monitoring selected performance measures can help an organization determine process stability and/or identify improvement opportunities. Specific criteria are used to define the organization's performance measures. Components of a good performance measure include:

- Documented numerator statement
- Documented denominator statement
- Description of the population to which the measure applies

$$\frac{\text{Numerator (number of times it occurred)}}{\text{Denominator (number of times it could have occurred)}}$$

In addition, the measurement period; baseline goal; data collection method; and frequency of data collection, analysis, and reporting must be identified. One important outcome that hospitals are required to continuously monitor is the documentation appropriateness rate. The criteria used to establish this performance measure include:

$$\frac{\text{Number of patient records with appropriate documentation}}{\text{Number of patient records reviewed}}$$

This measure would be collected through patient record review or from reports the health information (HI) department generates from the electronic health record (EHR). The HI department would send results to a medical staff committee responsible for documentation oversight. A baseline goal might be 90 percent of documentation being deemed appropriate (contains all required information).

The populations included in this performance measure are the medical staff and inpatient health records staff. Tracking this outcome allows the hospital to continuously monitor its compliance with appropriate documentation. (See figure 2.2. to review this process.) If the appropriateness of documentation does not meet the hospital's established performance standards (an internal comparison) or nationally established performance standards (an external comparison), this constitutes an opportunity for improvement (step 4 in the PI process in figure 2.2). An **opportunity for improvement** is defined as a healthcare structure, product, service, process, or outcome that does not meet its customers' expectations and, therefore, could be improved. In this case, not meeting the established performance standard signifies an opportunity for improvement. Following this conclusion, a team-based PI process, shown in figure 2.3, may be initiated to investigate the reasons for noncompliance with the standard.

When an organization compares its current performance with its own internal historical data, or uses data from similar external organizations across the country, it establishes a **benchmark**, also known as a *standard of performance* or *best practice*, for a particular process or outcome. Establishing a benchmark for each monitored performance measure assists the healthcare organization in setting performance baselines, describing process performance or stability, and identifying areas for more focused data collection. Accreditation standards are appropriate external resources that can be used to establish the performance measure of the average monthly health record delinquency rate (health records documentation not completed within required timeframes). Accrediting bodies will cite the healthcare organization when their health record documentation delinquency rate does not meet their established threshold. Hospitals commonly set the benchmark for their health record delinquency rate at less than 50 percent.

Once a benchmark for each performance measure is determined, analyzing data collection results becomes more meaningful. Results that fall outside the established benchmark often trigger further study or more focused data collection on a performance measure. When variation is discovered through **continuous monitoring**—the regular and frequent assessment of healthcare processes and their outcomes and related costs, the variation may represent an opportunity for improvement to change processes or services to better meet customer needs (AlTaweel and Al-Hawary 2021).

An example of the PI model in use for an improvement opportunity identified from ongoing data collection at Community Hospital is shown in figure 2.5. The hospital administration had previously identified the employee turnover rate as an important performance measure to monitor and had collected a number of years of historical internal data on this performance measure. In addition, it researched external comparison data from other hospitals in the community and throughout the state and determined that the best-practice rate for employee turnover in its area should be 5 percent. Accordingly, the administration set its employee turnover rate benchmark at less than 5 percent.

Figure 2.5. Community Hospital employee turnover rate

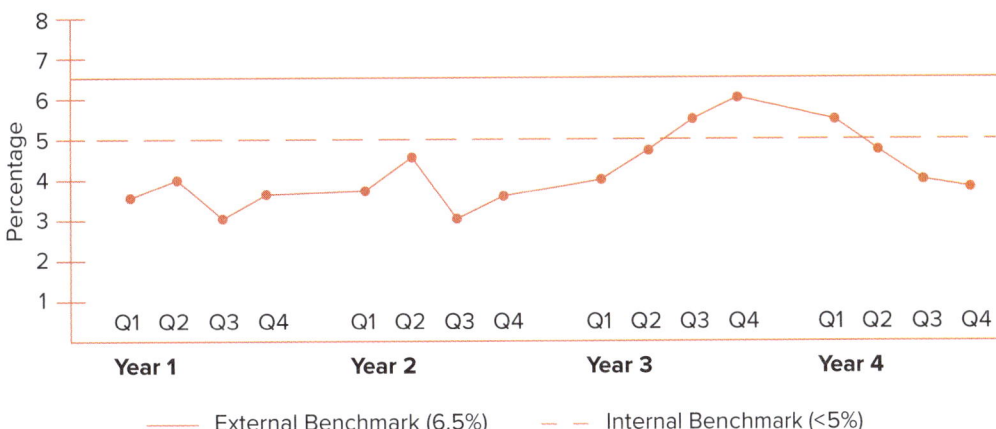

During the third year, the employee turnover rate began to steadily increase from 3 percent to 6 percent. After receiving third-quarter data that showed a continued increase in turnover, the Performance Improvement and Patient Safety Council recommended further data analysis by job class. The findings from this analysis showed a pattern in employee turnover within nursing. Exit survey data received from nursing staff were also studied, with reasons for leaving linked to salary and benefits. The council immediately recommended that the human resources department research community salary and benefits packages offered to nurses. The results of the research revealed that Community Hospital's salary and benefits package had not remained competitive, and nursing personnel were being recruited by hospitals with more attractive benefits packages. Once Community Hospital redesigned, implemented, and advertised its benefits package for nurses, the turnover rate decreased to below the established benchmark. Figure 2.6 shows how the PI model was applied in this situation.

Figure 2.6. Community Hospital PI model for reducing nursing turnover

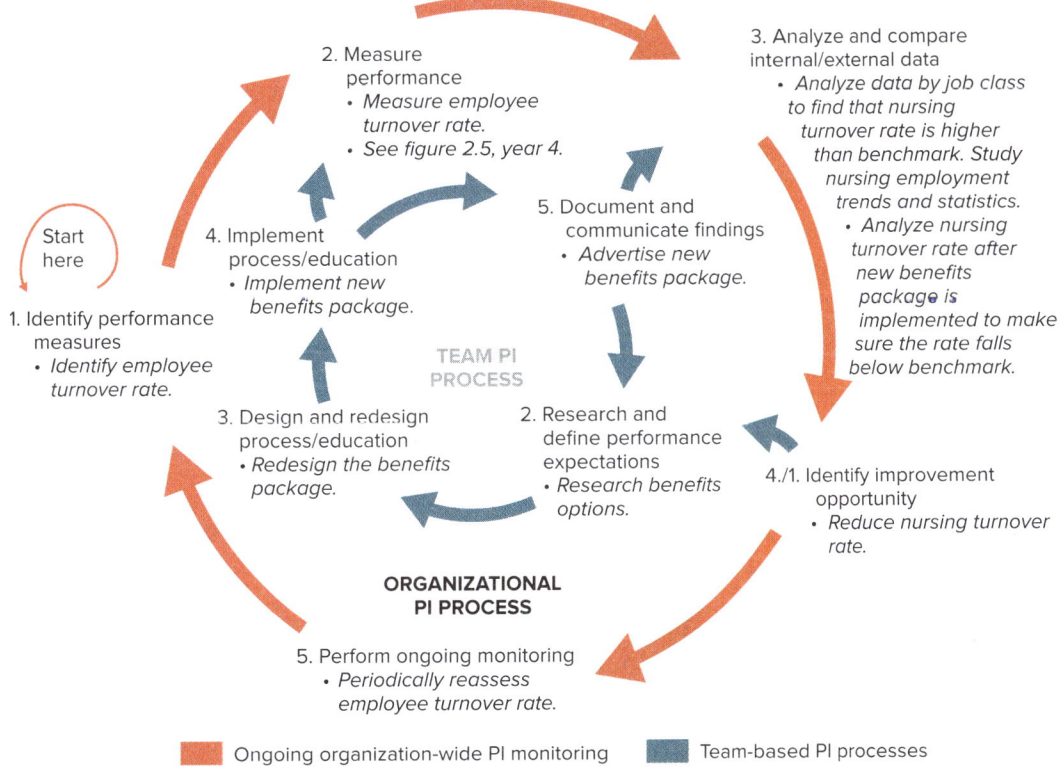

It is common practice in healthcare organizations to appoint a **leadership group** to oversee organization-wide PI activities. The leadership group is composed of the senior governing, administrative, and management groups of a healthcare organization that are responsible for setting the mission and overall strategic direction of the organization. This leadership group (sometimes named the Performance Improvement and Patient Safety Council or Quality Council) is responsible for defining the organization's PI program. Establishment of a PI program includes the following steps:

1. Define and implement the organization-wide PI model.
2. Establish a staff education plan to train employees in PI.
3. Prioritize and define PI measures.
4. Define data collection and reporting responsibilities.
5. Appoint PI teams when process variation exceeds established benchmarks.
6. Maintain a process of reporting significant findings and corrective actions to the board of directors and other stakeholders.

The person or group charged with identifying opportunities for improvement depends primarily on leadership's commitment to establishing a culture of continuous improvement. Ideally, PI opportunities should be identified by those closest to care or service processes.

Once an improvement opportunity has been identified, the leadership group can respond in a variety of ways. When the improvement opportunity is believed to be the result of a lack of knowledge or experience, an educational program may be recommended. When the improvement opportunity is the result of inefficiency or ineffectiveness in a work process, the leadership group may convene a **performance improvement (PI) team**—members of the healthcare organization who have formed a functional or cross-functional group to examine a performance issue and make recommendations with respect to its improvement—to examine the process. (The relationship between organization-wide performance monitoring and team-based PI processes is illustrated in figure 2.4.)

Team-Based PI Processes

Once an improvement opportunity has been identified and a team that consists of staff involved in the process under study has been assembled, the first task is to research and define performance expectations for the process targeted for improvement. The first steps may include the following:

1. Create a flow chart of the current process.
2. Brainstorm problem areas within the current process.
3. Research any regulatory requirements related to the current process.
4. Compare the organization's current process with performance standards or nationally recognized standards.
5. Conduct a survey to gather input on customers' needs and expectations.
6. Prioritize problem areas for focused improvement.

Process redesign incorporates the knowledge gained from data collection to change the process and involves the following steps:

1. Incorporate findings or changes identified in the research phase of the improvement process.
2. Collect focused data from the prioritized problem areas to further clarify process failure or variation.
3. Create a flow chart of the redesigned process.
4. Develop policies and procedures that support the redesigned process.
5. Educate involved staff about the new process.

PI teams can use a variety of tools to accomplish their goals. This textbook calls these quality improvement tools collected from traditional quality improvement practice and theory **QI toolbox techniques**. These tools make it easier to gather and analyze information, and they help team members stay focused on PI activities and move the process along efficiently.

After implementing a new process, the team continues to measure performance against customers' expectations and established performance standards. The team may need to redesign the process or product if measurements indicate that there is room for further improvement. When measurement data indicate that the improvement is effective, ongoing monitoring of the process is resumed (as shown in figure 2.2). The team documents and communicates its findings to the leadership group and other interested parties in the organization. Results may also be communicated to interested groups in the community.

The team is often disbanded at this point in the cycle, and routine organizational monitoring of the performance measures is resumed. If another opportunity for improvement arises, the team-based improvement process may be reinstituted.

 Check Your Understanding 2.1

1. Explain the assumptions that support the following statement: PI models used in healthcare today are always cyclical in nature.
2. A large hospital wants to reduce patient wait times in the emergency department. Using the PDCA cycle model, identify some tasks or activities that would need to be accomplished at each stage of the model (Plan, Do, Check, Act).

Systems Thinking

Systems thinking is an objective way of looking at work-related ideas and processes with the goal of allowing people to uncover ineffective patterns of behavior and thinking and then finding ways to make lasting improvements. A critical element of systems thinking is viewing an organization as an open system of interdependencies and connectedness rather than a collection of individual parts and professional enclaves. This approach sees interrelatedness as a whole and looks for patterns rather than snapshots of organizational activities and processes. Because so much of what is done in healthcare is related, the method of solving one problem and then going on to solve the next problem without understanding the connection between them will prove to be counteractive over time. This approach may work in a field where there is little change, but healthcare systems are often changing and require a systems thinking approach to ensure strategic alignment throughout the organization (McNab et al. 2020).

For example, many subsystems of a healthcare organization are dependent on accurate patient identification and demographic data collection at the time of admission or encounter registration. If the patient information is not entered correctly during the registration process, this could have a negative impact on many other processes that are dependent on this information. Some of these processes include coding accuracy, accurate billing for patient services, data abstraction for indexing and other databases, and accuracy of the master patient index and the EHR.

Process orientation traditionally has relied on measurements of cost, productivity, quality, and time to improve processes. There is a tendency to approach processes in a linear fashion, fixing one process at a time in a piecemeal approach. The challenge with this approach is that it is rarely effective in complex systems. Healthcare is a complex system because it has many interacting elements and parts (McNab et al. 2020). Anyone who has worked in a hospital or an integrated healthcare system should intuitively understand how systems thinking is more appropriate for managing complex organizations with diverse professional staff. PI efforts, such as quality control and QA, have focused heavily on structure and compliance standards. However, as PI efforts became focused on process and outcomes, the need to understand and embrace systems thinking became more apparent. Focusing on the outcome of a patient encounter forces all members of the healthcare team to work together rather than to operate as individuals who only contribute their expertise and energies to patient care in an episodic and isolated manner. This allows for a shared vision and supports a team working as a cohesive unit.

Systems thinkers consider the world around them from a holistic point of view and are an integral part of ensuring patient-centered care (Henry 2023). The physician's role has always been crucial to healthcare delivery. In the past, healthcare organizations operated under the assumption that physicians possessed all the necessary medical knowledge and that all other healthcare professionals should respond to their instructions. Then, schools of nursing began to specialize, and nursing began to develop a body of unique knowledge and skills. Other areas of specialization, such as medical laboratories, pharmacy, radiology, physical therapy, and health information, have also developed their own unique bodies of knowledge. Few individuals, including physicians, are capable of retaining the extensive knowledge and understanding of all specialized areas in health services organizations. Out of necessity, a greater degree of interdependence emerged among health professions. There is a need for information to flow in many directions rather than just from the physician to all others in the organization.

Systems Analysis Tools

Systems analysis can be applied at the work team, organizational, and healthcare setting levels. It involves four groups of analysis tools, shown in table 2.1.

Table 2.1. Systems analysis tools and sample uses

Tool	Example(s)	Application
Modeling and simulation	Queuing methods	Queuing is a term for waiting in line (e.g., waiting for a blood draw in the lab, waiting to be registered). This tool has enormous applicability to the healthcare system.
Modeling and simulation	Discrete-event simulation	Discrete-event simulation analyzes the independent variable of time against dependent variables such as patients, caregivers, administrators, inventory, capital equipment, and others.
Enterprise management	Supply-chain management Game theory and contracts Systems dynamic models Productivity measuring and monitoring	The complexity of business in the healthcare system lends itself to the application of mathematical tools used in other industries to manage networks of suppliers, distributors, and service providers.
Financial engineering and risk management	Return on investment Reduce risk Increase efficiency	The inherent risks of using these tools in healthcare involve the patient, the organization, and the environment. Healthcare organizations can use stochastic analysis (statistical forecasting) and risk models to predict the risk of financial losses.
Knowledge discovery	Data mining Predictive modeling Neural networks	Four different types of information can be retrieved through data mining: classifications, estimations, variability, and predictions. The information obtained through data mining also can be used to predict outcomes for a variety of actions through predictive modeling or neural networks.

Source: Adapted from Reid et al. 2005, 37–44.

Systems Control Tools

Statistical process control and scheduling are system control tools used to monitor and ensure that processes are performing as expected. Statistical process control is a type of run chart (line graph of data plotted over time) that indicates both upper and lower control limits to illustrate whether a process is stable or unstable. Scheduling involves ensuring that the right amounts of resources are in the right place at the right time. Although this sounds simple enough, scheduling can be difficult to implement. Forecasting demand, assessing workforce size and skill mix, and setting service standards depend on good data analysis. Sufficient information technology support, however, is necessary to implement these kinds of tools for everyday use. An example of this control tool might be scheduling enough staff, either on site or on call, that is available for an unexpected event, such as an emergency surgery.

 Check Your Understanding 2.2

1. Describe how the shift in healthcare to focus on outcomes has required healthcare organizations to adopt systems thinking.

2. When a healthcare organization seeks to determine how many patients were seen in the gastroenterology clinic in the past year and use this patient data to predict how many may be seen in future years, which knowledge discovery systems analysis tool should they use?
   a. Data mining
   b. Discrete-event simulation
   c. Exit survey
   d. Return on investment

Performance Improvement Frameworks

Healthcare organizations have adapted PI concepts and frameworks that have been successfully adopted in other industries. These frameworks include Six Sigma, Lean, and high reliability organizations (HROs), which provide the potential to improve efficiency and eliminate errors.

Six Sigma

Benchmarking has long been practiced within the domain of the healthcare system. However, some healthcare organizations have begun to benchmark against other industries and are selecting models that may be adapted to the healthcare industry. One example is applying the **Six Sigma** philosophy to PI programs in healthcare organizations. The Six Sigma goal is to satisfy customers by producing quality products, with a focus on variation reduction, waste elimination, and improved efficiency (Hessing n.d.). For example, the surgical unit at Community Hospital is experiencing a higher-than-normal rate of hospital-acquired infections (HAIs) among surgical patients. This problem is not only a patient safety issue, but can also lead to extended hospital stays, increased healthcare costs, and potential long-term health complications. This is creating inefficiencies with the system that will ultimately impact patient care.

Six Sigma uses statistics for measuring variation in a process with the intent of producing error-free results. Sigma refers to the standard deviation (*SD*) used in descriptive statistics to determine how much an event or observation varies from the estimated average of the population sample. For example, a student who scores 130 on an IQ test would be considered to have a higher IQ than 97.5 percent of the population. The average IQ is considered to be 100, and the *SD* for IQ is 15 points. Thus, a score of 130 is a variation of 2 *SD*s above the average. Only 2.5 percent of the population is estimated to have scores above 2 *SD*s.

Using this kind of statistic to measure quality variation in healthcare requires some refinement of Six Sigma. The ultimate goal of any PI program is to minimize error and, by extension, to decrease the number of errors occurring in any observation of a number of encounters or activities. Many healthcare organizations have embraced a more stringent culture of zero harm. As organizations create this culture they are less satisfied with the possibility of error and expect a climate of continuous patient safety leading to zero harm (Gandhi et al. 2020).

The Six Sigma measure indicates no more than 3.4 errors per 1 million encounters. Consider the challenge of achieving no more than 3.4 errors per 1 million prescriptions, surgeries, or diagnoses. Six Sigma was chosen as a target statistic because even 2 or 3 *SD*s would not be acceptable in certain scenarios. A 2.5 percent error rate for making correct change at a movie theater may be acceptable, but that error rate for airlines avoiding fatal crashes is completely unacceptable because airlines have hundreds of flights in the air on any given day. Even if there were only 100 flights per day, two or three fatal crashes per day would be devastating to the airline industry, not to mention the population as a whole. Similarly in healthcare, one unexpected death of a seemingly healthy patient with a low risk of mortality would be unacceptable, while a 2.5 percent registration error rate for patient type (e.g., inpatient, outpatient) may be inconvenient but not life-threatening for the patient. Therefore, it is important to keep this PI approach in proper perspective when it is applied to healthcare.

Six Sigma started in the electronics industry at Motorola and has gained a substantial foothold in manufacturing. The healthcare industry has adopted these techniques to improve processes and delivery of care. Deploying Six Sigma in healthcare requires the identification of elements of a product line that are "critical to quality" (CTQs). Focus groups or interviews can be used to elicit CTQs from customers. Typically, in healthcare, customers are patients, consumers, physicians, and other healthcare providers. All others involved—corporations, payers, accreditors, and licensers—are identified as stakeholders, entities with an important interest in the product (service) that do not have consumer relationships to it.

Underpinning the CTQs are elements "critical to process" (CTPs). These can be identified by such techniques as focus groups or interviews and represent those aspects of the living process that make the accomplishment of CTQs possible.

For example, the American Diabetes Association (ADA) and the National Committee for Quality Assurance (NCQA) have joined together to promote a CTQ "to provide clinicians with tools that support delivery of high-quality care to patients with diabetes" and to recognize those providers who are able to maintain the CTQ in their practices (NCQA n.d.). The CTPs supporting this CTQ include the first 10 evidence-based measures of the diabetes care rendered (see table 2.2). In addition, the program provides a computer application in which the provider can record the findings for each patient on a regular basis. The output of the application is forwarded to the ADA and the NCQA periodically, and when validated by them, the provider is placed on a public recognition list as meeting these evidence-based criteria and thus offering superior care for patients with diabetes mellitus. Patients win as customers. Providers win as customers. The ADA wins as a stakeholder in promoting better diabetes care. Payers win as stakeholders in identifying providers who use best practices in the management of this disease.

Table 2.2. Diabetes care CTPs

Diabetes Recognition Measure	Threshold (% of patients in sample)	Weight
HbA1c control >9.0%	≤15	15.0
HbA1c control <7.0%	40	10.0
Blood pressure control ≥140/90 mmHg	≤35	15.0
Blood pressure control <130/80 mmHg	25	10.0
LDL control ≥130 mg/dL	≤37	10.0
LDL control <100 mg/dL	36	10.0
Eye examination	60	10.0
Foot examination	80	5.0
Nephropathy assessment	80	5.0
Smoking status and cessation advice or treatment	80	10.0
Total points		100.0
Points needed to achieve recognition		75.0

Lean

Lean is a quality improvement technique often seen in the manufacturing sector. It has also been implemented in many other industries with great success. Toyota was one of the first and most visible organizations to implement this technique. Lean thinking is the concept of implementing value and eliminating waste. This technique has been adopted by some healthcare organizations as a way to streamline their processes in these seven areas:

- Overproduction (ordering duplicate tests)
- Wasting time (long wait times for patients)

- Waste of stock on hand (outdated or unused medications)
- Waste of movement (time spent walking from one location to another)
- Waste of defective products (expired vaccine)
- Waste in transportation (moving patients unnecessarily)
- Waste in processing (duplicate forms or redundant capture of information)

For example, a clinic may be ordering more vaccines than they can use before the expiration date. This is creating waste within the clinic and using resources that could be better spent on other necessities for patient care. Successful implementation of Lean techniques in a healthcare organization must include attention to the customer (patient-centered care), the customer's perspective, and efforts to reduce unnecessary waste. A key technique used in Lean thinking is root-cause analysis (Bharsakade et al. 2021).

Lean Six Sigma

Lean Six Sigma is a combination of the two methodologies, Lean and Six Sigma. Lean Six Sigma incorporates the attributes of Lean by focusing on the elimination of waste and removal of unnecessary steps in a process to increase the speed at which a process is done. Key attributes of Six Sigma are also incorporated to improve accuracy, such as the reduction of variation within processes, leading to increased optimization. By combining the two methodologies, the characteristics of each work together to decrease waste and eliminate variation, creating processes that have both speed and accuracy (see figure 2.7).

Figure 2.7. Lean Six Sigma

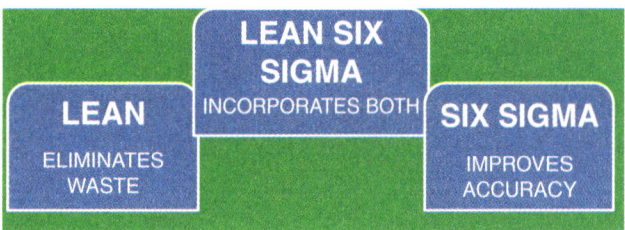

Let's look at an example of how the Lean Six Sigma methodology can improve an ineffective process. A hospital is experiencing delays and inefficiencies in the patient discharge process. These delays are causing patients to wait for longer periods of time to be discharged, resulting in reduced bed availability for patients needing to be moved to the inpatient setting. These issues negatively affect patient satisfaction and cause both waste and inefficiencies. The incorporation of Lean Six Sigma provides a framework for healthcare organizations to use both speed and accuracy to provide higher-quality care to patients. Customers are more satisfied because of the improved patient care and processes, and the environment created is also positive for employees. Organizations that use Lean Six Sigma are nimbler and can proactively respond to their environment to make necessary changes that can provide a competitive advantage for these organizations (ASQ 2023b). In the example involving the patient discharge process, the delays and inefficiencies would be considered waste. A QI team would analyze the process to determine the reasons for the delays and inefficiencies, and these processes would be redesigned to eliminate the waste. The redesigned processes would increase the speed at which patients are discharged and allow beds to be turned over in a timelier manner.

High Reliability Organizations

High reliability organizations (HROs) operate "under trying conditions and persistently have fewer than their fair share of crises" (Weick and Sutcliffe 2015, 7). HROs have learned to manage unexpected change, knowing that it can sometimes be prevented or at least anticipated and prepared for. The methodology of

HROs was seen initially in nuclear power plants, aircraft carriers, and wildland firefighting. These types of organizations have a high risk for error and failure, and the impact of those errors or failures is significant and can be catastrophic to the organizations and those around them. HROs have learned that mistakes and errors occur because of employees' mindlessness and distraction, which occur when employees are hurried or overloaded.

For example, during medication administration a nurse can lose focus if interrupted (as when another nurse asks a question about a different patient). Losing focus on medication administration is an example of mindlessness and a prime situation in which medical errors can occur. HROs are focused on mindfulness. In this context, mindfulness is defined as a keen awareness of the tasks and processes that enable employees to discover and correct errors that can escalate into a crisis before they occur. In an HRO, all employees are empowered to speak up and tell those who interrupt to wait their turn. Employees are encouraged to create an organizational culture that teaches all staff to respect certain high-risk tasks that need to be distraction-free to ensure patient safety. These organizations also pay close attention to weak signs of trouble to catch problems or errors in the earliest stage. Preoccupation with failure and sensitivity to operations are key traits of HROs. Because healthcare is an industry with a high potential for error and significant negative impact from these errors, many healthcare organizations are seeing the benefit of implementing the HRO methodology (Dupree 2015; Weick and Sutcliffe 2015, 45–47, 130).

Check Your Understanding 2.3

1. High reliability organizations (HROs) are concerned with mindlessness and distraction among healthcare employees. Mindlessness and distraction are more likely to occur when:
   a. Employees are the wrong fit for the job.
   b. Employees do not have enough to do.
   c. Employees are preoccupied, rushed, and overloaded.
   d. Employees are only concerned about caring for their patients.

2. University Hospital suspects that they are disposing of a high quantity of unused supplies in their outpatient surgery units because the supplies are past their expiration date. Which quality improvement technique has been used in other industries that could be used to investigate this issue?
   a. HRO
   b. Lean
   c. Six Sigma
   d. Systems thinking

Real-Life Example

Wildcat Hospital is a 400-bed acute-care facility offering a wide range of services. Dr. Jones is a cardiothoracic surgeon at the facility and has been practicing in the area for the past six years. Dr. Jones was performing a coronary bypass procedure on a 59-year-old patient. Although the procedure was going well, it took more time than usual to complete because the anesthesiologist needed extra time prior to surgery to ensure a safe experience with the anesthesia due to the patient's asthma and sleep apnea. The operating rooms had been especially busy, with a high number of unexpected trauma surgeries in addition to the already-busy OR schedule.

Dr. Jones was preparing to finish the procedure and close the incision when he noticed another physician looking in the window of the OR door. The physician looking in has been at the hospital for several decades. As he looked at Dr. Jones he lifted his arm and tapped on his watch to tell Dr. Jones that his surgery time had gone past what was scheduled. Although Dr. Jones is a confident and competent surgeon, this experience rattled him a bit and he was somewhat distracted by the other physician's behavior. He allowed himself to become a little "short-fused" and began to speed up his work, pressuring the other staff. Several days after the surgery, the patient returned to Dr. Jones's office with pain and issues with the surgical wound. After further workup, it was determined that a sponge was left in during the procedure.

The leadership team at Wildcat Hospital reviewed the situation surrounding the retained sponge and determined that the high reliability organization (HRO) methodology that was put into place in the hospital was not followed in this instance. The seasoned physician should have known that his behavior was unacceptable and caused an unnecessary distraction for Dr. Jones and the surgical team. Dr. Jones and the other staff members in the OR should not have allowed this physician's behavior to distract them. In an HRO culture, all employees should feel empowered to speak up in situations in which patient or employee safety is at risk.

Distractions and interruptions can occur during healthcare processes. Part of creating a culture of safety in a healthcare organization is training employees to be aware of distraction and how to manage it. Dr. Jones and the other OR staff should have used mindfulness to bring focus back to the patient on the table and avoid the unnecessary rush to conclude the surgery. Mindfulness is a key aspect of HRO culture. In this situation it would have helped to prevent this negative patient outcome. Instead of using the skill of mindfulness, Dr. Jones and the OR staff chose to let the seasoned physician distract them.

Case Study

The outpatient clinic at Memorial Hospital is experiencing a bottleneck in their appointment scheduling system. Patients are on hold for long periods of time when they call the clinic to make an appointment. There is no option for patients to make an online appointment, even though the scheduling tool allows for it. Employees often have trouble seeing available appointment slots for some providers.

Once patients make an appointment, they are not reminded of their upcoming appointment, and the clinic experiences many missed appointments (no shows). Patients are also not provided with the necessary documents and forms needed for their appointment and many spend a significant amount of time in the waiting room filling out forms on tablets, which leads to delays in treatment. These issues are resulting in delays, patient dissatisfaction, and increased administrative workload.

After review of the data and conversing with those involved in the process, the clinic leadership team decides to address this issue using Lean methodology. By applying Lean to this situation, the leadership team aims to reduce the waste caused by the ineffective processes and optimize the use of the appointment scheduling system.

The scheduling tool included in the clinic's information management system has not been fully utilized. The tool has functionality such as a centralized scheduling platform, online appointment capabilities, prioritization of urgent cases, and automated appointment reminders. The system also allows for distribution and online submission of registration forms. These tools are not currently being used. Employees who manage scheduling and patient check-in have not been asked about the issues they are experiencing related to workflow and patient delays. To begin to resolve the bottleneck, the leadership team has selected the front-office supervisor to use Lean methodology to create a plan for improvement.

Case Study Questions

1. Lean methodology is used in situations in which there is waste occurring in a process. Provide at least two examples of waste in the current patient scheduling processes at the clinic.

2. Using the two examples from question 1, provide two steps that can be taken by the front-office supervisor to establish a more standardized and efficient process for appointment scheduling.

3. Lean methodology is focused on patients and their perspective. In what ways is the current scheduling process not patient-centered? How will a system of continuous improvement and collecting regular feedback from both staff and patients improve the patient experience with the scheduling process?

Review Questions

1. Compare and contrast the use of Six Sigma, Lean, and HRO concepts with regard to quality in healthcare.
2. A healthcare organization is investigating the organization's compliance with the post-procedure patient education process. A performance measure will be used to assist in this investigation. Write this performance measure.
3. Community Hospital is concerned about their readmission rate for congestive heart failure patients in the last quarter. Which of the following methods would the hospital use to determine if their readmission rate is in line with similar-size hospitals?
   a. Write a performance measure.
   b. Perform benchmarking.
   c. Identify an improvement opportunity.
   d. Create a data measure.
4. As part of their HRO and Zero Harm initiatives, University Medical Center introduced a new protocol for medication administration and conducted extensive training sessions for all staff. As part of the new protocol, staff must verify all details of the medication and its administration instructions prior to giving it to the patient. A nurse preparing to administer medication to a patient following the new protocol notices that the dosage seems unusually high for the patient's condition. What should the nurse do?
   a. Administer the medication as prescribed, assuming the dosage is correct.
   b. Skip the medication administration and inform the patient's physician later.
   c. Double-check the medication dosage with a colleague or supervisor before administration.
   d. Ask the patient what their typical dose is for this medication.
5. A team may redesign a process or product if:
   a. Measurement indicates there is room for further improvement.
   b. New board members are appointed.
   c. The team adds a new member.
   d. Data cannot be collected on the process.

References

AHRQ (Agency for Healthcare Research and Quality). 2020. "Health Literacy Universal Precautions Toolkit, 2nd ed." https://www.ahrq.gov/health-literacy/improve/precautions/tool2b.html

AlTaweel, I. R. and S. I. Al-Hawary. 2021. The Mediating Role of Innovation Capability on the Relationship between Strategic Agility and Organizational Performance. *Sustainability* 13(14): 7564

ASQ (American Society for Quality). 2023a. "What Is The Plan-Do-Check-Act (PDCA) Cycle?" https://asq.org/quality-resources/pdca-cycle .

ASQ (American Society for Quality). 2023b. "What is Six Sigma?" http://asq.org/learn-about-quality/six-sigma/overview/overview.html.

Bharsakade R.S., P. Acharya, L. Ganapathy, and M.K. Tiwari. 2021. A lean approach to healthcare management using multi criteria decision making. *OPSEARCH*. 58(3):610–635, https://doi.org/10.1007/s12597-020-00490-5. Epub 2021 Jan 1. PMCID: PMC7775731.

CMS (Center for Medicare and Medicaid Services). n.d. "Glossary." Accessed November 3, 2023. https://www.cms.gov/glossary?items_per_page=10&term=performance%20measure&viewmode=grid

Dupree, E. S. 2015. Zero harm is the goal. *Patient Safety and Quality Healthcare* 10: 14, 16. https://www.jcrinc.com/products-and-services/high-reliability/-/media/cth/documents/what-we-offer/psqh_nov-dec_2015_issue_dupreepdf.pdf

Gandhi, T, D. Feeley, and D. Schummers. 2020. Zero harm in health care. *NEJM Catalyst Innovations in Care Delivery* 1(2).

Henry, T. 2023. AMA ChangeMedEd Initiative. "Why you need to be a systems thinker in health care." https://www.ama-assn.org/education/changemeded-initiative/why-you-need-be-systems-thinker-health-care.

Hessing, T. n.d. "What is Six Sigma." Accessed June 24, 2024. https://sixsigmastudyguide.com/what-is-six-sigma/

Institute for Healthcare Improvement (IHI). n.d. "Plan-Do-Study-Act (PDSA) Worksheet." Accessed November 3, 2023. https://www.ihi.org/resources/Pages/Tools/PlanDoStudyActWorksheet.aspx.

McNab D., J. McKay, S. Shorrock, S. Luty, and P. Bowie. 2020. Development and application of 'systems thinking' principles for quality improvement. *BMJ Open Quality* 9(1): e000714, https://doi.org/10.1136/bmjoq-2019-000714. PMID: 32209593; PMCID: PMC7103793.

NCQA (National Committee for Quality Assurance). n.d. "Diabetes Recognition Program." Accessed December 20, 2023. https://www.ncqa.org/programs/health-care-providers-practices/diabetes-recognition-program-drp/.

Reid, P. P., W. D. Compton, J. H. Grossman, and G. Fanjiang, eds. 2005. *Building a Better Delivery System: A New Engineering/Health Care Partnership*. Washington, DC: National Academies Press.

Vietze, J. 2013 (June). "PDCA_Process.png." Digital Image. Wikimedia Commons. https://upload.wikimedia.org/wikipedia/commons/a/a8/PDCA_Process.png.

Weick, K. and K. M. Sutcliffe. 2015. *Managing the Unexpected: Sustained Performance in a Complex World*, 3rd ed. San Francisco: Jossey-Bass.

Resources

Ilin M, and J. Bohlen. 2023. *Six Sigma Method*. Treasure Island (FL): StatPearls Publishing. https://www.ncbi.nlm.nih.gov/books/NBK589666/

Rathi, R., A. Vakharia, and M. Shadab. 2022. Lean six sigma in the healthcare sector: A systematic literature review. *Mater Today Proc*. 50:773-781, https://doi.org/10.1016/j.matpr.2021.05.534. Epub 2021 Jun 7. PMID: 35155129; PMCID: PMC8820448.

Weick, K. and K. M. Sutcliffe. 2007. *Managing the Unexpected: Resilient Performance in an Age of Uncertainty*, 2nd ed. San Francisco: Jossey-Bass.

Willminton, C., P. Belardi,, A. M. Murante, and M. Vainieri. 2022. The contribution of benchmarking to quality improvement in healthcare. A systematic literature review. *BMC Health Services Research* 22:139.

Identifying Improvement Opportunities Based on Performance Measurement

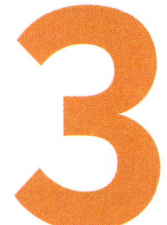

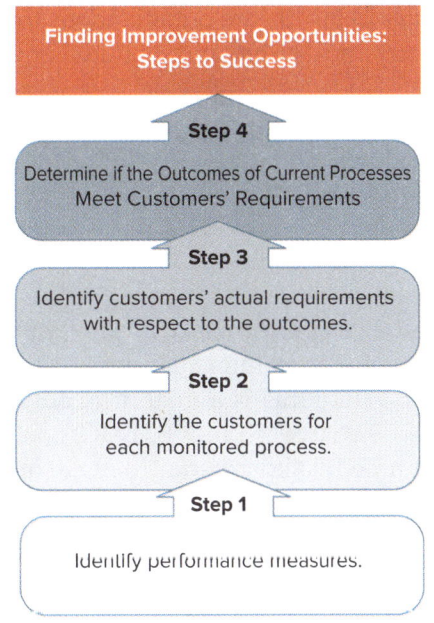

Learning Objectives

- Demonstrate how the principal aspects of healthcare are targeted for performance measurement
- Assess the significance of outcomes and proactive risk reduction in performance improvement methodology
- Apply brainstorming and the nominal group technique to performance improvement activities

Key Terms

Affinity diagrams
Benchmarking
Brainstorming
Goal
Nominal group technique
Outcome measure

Performance measurement
Process measure
Sentinel events
SMART goal
Systems

The US healthcare system is extremely complex. The idea of improving even a tiny element of the system may seem daunting to students new to the concept of performance improvement (PI). Where does the process begin? How are potential areas for improvement identified? To answer these questions, it is important to first develop a general understanding of the areas of healthcare services that are the focus of PI efforts.

Performance measurement in healthcare provides an indication of an organization's performance in relation to a specified process or outcome. Healthcare PI philosophies most often focus on measuring performance in the following areas:

- *Systems*: The foundations of caregiving, which include buildings (environmental services), equipment (technical services), professional staff (human resources), and appropriate policies (administrative systems)
- *Processes*: The interrelated activities in healthcare organizations that promote effective and safe patient outcomes across services and disciplines within an integrated environment
- *Outcomes*: The final results of care, treatment, and services in terms of the patient's expectations, needs, and quality of life, which may be positive and appropriate or negative and diminishing

Most PI projects address the organization's performance in at least one of these areas. The healthcare organization first sets a **goal** or aim for the system, process, or outcome that it wants to achieve. A goal is the level of attainment or result that you wish to accomplish. Once a goal is established, the PI project team then identifies the strategies or tasks to attain the goal.

Each healthcare organization will establish performance improvement goals that align with their strategic initiatives and the organization's mission. For example, an organization may set a goal to reduce hospital readmissions of heart failure patients. While this is a goal, it is not well defined. One technique used to effectively define a goal is to develop a **SMART goal**. A SMART goal defines the goal in terms of specific, measurable, achievable, relevant, and time-related criteria. To make our original goal SMART it needs to be defined in greater detail:

Specific: Reduce the 30-day readmission rate of heart failure patients by 20 percent within the next 12 months.
Measurable: Measure the baseline 30-day readmission rate for heart failure patients and track progress quarterly. Aim for a 20 percent reduction from the baseline rate by the end of the 12-month period.
Achievable: The goal is challenging but realistic, considering the implementation of evidence-based practices, improved patient education, and enhanced post-discharge follow-up procedures, with the support and collaboration of relevant healthcare teams.
Relevant: This goal aligns with the hospital's mission to provide high-quality patient care and addresses a critical issue in healthcare—reducing readmissions, which can improve patient outcomes and reduce healthcare costs.
Time-bound: Achieve the 20 percent reduction in the 30-day readmission rate for heart failure patients within the next 12 months, with progress monitored and reported quarterly.

Goals should be defined as *entry* (your starting point), *target* (realistic level to achieve), and *stretch* (optimistic level to achieve). An entry goal might be to optimize the treatment of heart failure patients across the continuum of care to improve care and reduce hospital readmissions by 20 percent within the next

12 months. A target goal might be to optimize the treatment of heart failure patients across the continuum of care to improve care and reduce hospital readmissions by 40 percent within the next 12 months. And the stretch goal might be to optimize the treatment of heart failure patients across the continuum of care to improve care and reduce hospital readmissions by 60 percent within the next 12 months.

Continuous Improvement Builds on Continuous Monitoring: Steps to Success

To discover which **systems**, processes, or outcomes need to be improved, a healthcare organization must first find out what is and what is not working with respect to customer needs and expectations. One way this can be accomplished is by using the results of customer satisfaction surveys and customer complaints. Most PI methodologies recognize that the organization must identify and continuously monitor the important organizational and patient-focused functions they perform, with special emphasis on high-volume (procedures that are performed often and routinely), high-risk (procedures with a greater risk for complications), and problem-prone (complicated processes that have potential for error) outcomes. (See figure 3.1 for an illustration of the process.)

Figure 3.1. Process of identifying improvement opportunities

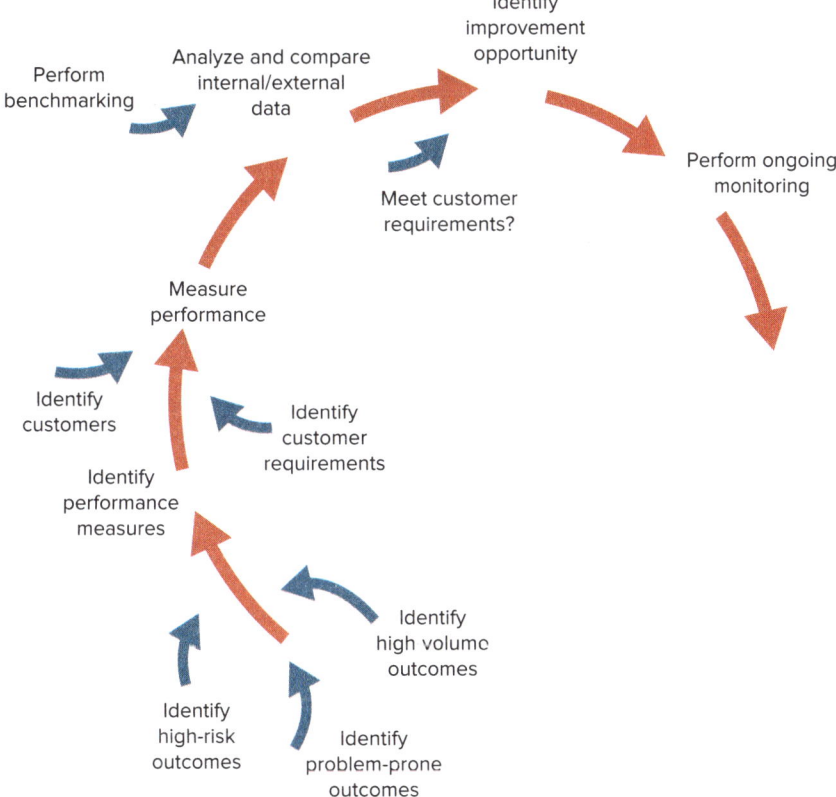

Step 1: Identify Performance Measures

Performance measures are a "gauge used to assess the performance of a process or function of any organization" (CMS 2023). Performance measures can be stated as process measures or outcome measures (see table 3.1):

- A **process measure** focuses on a way of delivering services that leads to a certain outcome.
  A scientific or experiential basis must exist for believing that the process, when executed as designed,

Table 3.1. Examples of process versus outcome measures

Measure	Type	Formula
C-section rate	Outcome	# of C-sections performed / # of deliveries
Transfusion report documentation completed	Process	# of documentation completed / # of patients receiving transfusions
Patient billing complaints	Outcome	# of complaints / # of patient days
Patients receiving info about advance directives	Process	# of patients receiving AD info / # of patients 18 or older

will increase the probability of achieving a desired outcome. Examples of process measures are the percentage of antibiotics administered immediately prior to open reduction internal fixation (ORIF) surgeries or the decision to incision time for cesarean sections. These process measures are monitored irrespective of specific patient outcomes if the medical staff were attempting to move staff practice to a model demonstrated to be more effective in the scientific literature and in the community in which the medical staff was based.

- An **outcome measure** is the result of systematically tracking a patient's clinical treatment and responses to that treatment, including measures of morbidity and functional status, for the purpose of improving care. An outcome measure may be the effect of care, treatment, or services on a customer, such as an unanticipated adverse event or, as in the previous example, the incidence of postoperative wound infections occurring in ORIF procedures in which antibiotics were and were not administered.

Many facilities develop measurable criteria to determine whether customer care, treatment, or services produce desirable or undesirable outcomes. The organization must then develop a data collection process or tool to track information on customer care, treatment, and services.

In addition, the processes, end products, and outcomes of every organizational unit may affect other organizational units. This means that in addition to the patients, the members of the organization may be one another's customers. For each process, the end products must first be identified, including those received by patient customers as well as other members of the organization.

Benchmarking is another means of identifying systems, processes, and outcomes for improvement. Benchmarking is the systematic comparison of the products, services, and outcomes of one organization with those of a similar organization (external benchmarking), or the comparison of one unit to another unit within the same organization (internal benchmarking). Benchmarking comparisons also can be made using regional and national standards if the data collection processes are similar. This process of benchmarking against an organization's established norm, which may be based on best-practice, state, or national standards, or some combination of these thresholds, helps the organization determine whether its processes fall within acceptable standard deviations of the norm. Items that fall outside the norm may be appropriate for PI projects.

Organizations sometimes receive dramatic information about the ineffectiveness of a care process through a **sentinel event**. Sentinel events usually involve significant injury to or the death of a patient or an employee through avoidable causes. The Joint Commission defines a sentinel event as a "patient safety event (not primarily related to the natural course of the patient's illness or underlying condition) that reaches a patient and results in death, severe harm (regardless of duration of harm), or permanent harm (regardless of severity of harm)" (Joint Commission 2024, GL-38). The event is called "sentinel" because it should trigger the staff's immediate attention.

Examples of sentinel events include a patient suicide in a setting where the patient received 24-hour care, infant abduction or discharge to the wrong family, rape, hemolytic transfusion reaction involving administration of blood or blood products having major group incompatibilities, and surgery on the wrong patient or wrong body part. Figure 3.2 shows the most frequently reported sentinel events for the first six months of 2023. Such outcomes get the organization's attention very quickly.

An analysis of the causes of a sentinel event usually allows the organization to make significant improvements in a process. The Joint Commission publishes Sentinel Event Alert newsletters that contain

Figure 3.2. Six most frequently reported sentinel events for the first half of 2023 (Joint Commission)

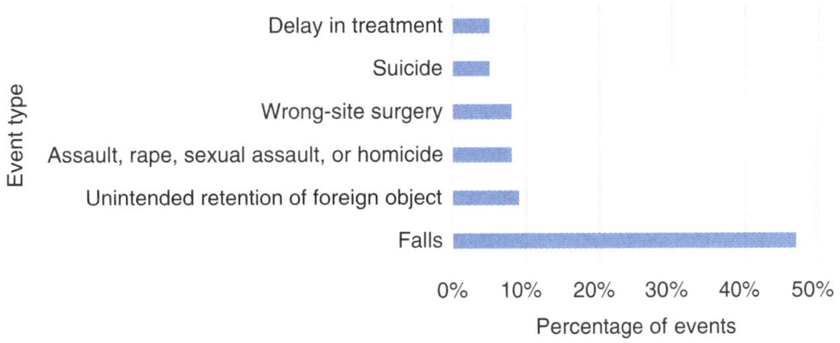
Event type
Delay in treatment
Suicide
Wrong-site surgery
Assault, rape, sexual assault, or homicide
Unintended retention of foreign object
Falls
0%
10%
20%
30%
40%
50%
Percentage of events

Source: Adapted from Becker's Clinical Leadership, 2023.

information related to sentinel events and outcomes (Joint Commission 2023). This information outlines risk-reduction strategies for many common sentinel events based on root-cause analysis from different organizations. Review of this information allows the organization to measure its own performance against the performance of other organizations.

The most important performance measures are those identified as strategically important to the organization's overall mission. Some organizations use the criteria of *high* or *low volume*, *high risk*, and *problem prone* to identify the performance measures that should receive the most scrutiny:

- Processes related to high- or low-volume outcomes affect numerous customers. High-volume processes increase the risk of incidents through the sheer number of processes performed. Low-volume processes increase the risk because they may be performed infrequently or be unfamiliar to staff, creating the opportunity for increased errors or patient safety risks.
- Processes related to problem-prone or high-risk outcomes can result in patient injury or negative outcomes that might expose the organization to malpractice suits or other legal actions. Either of these process outcomes increases the long-term cost to the patients, payers, or the organization due to increased length of stay required for additional procedures or costly malpractice fees.

The processes and outcomes related to strategically important services and to the organization's overall mission become the organization's performance measures—those measures by which the performance of the organization and its work units will be monitored by internal and external customers.

Step 2: Identify the Customers for Each Monitored Process

Who receives the outcomes or end products? During this step, the PI team should identify each customer category for the process under consideration. The list must be exhaustive and should include internal and external customers. Identifying all customers will be easier for some work areas than others. For example, a PI team in the radiology scheduling area may easily identify its customers as patients, patients' family members, providers and their office staff, and possibly others. However, in areas such as the health information services department, it may be more difficult to recognize customers, who include patients, patients' family members, providers, all other departments in the facility, administrators, accrediting bodies, internal or external auditors, and more. The PI team can create this list of customers through a brainstorming process. Steps 2 through 4 are initiated when a performance measure shows undesirable trends or outcomes requiring the formation of a PI team.

Step 3: Identify Customers' Actual Requirements with Respect to the Outcomes

Actual requirements must be identified from the customers' perspective. The objective is to identify the factors that the organization's internal and external customers value most. Organizations use a variety of methods to determine these customer requirements, including survey results, observation, and customer complaints.

Step 4: Determine if the Outcomes of Current Processes Meet Customers' Requirements

When the outcomes of current processes *do* actually meet customers' requirements, the organization should continue ongoing monitoring of the processes. The frequency of this monitoring would depend on the process under consideration. When the outcomes *do not* meet customers' requirements, a PI team should be formed to examine the processes in greater detail. Alternatively, the organization should develop an educational program to fine-tune staff members' ability to execute the processes effectively.

Check Your Understanding 3.1

1. Each healthcare organization will establish performance improvement goals that align with their strategic initiatives and organization mission. SMART goals are established to set clear expectations for all members of the organization regarding the goal the organization is trying to achieve. What does the "R" in the term SMART represent?
   a. Reasonable
   b. Relevant
   c. Recognizable
   d. Rational

2. The Northwest Hospital Corporation's Health Information (HI) Director wants to compare the time each of the hospitals in the corporation are spending on chart analysis, and determine how they are performing against the best-practice standard. The HI Director generated the following data to make this comparison. What is this comparison process called?
   a. Benchmarking
   b. Comparing
   c. Outcome comparison
   d. Process comparison

Northwest Hospital Corporation

HIM Corporate Dashboard

November, 20xx

	Analysis Days			Delinquency Rate
	IP	SDS	ED	
Community Region Facilities				
Hospital A	3.0	3.0	2.0	5%
Hospital B	1.0	2.0	1.0	0%
Hospital C	1.0	3.0	1.0	8%
Urban Region Facilities				
Hospital D	4.0	1.0	0.0	12%
Hospital E	2.0	32.0	30.0	23%
Hospital F	3.0	7.0	4.0	8%
Corporate Average	2.33	8.00	6.33	9%
Best-Practice Standard	2.0	2.0	1.0	<15%

QI Toolbox Techniques

 The most common toolbox techniques that PI teams use to determine performance measures, identify customers, identify customers' requirements, and identify whether customers' requirements are met include brainstorming, affinity diagrams, and the nominal group technique.

Brainstorming

Brainstorming can be conducted in a structured or an unstructured way. In *structured* brainstorming, the leader solicits input from team members by going around the table or room. Each team member comments on the issue in turn or passes until the next round. This process continues until participants have no new ideas to suggest or until the time period set in the meeting agenda has elapsed. In *unstructured* brainstorming, members of the team offer ideas as they come to mind. Some members may have no ideas to offer, and others may contribute a number of ideas. In either method, several general rules are followed:

- Everyone agrees on the issue to be brainstormed.
- All ideas are recorded in the team member's own words, using a white board, flip chart, or brainstorming software.
- Ideas are never criticized or discussed during the brainstorming period.
- The process is limited to the time allotted, 5 to 15 minutes at most per topic.

Affinity Diagrams

Affinity diagrams are used to organize and prioritize ideas after the initial brainstorming session. This type of diagram is useful when the team generates a large amount of information. The team members agree on the primary categories or groupings from the brainstorming session, and secondary ideas are listed under each primary category. An example is shown in figure 3.3. This process allows the team to tackle a large problem in a more manageable way (ASQ n.d.a) This process may be completed manually using sticky notes or with a software tool. Both methods ensure that all ideas can easily be transferred from one category or grouping to another as team members work to group or rank ideas.

Figure 3.3. Example of an affinity diagram

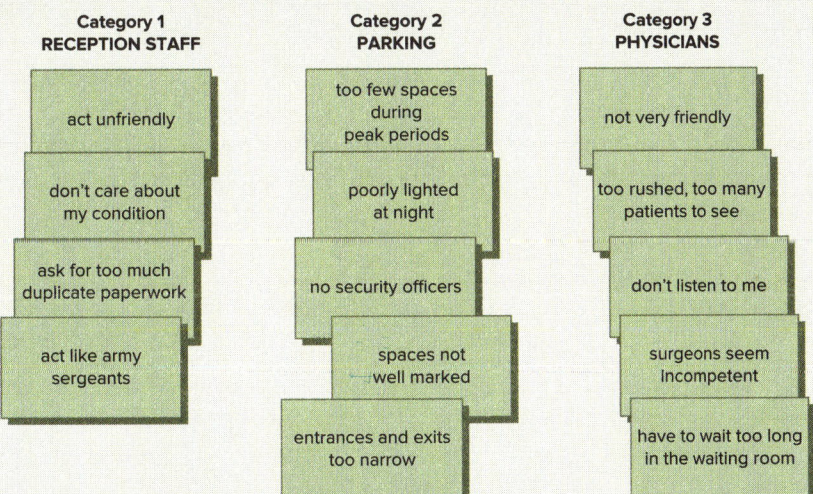

Nominal Group Technique

The **nominal group technique** gives each member of the team an opportunity to select the most important ideas from the affinity diagram. As discussed by Nancy Tague in *The Quality Toolbox*, 3rd edition (Tague 2024), this technique allows groups to narrow the focus of discussion and to make decisions without getting involved in extended, circular discussions during which the more vocal members dominate. All the ideas obtained during an earlier brainstorming session are written in a place where everyone can see them. Teams usually use white boards, flip charts, or software tools for this purpose.

Next, team members vote on the various issues or ideas to determine which should be considered first. The facilitator writes the numeral 1 by the idea that each team member chooses as most important. This process continues until all of the team members have ranked all the issues or ideas on a numerical scale. For example, if five issues were listed, each team member would rank them from 1 to 5, with 1 being the most important and 5 being the least important. The facilitator then adds up the rankings for each issue. The issue with the lowest sum is selected as the team's choice for most important. The team will work on this issue first, followed by the other four issues in ranked order.

Another way to vote is to use adhesive dots in various colors. Each team member chooses a color, and the members affix their dots to the five issues they think are most important. The issue that has the most dots is the most important. This method works well because members can be influenced by other members' placement of votes, thus allowing consensus to begin to develop during the voting process (ASQ n.d.b).

Check Your Understanding 3.2

1. Sue has been trying to understand why the coding staff has not been meeting its productivity standards in the past three months. At a recent department meeting, she asked the coding staff in attendance to help her think of all the possible reasons for the drop in productivity. As the ideas were generated, Sue recorded each of them on a whiteboard. This is an example of _____.
   a. Team input
   b. Benchmarking
   c. Systematic input
   d. Brainstorming

2. After Sue had recorded all the ideas from the coding staff on the whiteboard, she asked each of the coders to group the ideas into like categories. After this grouping had taken place, Sue then created a graphic display of the grouping. This graphic display is called a(n):
   a. Brainstorming diagram
   b. Cause-and-effect diagram
   c. Affinity diagram
   d. Sentinel diagram

3. Finally, after Sue created the graphic display of all the idea groupings, she asked the coding staff to prioritize each of the groups from most important to least important. This process is called:
   a. Nominal group technique
   b. Benchmarking
   c. Decision-making technique
   d. Brainstorming

Real-Life Example #1

At one hospital, data from customer satisfaction surveys indicated an increase in patient complaints about having to come to the facility two or three times for preoperative testing. The PI team assigned to explore the problem identified the following performance measures, customers, and customers' requirements and determined whether the customers' requirements were met:

Step 1: *Performance measures?*
- Registration information provided and surgery scheduled by physician's office
- Number of visits required to complete preoperative testing
- Preoperative workup completed by day of surgery

Step 2: *Customers for monitored process?*
- Patient and patient's family
- Physicians and office staff
- Surgery staff
- Registration staff

Step 3: *Customers' requirements?*
- One-time communication of registration information
- Preoperative workup completed prior to day of surgery and coordinated in one visit

Step 4: *Customers' requirements met?*
- Patient satisfaction surveys showed only 76 percent satisfaction with same-day surgery registration and preoperative workup processes.
- Registration staff and physicians' office staff were hearing complaints from patients that the registration process was cumbersome and not user-friendly.
- Duplicate data collection occurred between physician office registration and same-day surgery registration.

The data collection process indicated patient dissatisfaction with services. Several problems were clearly identified that could lead to an improved outcome for patients through a PI process with a combined team approach (example of outcome as a performance measurement).

Real-Life Example #2

In another hospital, the number of accounts waiting to be billed had increased over the past six months. The business office and HI department decided to look at the timeliness, appropriateness, and effectiveness of their information-processing procedures. A PI team assigned to examine the process developed the following information (example of process as performance measurement):

Step 1: *Performance measures?*
- Patient insurance and benefits information received at time of registration
- Health record documentation complete at time of discharge
- Clinical codes assigned and transmitted within 72 hours of patient discharge
- Unbilled accounts less than $1 million

Step 2: *Customers for monitored process?*
- Patients
- Physicians and other clinical staff
- Business office staff
- Health information staff
- Administration
- Third-party payers

Step 3: *Customers' requirements?*
- Unbilled accounts continuously below $1 million
- Health record delinquency rate less than 50 percent
- HI health record completion standards met
- Business office benefits verification standards met

Step 4: *Customers' requirements met?*
- Actual unbilled accounts greater than $3 million
- Actual health record delinquency rate greater than 50 percent
- HI backlogs in all chart completion areas
- Business office verifying benefits at admission only 48 percent of time

Case Study

Due to increased patient volumes in the facility, the coding manager at Community Hospital is faced with an increased discharged not final billed (DNFB) rate. The management staff of the HI department has brainstormed the following list of potential solutions to rectify this problem:

- Implement computer-assisted coding (CAC)
- Send coders home to work remotely
- Implement flex time
- Perform a time study to see how coders are spending their time
- Hire a coding support person to handle clerical activities
- Have all coders code only one patient type (e.g., inpatients, outpatients, emergency room, ancillary)
- Hire more coders
- Provide more coding training
- Change encoders
- Change the coding workflow
- Train coders to code more than one patient type
- Send all coders to a regional coding meeting

Case Study Question

1. Using the potential solutions listed above, determine common themes for the brainstormed solutions. Next, create an affinity diagram using the categories and potential solutions.

Review Questions

1. Which of the following would be a customer for the release of information function in a hospital HI department?
   a. Attorneys representing malpractice claims
   b. Housekeeping
   c. Central supply
   d. Former employers of personnel

2. Categorize the following as either a process measure or an outcome measure by completing column 2 (Type: Outcome or Process) in the table below:

Measure	Type: Outcome or Process	Formula
Total incidences of inpatient falls		# of inpatient falls / # of patient days
Utilization management: # of patients for whom discharge planning was completed		# of patients who had discharge planning completed / # of patients discharged
Procedure appropriateness: Surgical criteria not met		# of appropriate surgical cases / # of surgical cases
Transfusion form not completed		# of transfusion forms completed / # of patients receiving transfusions
Mortality rate		# of deaths / # of discharges

3. Hospital administration has been receiving customer complaints about the level of service provided during the registration process. Patients complain that it takes too long to complete the registration process for their outpatient procedures. What should this hospital's next step be?
   a. The organization should compare registration time data to similar organizations to determine if their registration time is in line with other organizations.
   b. The organization must contact their accrediting organization immediately to report the complaints.
   c. The organization is on target; the administration should ignore the customer complaints.
   d. The organization should benchmark the registration process against the hospital's accounts receivable process.

4. How can healthcare organizations use customer or patient complaint data to improve processes?

5. Performance improvement activities are often focused on high-volume processes (for example, procedures that are performed often and routinely within the organization). This focus of PI activities exists so that complacency or routineness does not occur and result in errors or complications. Why should healthcare organizations equally focus their PI activities on low-volume processes (for example, procedures that are only performed once in a while)?

References

ASQ (American Society for Quality). n.d.a. "What is an Affinity Diagram?" Accessed December 8, 2023. https://asq.org/quality-resources/affinity.

ASQ (American Society for Quality). n.d.b. "What is Nominal Group Technique?" Accessed December 8, 2023. https://asq.org/quality-resources/nominal-group-technique.

Becker's Clinical Leadership. 2023. "Most common sentinel events in first half of 2023: Joint Commission." https://www.beckershospitalreview.com/patient-safety-outcomes/most-common-sentinel-events-in-first-half-of-2023-joint-commission.html.

CMS (Center for Medicare and Medicaid Services). n.d. "Glossary." Accessed November 3, 2023. https://www.cms.gov/glossary?items_per_page=10&term=performance%20measure&viewmode=grid

Joint Commission. 2024. *Glossary in Hospital Accreditation Standards*. Oakbrook Terrace, IL: Joint Commission Resources.

Joint Commission. 2023. "Sentinel Event Alert Newsletters." https://www.jointcommission.org/resources/sentinel-event/sentinel-event-alert-newsletters/#sort=%40z95xz95xcontentdate%20descending.

Tague, N. R. 2024. *The Quality Toolbox*, 3rd ed. Milwaukee, WI: ASQ Quality Press.

Resources

AHRQ (Agency for Healthcare Research and Quality). n.d. "Patients and Consumers." Accessed December 11, 2023. https://www.ahrq.gov/patients-consumers/index.html.

IHI (Institute for Healthcare Improvement). 2023. "Improvement Areas." https://www.ihi.org/improvement-areas

Oachs, P. K. and A. L. Watters, eds. 2020. *Health Information Management: Concepts, Principles, and Practice*, 6th ed. Chicago: AHIMA.

Using Teamwork in Performance Improvement

4

Learning Objectives

- Demonstrate the effective use of teams in performance improvement activities
- Compare and contrast the role of the performance improvement team leader and the role of team members
- Explain the contributions that team charters, team roles, ground rules, listening, and questioning can make to improve the effectiveness of performance improvement teams

Key Terms

Action plan
Agenda
Cross-functional
Functional
Ground rules
Kaizen event
Mission statement
Performance improvement council
Rapid improvement event

Team charter
Team facilitator
Team leader
Team member
Team recorder
Timekeeper
Values statement
Vision statement

Performance improvement (PI) teams involve a number of people working over long periods of time. They are costly in terms of both time and money. Therefore, PI teams should be considered an organizational resource to be used appropriately and prudently.

The early quality improvement philosophies of W. Edwards Deming, J. M. Juran, and Philip Crosby were based on team processes. Therefore, when quality improvement methodologies were first applied to healthcare organizations, it was assumed that PI activities were best accomplished by PI teams. Experience with PI processes in healthcare settings, however, has shown that PI teams are not always required.

Today, when an improvement opportunity is identified, the organization's leadership or PI council can initiate one of three approaches:

- Initiate a rapid improvement event.
- Disseminate information or develop an educational training program.
- Develop a functional or cross-functional PI team.

Sometimes the leaders of an organization may decide that they already have all the facts they need about an improvement opportunity and that the changes required are "quick fixes." In such cases, they may decide to initiate a rapid improvement. The **rapid improvement event**, also called a **Kaizen event**, involves relatively simple fixes that improve work processes without going through the whole PI process and without the need to involve other departments. Specifically, Kaizen is a Japanese term meaning continuous improvement (Lean Enterprise Institute 2024). In a rapid improvement event, an improvement can be implemented without a major investment of time, personnel, and resources. A rapid improvement event team does not spend a lot of time gathering data and reengineering processes. A team is usually composed of individuals from a similar group who are very familiar with the processes or end products that need improvement (Juran 2019). For example, the members of the health information (HI) department may want to increase response time to record authentication. The HI department may plan several ways to remind providers to complete necessary record authentication to facilitate timely documentation.

Some improvement opportunities involve only the dissemination of information or better individual training. An example of this might be when the privacy officer of the organization notices an increase in unattended workstations. A training session to reeducate and remind employees to lock their workstations before they leave them to ensure the security of patient information would be a quick fix. Again, this approach to implementing an improvement can be accomplished without expending large amounts of resources.

However, when the improvement opportunity is complex, or involves multiple departments or multiple work units within a department, the team-based approach should be considered. A PI team is instituted to research, plan, and implement the improvement. PI teams may be **functional** or **cross-functional**. A functional team involves staff from a single department or service area. A cross-functional team (also called a multidisciplinary or interprofessional team) involves more than one department, service area, or discipline. For example, a cross-functional team may be needed to address a shortage of blood or blood products in a hospital that cares for emergency, surgical, and obstetrics patients, any of whom may need blood at any time during their hospital stay. Individuals from all involved areas, including the laboratory, administration, surgery, obstetrics, and the emergency department (ED), may need to help set priorities and explain the particular needs of their own areas.

This chapter discusses the composition of PI teams and the roles of individual members. It explores the purpose of team charters, mission statements, and vision statements; ground rules for meetings; and the skills needed to develop effective teams.

Effective Teams and Team Composition

Effective team function is crucial to the success of PI programs in healthcare organizations. An organization's leaders can implement a variety of initiatives to help teams function more effectively. However, one major issue appears to predict the likelihood of team effectiveness in the PI realm: the organization's expectations.

Some consultants believe that every team needs development and, consequently, many use team-building exercises as a matter of course. The single most important way for an organization to achieve effective teams is to make team problem solving and team PI part of the organizational culture. From the moment an individual is hired to work within a healthcare organization, the message should be overtly communicated by the organization that the individual is expected to participate in team projects and that this is part of everyone's job description. By making team participation part of the organizational culture, employees will understand that they are expected to cooperate with and participate in team approaches to organizational issues.

That said, there may be individuals on a team who are uncooperative or have their own agendas. However, a knowledgeable and experienced PI team can direct individuals who are not team players into positive team production. People issues are discussed later in this chapter.

When convening a cross-functional PI team is appropriate, the organization's leaders must determine the composition of the team. The PI team should be made up of individuals close to the process to be improved because they are best qualified to accomplish the process review. This may mean that some teams will include more staff than managers. Questions that should be asked to identify team members include the following:

- Which departments or disciplines are involved in the process?
- Who are the customers of the process? Customers include all who will receive the product or service that the process produces.
- Who supplies the process? That is, who provides (supplies) a product or service that begins or supports or sustains the process to be improved?

Applying this line of questioning to the example of the multidisciplinary team addressing a hospital's blood supply shortage, the departments and disciplines identified in the process include the laboratory, administration, surgery, obstetrics, and the ED. Some of the disciplines and departments identified on the team are the customers of the process; for example, the patient care areas and the patients requiring the blood products. The suppliers of the process are the laboratory and administration areas, both of which are responsible for coordinating the availability of blood products to the hospital's patient care areas.

Limitations on the number of people who can participate on a team and other factors sometimes mean that all the people involved in a process to be improved cannot participate directly on the PI team. When this happens, the team must make provisions to contact the other individuals affected by the improvement initiative. Because their perspectives and information are of critical importance, the team must develop some means for obtaining their input.

It is important to keep teams small and manageable. The general rule of thumb is that teams should be made up of 8 to 10 members. Once the team has been formed, the team members should determine which individuals, departments, and disciplines are key players in the process. Then they can bring other individuals, departments, and disciplines into the process on an ad hoc basis.

Team Roles

After the team has been selected, a **team leader** should be chosen. Having a leader is necessary to get the team organized. The organization's leaders may select the team leader, or the team may select its own leader.

The team leader should be someone the team respects as well as someone who is organized and will take the initiative to see the team through the process. This person should also know or understand the PI process and clearly understand the process to be improved. The team leader is primarily responsible for championing the effectiveness of the process in meeting customers' needs. The leader is also responsible for the *content* of the team's work and for the following specific activities:

- Preparing for and scheduling meetings (standard meeting day, time, and location)
- Sending out meeting announcements, other necessary materials, and team assignment reminders

- Conducting meetings (the importance of following an agenda is discussed later in the QI Toolbox Technique section of this chapter)
- Focusing the group's attention on the task at hand
- Ensuring group participation and asking for facts, opinions, and suggestions
- Providing expertise in the organization's PI methodology, tools, and techniques
- Coordinating data collection
- Assigning tasks
- Facilitating implementation of **action plan** (a set of initiatives to be undertaken to achieve a performance improvement goal) items
- Critiquing the meetings
- Serving as the primary spokesperson and presenter for the team
- Keeping attendance records
- Contacting absent members to review the results of the meeting and provide any materials that were distributed during the meeting

The PI team also may want to identify a **team facilitator**. The facilitator should be someone who knows the PI process well and has facilitated such a team in the past. The facilitator may be required to train the team in the PI process and quality improvement (QI) tools. This person must understand the process to be improved and is primarily responsible for ensuring that an effective PI process occurs. Some teams combine the roles of the leader and the facilitator and assign one person to both functions. The responsibilities of the team facilitator include:

- Serving as advisor and consultant to the team
- Acting as a neutral, nonvoting member
- Suggesting alternative PI methods and procedures to keep the team on target and moving forward
- Managing group dynamics, resolving conflict, and modeling compromise
- Acting as coach and motivator for the team
- Assisting in consensus building when necessary
- Recognizing team and individual achievements

The role of the **team member** includes the following functions:

- Participating in decision-making and plan development for the team
- Identifying opportunities for improvement
- Gathering, prioritizing, and analyzing data
- Sharing knowledge, information, and data that pertain to the process under study

The role of **team recorder** (also called team scribe) is vital to the team's success. This team member keeps minutes of the team's work during the meetings, including any documentation required by the organization. The recorder performs the following functions:

- Recording information for the group
- Creating appropriate charts and diagrams
- Assisting with notices and supplies for meetings
- Distributing notices and other documentation to team members in a timely manner, along with scheduled meeting times

- Developing meeting minutes within the facility policy timeline and using a reporting format that assigns duties with time frames
- Producing an agenda for new meetings with assignments for team members from the previous meeting

Teams may also assign someone to be a timekeeper. The **timekeeper** helps the team manage its time and notifies the group during meetings of time remaining on each agenda item to keep the team moving forward on its PI project.

Team Charters

In many healthcare organizations, the initiation of a PI team begins with the ongoing data review of performance measures identified by the **performance improvement council**, the leadership group that oversees performance improvement activities in the healthcare organization. The PI council generally makes a recommendation for the implementation of a PI team when a performance measure shows a negative or downward trend in the performance of a process or outcome. This can then be formalized with a **team charter**.

Team charters explain the issue(s) the team was initiated to address, describe the team's goal or vision, and list the initial members of the team and their respective departments. Team charters are helpful because they keep the team's objective in focus. Usually, team charters also identify any mitigating factors that may limit the PI process, such as financial limitations, full-time employee restrictions, or time constraints. They keep the organization focused on the opportunity for improvement and the team focused on its mission. Team charters may also include the ground rules that outline the expected behaviors of team members. See figure 4.1 for an example of a team charter.

Check Your Understanding 4.1

1. The HI department is concerned about a backlog of release of information (ROI) request processing. The HI manager assembles a team from the ROI staff to work on this issue to improve the ROI process and performance. This is an example of which type of team?
   a. Rapid improvement event team
   b. Functional team
   c. Cross-functional team
   d. Total quality management (TQM) team

2. The HI manager creates a document that explains the ROI issues the team was implemented to improve, describes the goals and objectives the team wants to accomplish, states the team vision, and lists the initial members of the team from the department. She then sends this document to the quality and performance improvement council to report on the department's PI activities. This document is called the:
   a. Team charter
   b. Team mission
   c. Team charged
   d. Team vision

3. A hospital emergency department is experiencing prolonged waiting times for patients before they can see a healthcare provider, leading to patient dissatisfaction and potential delays in critical care. Which type of team would be created to investigate this situation and devise an immediate solution?
   a. Rapid improvement event team
   b. Functional team
   c. Cross-functional team
   d. Total quality management (TQM) team

Figure 4.1A. Example of a team charter

PERFORMANCE IMPROVEMENT TEAM CHARTER
(Page 1 of 2)

Team Name	Date Submitted to Performance Improvement Council
Clinical Laboratory Services	February 15th

Statement of the Problem, Issue, or Concern to Be Addressed by the PIT

Safety issues or other problems concerning the hospital labs increased 207% over a one-year time frame.

Statement of the Goals, Objective, and Desired End State

Identify specific problem areas within laboratory services, conduct a baseline study to assess each area, analyze results, develop an action plan, implement improvements, and evaluate results.

Proposed Team Members

Name	Title	Department
Roger Jones	Chief Clinical Officer	Administration
Jill Andrews	Lab Manager	Laboratory
Ben Carlson, M.D.	Emergency Physician	E.R.
Sandy Johnson	Director of Clinical Ser.	Administration
Kathy Smith, R.N.	Director of Nursing	Nursing
John Rasmussen	Lab tech	Laboratory
Sue Hol	Lab tech	Laboratory
Pam Richards	Coordinator	Quality Management

Project Resources

Planned Start Date	Planned Completion Date	Planned Frequency of Meetings
February 20th	June 1st	weekly
Administrative/PIC Support Needed (if any)		Estimated Cost of Team's Work
		$3,500.00

Figure 4.1B. Example of a team charter (*Continued*)

PERFORMANCE IMPROVEMENT TEAM CHARTER
(Page 2 of 2)

What important organizational or patient care functions will the project measure or improve? (Check all that apply.)

- ☐ Ethics Rights, Responsibilities
- ☑ Provision of Care, Treatment, and Services
- ☑ Improving Organizational Performance
- ☐ Leadership
- ☑ Management of the Environment of Care
- ☐ Management of Information
- ☑ Management of Human Resources
- ☐ Surveillance, Prevention, and Control of Infection
- ☐ Medication Management

Project Benefits
How will the project support the mission/values and/or achieve the organization's strategic goals?

- ☐ Improved Patient Outcomes
- ☑ Cost Savings
- ☑ Improved Service
- ☐ Time Savings
- ☐ Other _____

How? *reduce safety violations in the laboratory and rework*

_____

Signature of Applicant: *Jill Andrews*   Date: *Feb. 15th*

To Be Completed by Performance Improvement Council

Comments

_____

Performance Improvement Council Recommendations

_____

Signature   Date

Mission, Vision, and Values Statements

Healthcare organizations may use a mission statement, vision statement, and values statement at many different levels. The corporation as a whole may have a mission and vision statement, as may the separate divisions of the corporation. Departments within facilities may also have mission and vision statements.

To be effective, mission, vision, and values statements of a PI team should be developed in concert with the overall goals as outlined in the organization's strategic plan. The statements should reflect the mission and vision of the organization as well as the goals of the individual PI team.

After the team has been assembled and the leader has been chosen, the team should establish its mission. The **mission statement** identifies the PI team, what it does, and whom it serves. For example, the mission of the PI team might be "to provide quick, accurate billing to all clients and third-party payers in an honest, efficient, and user-friendly manner." Developing a mission statement can help both the team and the larger organization identify the goals and purpose of the PI initiative. The team's mission statement should answer the following questions:

- What process is to be improved?
- For whom is the process performed?
- What products does the process produce?
- What is not working with the current process?
- How well must the process function?

The team should articulate its vision for the process. A **vision statement** describes what the organization or PI team initiative will look like or be in the future, or it describes some milestone the organization or PI team will reach in the future.

The team's vision for a process may not be validated by existing data and observations of the process. In such cases, disharmony between the vision and reality becomes apparent. And because humans have a natural tendency to resolve disharmony, the team has an opportunity to improve the process. The more clearly the group maintains its focus on "what should be" and acknowledges "what is," the more focused it will be on implementing its vision of the desired outcome.

Quite often, organizations give up their vision because of the large gap between their vision and the current reality. Some organizations focus on their vision and ignore the way things are, or they believe the current situation is better than it really is. In either case, the natural tendency for resolution or change dissipates.

The team that focuses on "what should be," while at the same time maintaining an accurate perception of the current state of the process, takes a powerful step toward creating the results it envisions. When the PI team focuses clearly and consistently on its mission and vision, it naturally and almost effortlessly senses what still needs to be done. New processes present themselves, and the group becomes increasingly aware of additional opportunities for continuing improvement.

In addition to defining the team and organizational mission and vision, the values of each should be defined. A **values statement** is a short description that communicates an organization's social and cultural belief system. An example of a PI team values statement is "honesty, efficiency, and user-friendliness."

At the organizational level, values statements represent the core practices and inform all stakeholders (e.g., employees, patients and their families, members of the community) of their commitment to those core practices. In healthcare, values might include a commitment to patient safety, error reduction, service excellence, and compliance (see figure 4.2 for an example of mission, vision, and value statements).

Figure 4.2. Sample PI team mission, vision, and values statements

Mission statement:	Evaluate hospital laboratory services for patients with regard to safety issues, error-reduction processes, and delivery of services while maintaining 94% compliance with these services.
Vision statement:	Safe, timely, and compliant laboratory services are provided 98% of the time.
Value statements:	Patient safety: We prioritize the safety of our patients by ensuring the accuracy, reliability, and security of laboratory services. Every action we take is guided by our unwavering commitment to minimizing harm and promoting well-being. Error Reduction: We relentlessly strive to identify, assess, and reduce errors within our laboratory processes. We embrace a culture of learning from mistakes to enhance the quality and reliability of our services. Service Excellence: We are passionate about delivering exceptional laboratory services that meet or exceed the needs and expectations of our patients and healthcare providers. We continuously seek to improve our processes and procedures to ensure seamless and timely service delivery. Compliance: We are resolute in our commitment to maintaining a 94% compliance rate with established quality and safety standards. This serves as a benchmark for our dedication to achieving excellence and accountability.

Ground Rules for Meetings

Establishing ground rules for meetings helps a team maintain a level of discipline. **Ground rules** are basic expectations for team members and include a discussion of attendance, time management, participation, communication, decision-making, documentation, room arrangements, and cleanup. The ground rules will not be the same for every team, because each team should decide how it wants to proceed, but the ground rules should be well known to everyone on the team, and everyone should have participated in their development. Most teams that use ground rules allow for periodic review and revision of those rules, particularly when team membership changes. New members must be brought up to speed on the ground rules when they begin attending team meetings. (See figure 4.3.)

Figure 4.3. Sample meeting ground rules worksheet

Ground Rules Worksheet

1. Every individual has a viewpoint that is valuable, every individual can make a unique contribution, and every individual can speak freely.

2. All team members must listen attentively and respectfully without interrupting. Only one person should speak at a time.

3. All team members must be willing to accept responsibility for assignments and complete any assigned tasks between meetings.

4. The organizational positions/levels of team members will not be recognized during team meetings. Every member of the team is an equal participant.

5. Solutions must be created with resources that are currently available. Money and additional staff are not considered issues.

6. _____
7. _____
8. _____
9. _____
10. _____

The attendance discussion should establish who will schedule meetings, arrange for a meeting room or schedule a virtual meeting, and notify members. The ground rules should include the team's expectations regarding absences, including whether team members can be removed for absenteeism and whether substitutes can attend meetings.

Cancellation of meetings should be discussed, as well as how the team will address issues of tardiness. This discussion should also include how the time allotted to agenda items will be monitored. For example, will the team assign a timekeeper at the start of each meeting?

Discussion of team member participation should include the team's expectations regarding advance preparation. The team should have a plan for encouraging all members to make equal contributions, determining how activities will be monitored to ensure productive meetings, deciding how assignments and expectations for their completion will be made, and deciding how ad hoc members will be invited and prepared for their input.

Ground rules for communication are imperative for team effectiveness, particularly regarding how candid members may be and whether information discussed in the team process must remain confidential. PI data are considered confidential in most facilities and may be legally protected from reproduction or use outside the facility or agency. The team needs to clearly define how information will be managed and protected during the project.

The team should decide what will happen when discussions get off track, how interruptions or side conversations will be handled, what listening skills are expected, how differences of opinion and conflict among members will be expressed and resolved, and how creativity will be encouraged and negative thinking discouraged. Finally, the team must decide whether consensus or majority decisions will be taken on issues that require a vote. Other questions that may require discussion include:

- Will there be meeting breaks, and if so, how will they be handled?
- Who is responsible for setup and cleanup of the meeting room?
- Does the team require information technology support? If so, who will coordinate it?
- How, when, and why should administration be involved?
- How will department managers be notified of the need for department employees to participate on a team?
- Is overtime necessary for this team to complete its assignment?

Problem-Solving Techniques, Listening, and Questioning

Encouraging team productivity can be a major issue in many organizations. This is an outgrowth of the two common management styles that most organizations tend to gravitate to. One style is inclusive: all viewpoints are considered with respect to their potential contribution to solving the PI issue at hand. The other style is exclusive: its goal is to get to a result as quickly as possible. Each style has positive and negative aspects. People who operate by the inclusive style can get mired in details and discussion and achieve results only after extensive processing. People who operate by the exclusive style can fail to perceive important details in their rush to implement a solution. A combination of the two styles is more effective than either style alone. Each style can be employed at appropriate points in the development of a team process.

The management style employed will depend on the maturity of the team and its effectiveness. To improve PI team effectiveness, the cyclical PI methodology was developed to give teams a structure to follow in problem solving. QI toolbox techniques were developed to give teams an easy way to organize and analyze data, and the concept of facilitation was developed to help move teams along.

Another area that is extremely important in the development of good team interaction and functioning is the ability to listen and question. PI team members need to be able to do both, and team leaders may need to work with team members to develop this skill. Individuals tend to be either active communicators or passive listeners. Active communicators can quickly dominate a team meeting. They are accustomed to expressing themselves and being heard. Sometimes their listening skills are eclipsed by their own volubility. These team members may need to be reoriented by the team leader or facilitator to practice listening more often, allowing the quieter individuals on the team an opportunity to express their perspectives. Similarly, the quieter members may have become accustomed to listening to other people and not voicing their opinions. They may have to be reoriented to contribute by sharing their knowledge and expertise with the group so that important details are not overlooked.

Often in human communication in organizations, individuals become invested in their own perspectives and ways of seeing and interpreting situations. This can happen with both active communicators and passive listeners. The active communicators often react by trying to persuade everyone else on the team of the justness of their perspectives. The passive listeners may say nothing but internally retain their commitment to their own perspectives. Neither of these tactics moves the team toward resolving the problem. Team members may have to be reoriented to listen carefully to others' perspectives and to seek a common understanding of those perspectives using questioning techniques.

The power of the question lies in the fact that it compels an answer. When the right questions are asked, the information, experience, reactions, perspectives, and attitudes that they prompt provide important answers. Not asking questions may result in only one perspective, which may or may not reflect the reality of various situations. One individual can never know as much about an opportunity for improvement as the collective members of the team. Trying to make decisions without sufficient information decreases the likelihood that a new solution will solve the problem, so it is important for PI team members to use effective questioning techniques.

When using questioning methods, team members should maintain a positive attitude about the importance of asking rather than telling and remember that each person's unique experience, background, and training allows them to contribute unique information. It is also important to recognize that there is more than one type of questioning. Different styles of questioning can be used to gather different types of information.

People Issues

In discussing the effectiveness of PI teams, we must specifically recognize the effects that individuals have on PI processes. In reality, all the team-development techniques are intended to help teams function *through* the people issues and become effective teams. Effective teams typically succeed in the following objectives:

- Establishing goals cooperatively, with all members who have perspectives on the issues contributing
- Communicating in a two-way mode, with all members participating; encouraging and holding responsible members who do not spontaneously communicate
- Valuing open expression of both ideas and feelings as important perspectives on organizational issues
- Distributing leadership and responsibility among all team members, with each member responsible for tasks that make important contributions to team accomplishments
- Distributing power among all team members on the basis of information, ability, and contribution to team activities, not on the basis of a team member's place in the formal organizational structure
- Matching decision-making techniques to the type of decision-making situation, and usually making important decisions through consensus, meaning that the group as a whole agrees on the appropriate course of action
- Viewing periodic controversy and conflict among team members as a positive aspect of team growth, and understanding that in working through the processes, the team has been initiated to improve
- Focusing on the issues that the team has been organized to address and keeping at the heart of its work the mission, vision, and values of both the overall organization and the PI team
- Making sure that the team's PI efforts and management of project design or tools are cost conscious

Even those new to the team concept generally can see the importance of these factors. However, in real situations there may be conflict between individuals' roles in the formal organizational structure and their roles in maintaining an effective team structure. Formal organizational roles often require authority for various functions and responsibilities. Effective teams share authority for team performance. Therefore, when individuals are new to the team concept or team approaches to problem solving, they will have to get reoriented; for some, this reorientation is difficult.

Most individuals coming to a PI team for the first time are unfamiliar with the data collection and analysis aspects of team functioning. Some may not want to be involved with such detailed activities and may not have the mathematical skills necessary to perform these activities with ease. The team may have to spend some time helping such individuals accomplish their tasks in specific areas.

Many individuals in healthcare, particularly clinicians, managers, and administrators, are comfortable with decision-making. However, effective teams make decisions as groups, often by consensus, acknowledging perspectives of all participants. For many, giving up the right to make individual decisions is difficult. The team or the leadership of the PI initiative may have to help such persons learn a new, team-oriented, decision-making style.

Conversely, people sometimes come to a team with little or no management experience. These individuals make few decisions in their work outside of day-to-day job procedures. Dealing with PI issues without carrying out someone else's orders may be difficult for them. Some team members may resist being empowered because they come from a culture where employees complain rather than look for solutions to a problem. Encouraging such individuals to participate and mentoring them through the process can help them develop new skills.

Check Your Understanding 4.2

1. After a PI team has defined their mission for the improvement process, their next step is to develop a statement that describes what the improvement process initiative will look like in the future. This statement is called the _____.
    a. Team charter
    b. Team mission
    c. Team charge
    d. Team vision

2. When a PI team first meets and discusses participation expectations, communication methods, and plans for decision-making techniques to be used, these are examples of team _____.
    a. Action plans
    b. Agendas
    c. Ground rules
    d. Mission statements

QI Toolbox Techniques

Agenda

An **agenda** is a list of the tasks to be accomplished during a meeting. For a meeting to be effective, the team must operate with a common purpose and specific goal. Communication of the meeting's common purpose and specific goal(s) is usually accomplished by establishing an agenda. Using an agenda ensures that every team member knows which items will be discussed or worked on. (See the sample agenda in figure 4.4.) The agenda should be sent to all team members before the meeting. This allows them to prepare to discuss specific agenda items. The agenda should indicate how long the team will spend on each item. Setting time frames for agenda items helps the team leader keep the group focused on the process and moving forward.

Figure 4.4. Sample meeting agenda

AGENDA	
Date: January 15	**Team:** Registration Process
Time: 10:00 a.m.	**Place:** Conference Room B
Time Allotted:	**Item:**
5 minutes	1. Review and approve minutes from last meeting
5 minutes	2. Review agenda and time frames
15 minutes	3. PI step: Registration process discussion on how the computer system affects the registration process
15 minutes	4. PI step: Registration process discussion on what happens now when the computer system is "down"
15 minutes	5. Brainstorm possible ideas to improve the computer system
10 minutes	6. Process (evaluate) meeting
10 minutes	7. Plan next steps, assign team members' duties, and set agenda for next meeting

Standard agendas typically begin with a review and approval of the last meeting's minutes. Once this has been accomplished, the PI team should review the agenda for the current meeting and approve the time frames that have been set. This allows the individual team members to have input on how long a certain agenda item should be discussed.

As a closing item of business, many teams find it helpful to evaluate the effectiveness of the meeting. Asking the following questions may be helpful:

- Did the team accomplish what it set out to accomplish during the meeting?
- Is the PI process moving forward?
- Does the team need to ask additional people to sit in on the process meetings?
- Did members participate appropriately, listen effectively to other members' suggestions, and stay focused on the agenda?

Finally, the next meeting's agenda and team member assignments should be agreed upon and tied to the current meeting's evaluation process and minutes. In other words, the next meeting should be structured based on the accomplishments of the current meeting.

Team Charter

Team charters explain those issue(s) the team was initiated to address, describe the team's goal or vision, and list the initial members of the team and their respective departments. Team charters are helpful because they keep the team's objective in focus. Usually, team charters also identify any mitigating factors that may limit the PI process, such as financial limitations, full-time employee restrictions, or time constraints. They keep the organization focused on the opportunity for improvement and the team focused on its mission. Team charters may also include the ground rules that outline the expected behaviors of team members. See figure 4.1 for an example of a team charter.

Real-Life Example #1

Customer satisfaction surveys indicated that the triage process in the ED of a small metropolitan hospital was inadequate. Communication was fragmented, precertification was not taking place in a timely manner, intake processing time had increased, the main patient waiting area was not private, and referral volume was increasing.

To address these problems, a PI team was chartered. The team charter included the following:

- **Team leader:** ED manager
- **Team members:** Representatives from the business office, health information, administration, utilization review, and finance
- **Ad hoc members:** Representatives from regulatory affairs, reception, nursing, and case management, and an ED physician
- **Team mission statement:** Evaluate the ED's clinical assessment process regarding patient privacy, data collection, and staff communication, while maintaining patient and employee satisfaction with this process
- **Team vision statement:** Design a centralized clinical assessment center to facilitate patient privacy, data collection, and staff communication to achieve 95 percent patient and employee satisfaction with this process
- **Team value statement:** Provide an engaging environment for employees that provides privacy for our patients and facilitates accurate data collection

Real-Life Example #2

An organization's HI department was experiencing an increase in physician chart delinquencies, delays in diagnosis and procedure coding, and delays in processing requests for patient information. In addition, the business office was experiencing delays in the billing process due to incomplete insurance information and an increase in accounts payable due to the chart completion problems occurring in the HI department.

To address these issues, a PI team was formed. The team was composed of the following individuals:

- **Team leader:** HI manager
- **Team members:** Representatives from the HI department, the business office, registration, and administration, and the physician chairman of the HI committee
- **Team mission statement:** Evaluate the physician chart completion and admission interview processes and their impact on coding, billing, release of information, and accounts payable, while providing support to organization-wide management of information, financial viability, and the billing and collection process
- **Team vision statement:** Achieve timely physician chart completion and a detailed admission interview, which will lead to timely and effective coding and billing of patient information
- **Team value statement:** Comprehensive documentation that supports accurate billing.

The HI department's vision was to "contribute and provide support to the effective organization-wide management of information." The business office's vision statement was to "give support to organization-wide financial viability and provide accurate and timely exchange of financial information that allows for an efficient and effective billing and collection process."

This team made a recommendation to the HI committee to change the physician chart completion policy from 30 days after discharge to 7 days after discharge. This change improved the coding turnaround time and processing of requests for patient information, which in turn improved the billing cycle. An additional process change was to have a business office representative interview patients upon admission. This eventually improved the accuracy of financial information needed for billing and collection.

Real-Life Example #3

Safety issues and other problems concerning the laboratory department at one hospital increased 207 percent over a period of one year. The objectives of the PI team were to identify specific problem areas within laboratory services, conduct a baseline survey to assess each area, analyze the survey results, develop an action plan to implement improvements, and evaluate the results of the changes. The team charter was made up of the following:

- **Team leader:** Chief of pathology
- **Team members:** The laboratory manager, an ED physician, the director of nursing, and a laboratory technician
- **Team mission statement:** Identify, analyze, and implement changes to improve safety issues and other problem areas within the laboratory department
- **Team vision statement:** Provide reliable, timely diagnostic services for the clinical staff
- **Team value statement:** Efficient and accurate laboratory services

The survey indicated that inappropriate techniques for specimen collection were being used, and the reference laboratory was slow to return results to the organization. Team recommendations included education and training on specimen collection and a change in the contract reference laboratory used by the organization.

Case Study

"Why can't admitting remember to change these patients to preadmit so we can see the information from the emergency room in their electronic record and view their current medications?" the scribe complained to the cath lab nurse. "I will never understand why it is so difficult to get cath lab patients transferred from an ED patient to preadmit." The scribe stops trying to record patient information in the electronic health record (EHR) and calls the admitting department. The scribe is frustrated because admitting has not updated the patient type listed in the EHR. The patient had come into Regional Medical Center with chest pain and was seen a few minutes ago in the ED for an acute myocardial infarction. An EKG was ordered and showed that the patient had a STEMI. Once this diagnosis was made, the patient was emergently transferred to the cath lab.

Although the EHR used by the facility has many features that allow care providers to access necessary patient information and input provider orders, the system has a few issues. The issue in the cath lab was the fact that cath lab personnel could not view important patient information or chart new information until the admitting department changed the patient type from "ED" to "preadmit." While there was a way to override the system to view the necessary information, this process was also concerning. There had been some instances where the latest information from the ED was not in the system if the system had been overridden. The hospital's quality measures and reporting requirements necessitate accurate times. Without the ability to chart in real time, the time of arrival to the cath lab and the time the vessel was opened are not accurately reflected in the system. Regional Medical Center collects data to determine how long it takes cath lab staff to open a vessel once the patient is in the cath lab.

The procedure in the cath lab is that a scribe or technician is responsible for documenting everything that happens during the encounter. Without the ability to document directly into the EHR, the scribe or technician spends precious time contacting admitting and documenting the encounter on paper. This information must then be transferred into the EHR (back charted).

The scribe calls the admitting department and states, "The patient from ED room five is here in the cath lab, and the patient type is still set at ED. You realize that I cannot do my job when you do not do yours, right? Why can't you admitting clerks figure out how to get these patient types changed faster and do your job so that I can do mine?" The admitting clerk responds, "I have been busy taking care of other patients and didn't realize this was the patient that was taken to the cath lab. I do have other patients to take care of besides the one you have in the cath lab. Just override the system so you can view the information until I get the type changed." The scribe replies, "Truly you don't understand the ramifications of what your job entails and the problems this can cause the patient. Just make the change. Now!" The patient type is changed, and the technician is now trying to document what has happened to this patient in the cath lab from memory.

Case Study Questions

1. In your opinion, is there an opportunity for improvement in this system? Why or why not?
2. If there is room for improvement, is a PI team appropriate in this context?
3. From your knowledge of hospital organizational structure, who should be on the PI team? Which departments should be represented? Which staff positions from these departments would you include? What is your rationale for including each individual?

Review Questions

1. Write a team-based mission statement that includes all five questions that a team mission statement should answer.

2. A healthcare organization posts the following statement on their website:
"As an organization we are honest, ethical, and strive to always do the right thing for the community, our employees, and the patients that we serve." This is an example of which type of statement?
    a. Mission statement
    b. Purpose statement
    c. Values statement
    d. Vision statement

3. You have been appointed as the new HI Manager at a local hospital. As part of your upcoming staff meeting, an agenda is needed to keep the meeting on track. Create an agenda for the meeting that includes the following items for discussion: performance appraisals, scanning backlog, and the new vacation leave policy. Be sure to adhere to good agenda techniques.

4. What is the primary purpose of a team charter?
    a. To assign hierarchical roles within the team
    b. To outline individual performance metrics
    c. To establish clear team goals and objectives
    d. To regulate patient scheduling and appointments

5. Sharon was upset at the conclusion of the last PI team meeting because all the other members just got up and left the room without cleaning up their lunch mess and paperwork. What team protocol must be missing for this situation to occur?
    a. Agenda
    b. Ground rules
    c. Project timeline
    d. Vision statement

References

Juran. 2024. "Kaizen (Rapid Improvement Event)." https://www.juran.com/blog/kaizen-rapid-improvement-event/

Lean Enterprise Institute. 2024. "Kaizen." https://www.lean.org/lexicon-terms/kaizen/

Resources

Hammond, K. M. and C. J. Morgan. 2022. Development of interprofessional healthcare teamwork skills: Mapping students' process of learning. *Journal of Interprofessional Care* 36(4): 589–598.

Schmutz, J. B., L. L. Meier, and T. Manser. 2019. How effective is teamwork really? The relationship between teamwork and performance in healthcare teams: a systematic review and meta-analysis. *BMJ Open* 9(9): e028280.

Aggregating and Analyzing Performance Improvement Data

Learning Objectives

- Explain how internal and external benchmarks differ
- Use common healthcare data collection tools
- Apply the concept of data aggregation in support of data analysis
- Choose the correct graphic presentation for a specific data type
- Design graphic displays for a given set of data
- Analyze the data for changes in performance displayed in graphic form

Key Terms

Absolute frequency
Artificial intelligence (AI)
Bar graph
Check sheet
Continuous data
Control chart
Data analysis
Discrete (count) data
Histogram
Likert scale
Line chart
Mean (*M*)
Median

Nominal data
Normal distribution
Ordinal data
Pareto chart
Pie chart
Pivot table
Predictive analytics
Relative frequency
Sampling
Scatter diagram
Skewing
Standard deviation (*SD*)

After the performance improvement (PI) team has administered its survey or collected data by abstracting information from other sources, it is ready to aggregate and analyze the data. In addition to survey results, sources of data may include health records, organization-wide incident reports, and annual employee performance evaluations and staff competency results. Abstracted data and survey results can provide invaluable information about a process and thereby point the team in a specific direction for improvement. Internal and external data comparisons—benchmarking—can provide additional information about why and how well the process works or does not work in meeting customers' expectations.

It is best to conduct an internal data comparison with data collected over a period of time. For example, collecting data over a three- to six-month time frame establishes an internal baseline for benchmark purposes. To establish the baseline, the organization averages all collected data. This internal baseline becomes the organization's benchmark to maintain or improve upon when external benchmark comparisons are not available. Organizations use internal benchmark data for provider performance comparisons, unit-to-unit comparisons, and facility-to-facility comparisons within a corporation.

Comparing an organization's performance with the performance of other organizations that provide the same types of services is known as *external benchmarking*. The other organizations need not be in the same region of the country, but they should be comparable in terms of size, services, and patient mix. The use of external benchmarks can be instructive when comparisons are made with an organization doing an outstanding job with a process similar to the process on which the PI team is focusing. For example, if the national standard for the average number of adverse drug reactions is X, then comparing an organization's number with the national average would give the team information about the effectiveness of the organization's medication program.

In figure 5.1, note the comparison of Western States University Hospital's physician specialty lengths of stay. This report allows the organization to do both internal and external comparisons. Internal comparisons can be performed on the mean length of stay observed (Mean LOS Obs) between specialties of practice. For instance, note the difference in mean length of stay between Family Practice and General Internal Medicine. External benchmarking also can be performed by comparing the mean length of stay observed and the mean length of stay expected (Mean LOS Exp). Note also the major differences in standard deviation (*SD*) for length of stay (*SD* LOS Obs) between the two services. Benchmarking on mortality can be performed using the columns % Deaths (Obs) and % Deaths (Exp). Where might Western States University Hospital want to focus attention on improving hospital lengths of stay (reducing the number of inpatient days)?

PI teams can use several tools for data aggregation, analysis, and presentation. These tools are discussed in more detail later in this chapter.

Figure 5.1. Length of stay (LOS) summary by physician specialty

Physician Specialty	Cases	Mean LOS (Obs)	SD LOS (Obs)	Mean LOS (Exp)	LOS Index	Savings Opp (Days)	% 30 Day Readmit	% With Comps	% Deaths (Obs)	% Deaths (Exp)	% Early Deaths
Cardiology	1	6.00	—	6.36	0.94	0	0	0	0	0.75	0
Endocrinology	1	3.00	—	3.93	0.76	–1	0	0	0	0.83	0
Family Practice	17	8.47	11.44	6.26	1.35	38	11.76	0	0	4.27	0
Infectious Disease	4	4.00	2.94	4.35	0.92	–1	0	0	0	1.13	0
General Internal Medicine	34	3.82	3.00	4.89	0.78	–36	0	0	5.88	4.39	2.94
Nephrology	3	3.67	0.58	4.99	0.73	–4	0	0	0	4.03	0
Neo/Perinatal Medicine	1	4.00	—	3.69	1.08	0	100.00	0	0	0.92	0
Prev/Occ Med	6	4.83	4.83	6.37	0.76	–9	16.67	0	33.33	16.57	16.67
General Pediatrics	7	3.43	2.15	3.55	0.97	–1	0	0	0	0.18	0
Pulmonary/Crit Care	2	17.50	21.92	14.65	1.19	6	0	0	50.00	61.46	50.00
General Diag/Interv Radiology	1	1.00	—	12.02	0.08	–11	0	0	100.00	80.25	100.00
Rheumatology	1	2.00	—	3.40	0.59	–1	0	0	0	0.39	0
Internal Med Heme/Onc	1	3.00	—	3.71	0.81	–1	0	0	0	0.90	0

Legend:

Comps = Complications
Crit = Critical
Diag = Diagnostic
Exp = Expected
Heme = Hematology
Interv = Interventional
LOS = Length of stay
Med = Medicine
Neo = Neonatal
Obs = Observed
Occ = Occupational
Onc = Oncology
Opp = Opportunity
Prev = Preventive
Readmit = Readmission
SD = Standard deviation

Data Collection Tools

Certain types of data and information need to be accumulated over time to support clinical and management functions. The organization must assess its need for aggregate data and information and define the types of required data and information to support individual care and care delivery, decision-making, management and operations, analysis of trends over time, performance comparisons over time within and outside the organization, and PI. Common types of data collection tools used in healthcare organizations include incident reports, safety and infection surveillance reports, employee performance appraisals, staff competency examinations, restraint use logs, adverse drug reaction reports, surveys, diagnosis and procedure indices, case abstracts, and peer review reports. Individually, these tools do not describe the quality of care provided by the healthcare organization. So the data from these reports must be aggregated to provide useful information about the organization's performance in key areas.

To aggregate data, the values of one data element over a set period of time (such as a month or quarter) are added together. These aggregated data are then compared with previous months or quarters to determine if there is a variance from the established benchmark.

Sometimes, the organizational characteristic or parameter about which data are being collected occurs too frequently to measure every occurrence. In this case, those collecting the data might want to use sampling techniques. **Sampling** is the recording of a smaller subset of observations of the characteristic or parameter, making certain that a sufficient number of observations have been made to predict the overall configuration of the data. (See White 2020 for additional reading.) Accrediting bodies may have defined sample size parameters based on the size of an organization's patient population. The organization should identify and adhere to these guidelines to comply with their given accreditation standards. Other approaches to sampling methodologies can be found in a standard statistics textbook.

When an organization needs to collect a new data element, a variety of data collection tools can be used, and these may be manual methods or electronic querying. First and also simplest is the check sheet.

Check Sheets

A **check sheet** is used to gather data based on sample observations to detect patterns. When preparing to collect data, a team should consider the four W questions:

- ***Who* will collect the data?** For example, when collecting data on tobacco use by patients, determining who will collect the data is vital to data accuracy. Most often, the individual(s) collecting the tobacco use information will be part of the clinical staff. A nonclinical person can be trained to look for specific documentation in the health record under clinical guidance.
- ***What* data will be collected?** The data elements might include tobacco use screening, tobacco use treatment offered or provided, tobacco use treatment offered or provided at discharge, and tobacco use assessment status after discharge.
- ***Where* will the data be collected?** Most often, data for the tobacco use will be abstracted or collected from the individual patient health record. However, some data may have to be collected from other sources.
- ***When* will the data be collected?** This question is defined by time parameters as defined by the research or PI team.

Once the team answers the four W questions, it can develop a check sheet to collect the data. (See figure 5.2.) Check sheets make it possible to systematically collect a large volume of data. It is important to make sure that the data are unbiased, accurate, properly recorded, and representative of typical conditions for the process.

Figure 5.2. Example of a check sheet

Problem	Day 1	Day 2	Day 3	TOTAL
A	II	III	II	7
B	I	I	I	3
C	IIII	II	IIII	10
TOTAL	7	6	7	20

A check sheet is a simple, easy-to-understand form used to answer the question, how often are certain events happening? It starts the process of translating opinions into facts. Constructing a check sheet involves the following steps:

1. The PI team determines who is responsible for collecting the data: a clinician, technician, or another person.
2. The PI team agrees on which event to observe.
3. The team decides on the time period (hours to weeks) during which the data will be collected.
4. The team determines the appropriate source from which the data will be collected. This may be health records, charge slips, and other sources.
5. The team designs a form that is clear and easy to use. The team should make sure that every column is clearly labeled and that there is enough space on the form to enter the data.
6. The team collects the data consistently and honestly. Enough time should be allowed for this data-gathering task.

Check sheets can also be used to tally survey responses. For example, if a survey included a question that asked for the days of the week on which patients had surgery, the results could be tabulated by using a check sheet that included each day of the week.

Healthcare organizations do not have to develop new data collection methods for every PI project. They must determine what they are already collecting and how those data can be used in future PI measurement processes.

Types of Data

Before a PI team can decide how to display performance data, it must determine which types of data have been collected. The four data categories are nominal, ordinal, discrete, and continuous.

Nominal data, also called categorical data, include values assigned to name-specific categories. For example, health insurance status can be subdivided into three groups, "yes," "no," or "don't know," or three categories, "1," "2," and "3." Nominal data are usually displayed in bar graphs (see figure 5.3) and pie charts (see figure 5.4).

74 Chapter 5 **Aggregating and Analyzing Performance Improvement Data**

Figure 5.3. Example of a bar graph

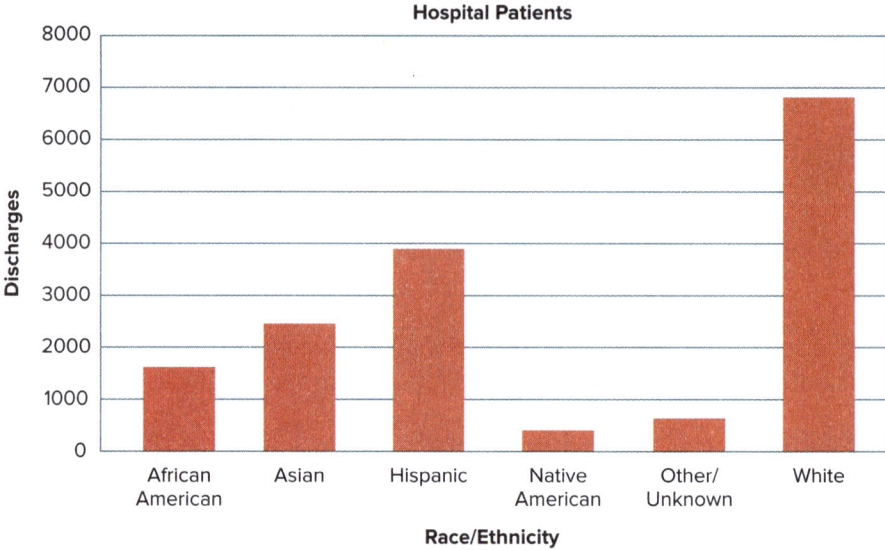

Figure 5.4. Example of a pie chart

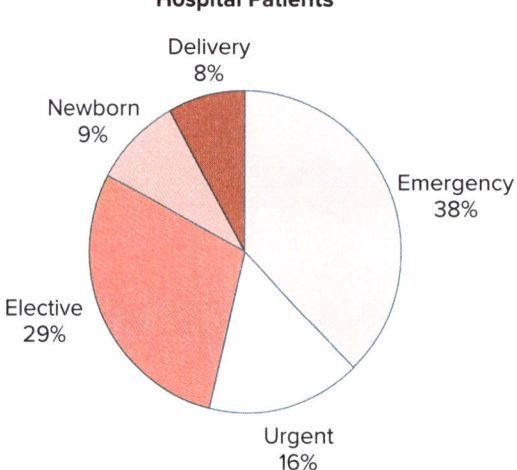

Ordinal data, also called ranked data, express the comparative evaluation of various characteristics or entities, and relative assignment of each to a class according to a set of criteria. Many surveys use a Likert scale to quantify or rank statements. A **Likert scale** allows the respondent to state the degree to which he or she agrees or disagrees with a statement. It typically ranges from 1 to 5. This type of scale allows the PI team to determine how respondents feel about issues. Ordinal or ranked data, like nominal data, are also best displayed in bar graphs and pie charts.

Discrete (count) data are numerical values that represent whole numbers; for example, the number of children in a family or the number of unbillable patient accounts. Discrete data can be displayed in bar graphs.

Continuous data assume an infinite number of possible values in measurements that have decimal values as possibilities. Examples of continuous data include weight, blood pressure, and temperature. Continuous data are displayed in histograms (see figure 5.5) or in a line chart (see figure 5.6).

Figure 5.5. Example of a histogram

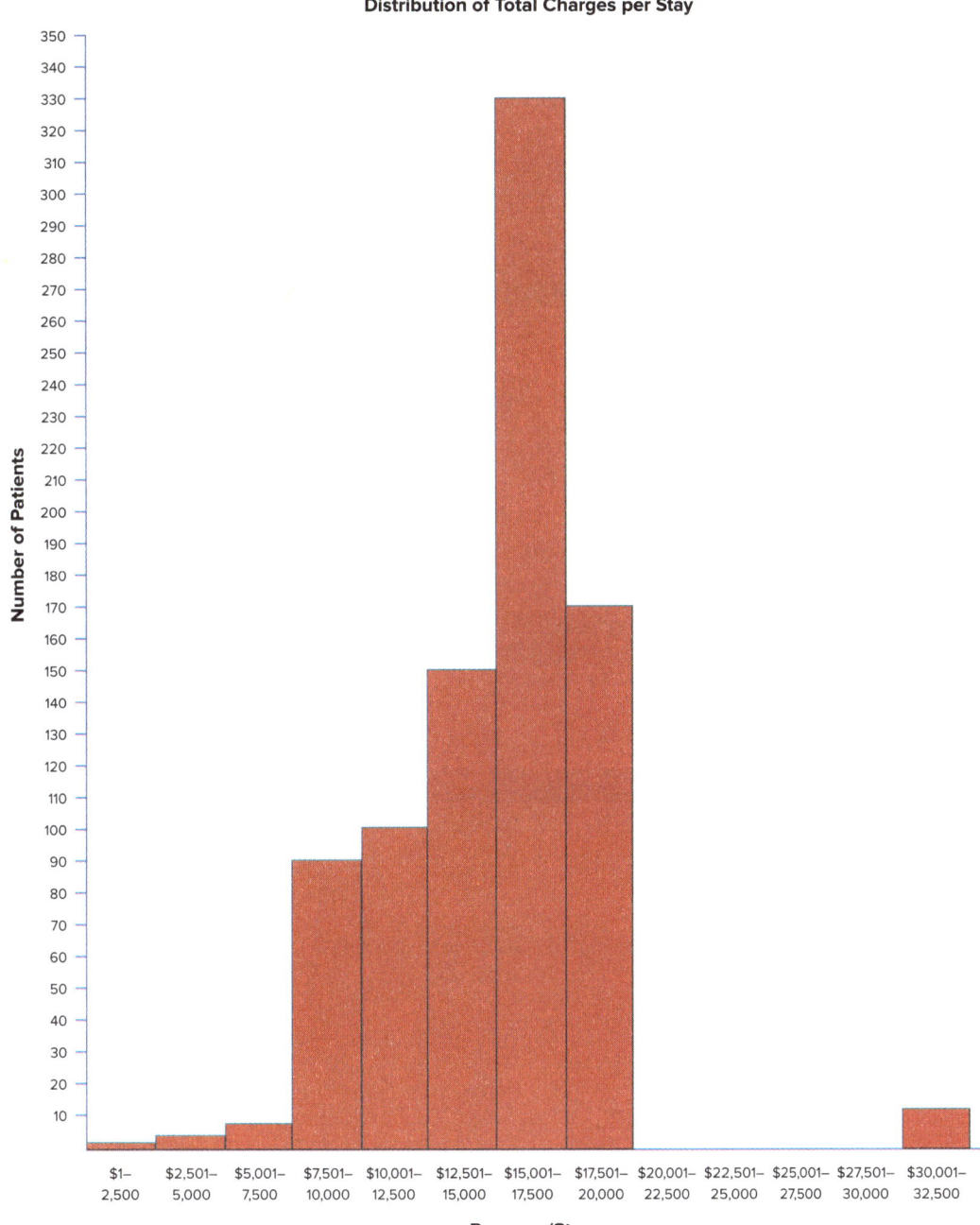

Figure 5.6. Example of a line chart

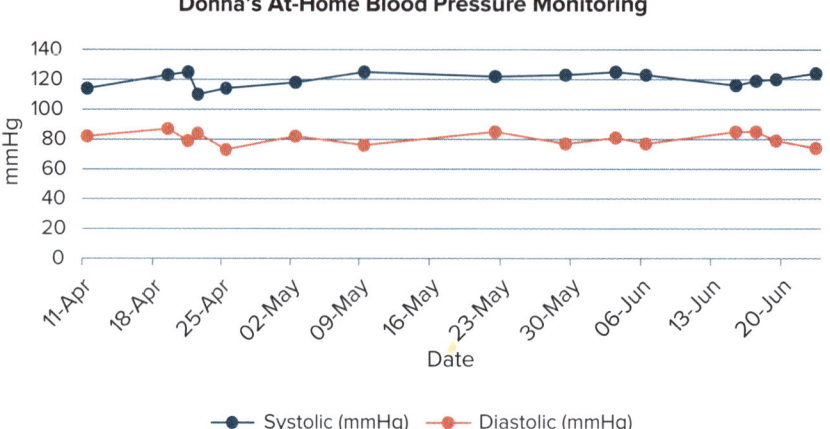

Two terms often used in data analysis are **absolute frequency** and **relative frequency**. Absolute frequency refers to the number of times a score or value occurs in the data set. For example, in the data set shown in table 5.1, the frequency of the score or value 25 is 3. Relative frequency is the percentage of the time a characteristic appears within a data set. In the example, the percentage of observations in which the respiration rate was 25 was 3:7, or 42.9 percent—its relative frequency.

Table 5.1. Sample data set

Date and Time	Respiration Rate Recorded
Jan. 5, 8:00 a.m.	22/min
Jan. 5, 12:00 noon	25/min
Jan. 5, 4:00 p.m.	25/min
Jan. 5, 8:00 p.m.	22/min
Jan. 5, 12:00 midnight	21/min
Jan. 6, 4:00 a.m.	23/min
Jan. 6, 8:00 a.m.	25/min

Check Your Understanding 5.1

1. A PI team is concerned with the time that it is taking for patients to get through the registration process. To better understand the causes or reasons for the delay in this process the PI team would like to gather observational data. Which data collection tool would be appropriate for this team to develop for this purpose?
   a. Check sheet
   b. Ordinal data tool
   c. Balance sheet
   d. Nominal data tool

2. The health information department wants to assess the overall satisfaction of their customer service to other departments throughout the hospital. They develop a survey using the following options: A) Very Dissatisfied; B) Dissatisfied; C) Neutral; D) Satisfied; E) Very Satisfied. The survey is using a _____ to evaluate their customer service.
   a. Bar chart
   b. Continuous data
   c. Likert scale
   d. Check sheet

Management of Data Sets

Healthcare organizations use information systems and other technology to support various aspects of their operations. These systems record all aspects of patient registration for service, type of service requested, dates and times the service was rendered, rendering providers, clinic or hospital census, bed utilized, and so on. Patient financial services manage the data associated with collecting charges, manifesting a bill, outputting the bill, receiving and recording payments from insurers or patients, and posting all those transactions as necessary to general ledger accounts. Clinical components capture the information associated with the condition of the patient and the clinical provision of service by the provider, deriving such data as blood pressure, temperature, findings on physical examination, and probable diagnosis. Provider order-entry systems communicate requirements for care provision to nursing and ancillary services staff, and each system maintains the data details for each order transaction. Individual departments or collections of departments in healthcare organizations, such as radiology, pharmacy, and clinical laboratories also use these systems as part of their workflow. Therefore, when working out the details of data collection, it is important to identify systems that may be a source of data that can be beneficial to the organization's PI activities and to use the systems' reporting tools to provide often very complex data sets to the PI teams for analysis and interpretation.

The use of data sets for PI purposes must be designed very carefully. First, examine the nature of the data to be sure they accurately reflect the subject under investigation. Reliability can be significantly influenced by the original sources of the data set when the data were created and how carefully data were derived from those original sources. Using data without a clear picture of these aspects may lead a PI team to make inappropriate interpretations.

An example of this type of complexity that occurred at Western States University Hospital was the request from an external public health monitoring agency for data regarding the hospital's experience with "severe sepsis." The cases appropriate for reporting to this agency would have to be retrieved using ICD-10-CM codes assigned at discharge by the health information (HI) staff. However, given the inconsistent usage of the term "sepsis" and its related terms by hospital house staff and attending staff, documentation in the health record could end up being coded as any of the following ICD-10-CM codes:

A40.0–A41.8	Sepsis due to a variety of bacterial organisms
R78.81	Bacteremia
R65.10	Systemic inflammatory response syndrome (SIRS) of non-infectious origin without acute organ dysfunction
R65.11	Systemic inflammatory response syndrome (SIRS) of non-infectious origin with acute organ dysfunction
A41.9	Sepsis, unspecified organism
R65.20	Severe sepsis without septic shock
R65.21	Severe sepsis with septic shock

Patients in any or all of these categories may have died, making the designation "severe" possible for any of them. Using only the cases coded with R65.20 might leave out many other cases relevant to the measure of "sepsis" in the hospital. Depending on the adequacy of the clinical documentation, a patient coded with bacteremia might also have met the other requirements for severe sepsis (bacterial blood or urinary tract infection as well as some type of organ failure due to the infection) without the word "sepsis" ever occurring in the health record. Therefore, in working up the reported data for a monitoring agency or a PI team, quality management staff must be very careful to work with infection control staff to identify appropriate cases. Such complexities, overlaps, and inconsistencies may be inherent in any data set used for PI and quality management purposes in healthcare.

Once the data set to be used by a PI team has been identified, the actual extraction and reporting of specific incidences must be considered carefully. The process of extraction of relevant cases from the entire data set is known as *querying*. If a simple case list is required for one or a few parameters or characteristics of a patient population similar to the previous sepsis example, the extraction probably will be fairly straightforward. However, if a multilevel query is involved, one that begins by extracting cases exhibiting one relevant characteristic and then creating one or two subsets against other relevant characteristics, the process of the query needs to be planned out carefully. In reality, the multilevel query is more common, so individuals involved in this work usually deal with a fair amount of complexity. An example built on the earlier discussion of sepsis would probably find a multilevel query defining a time period of interest, requesting the ICD-10-CM codes for sepsis to be extracted from the time period, and then perhaps further limiting that set by whether sepsis was present on admission or developed during hospitalization. The resulting three-level set would probably still require validation by infection control staff against infection control databases.

Analysis of Data

Healthcare organizations collect a significant amount of data through their electronic systems, and these data need to be used in a planned and meaningful manner. Decisions regarding quality of care and patient safety must be made after good data collection and analysis have been performed. **Data analysis** is primarily defined as the task of transforming, summarizing, or modeling data to allow the user to make meaningful conclusions. Data analysis may be characterized as turning data into information that may be used for operational decision making" (White 2021, 2). The data must meet standards related to data quality to ensure that decisions are being made based on reliable data.

Data Quality

In order for healthcare organizations to use their data in performance improvement activities, they must have quality data. As the old adage states, "garbage in, garbage out!" If organizations cannot rely on their data, there is no use collecting it and even less reason to base decisions on it. AHIMA defines data governance as, "the extent to which healthcare data are complete, accurate, consistent, and timely throughout its life cycle, including collection, application (including aggregation), warehousing, and analysis" (Buttner et al. 2021, 1). Healthcare organizations should apply the five components of the data lifecycle (capture, process, use, store, and dispose) as a means to ensure the quality of their data collection and use (see figure 5.7).

Figure 5.7. AHIMA data lifecycle

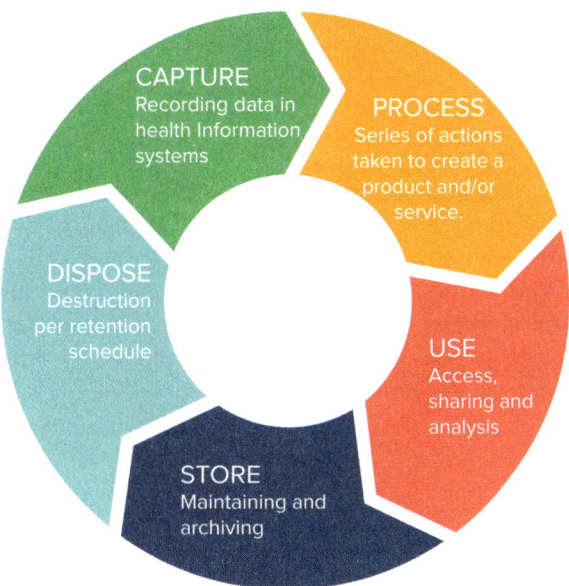

Source: Butltner et al. 2021

In addition to the data lifecycle, AHIMA also specifies 10 characteristics of data quality:

- Accuracy: The data should be free of errors, is correct
- Accessibility: Proper safeguards established to ensure data is available when needed
- Comprehensiveness: The data contains all required elements
- Consistency: The data is reliable and the same across the entire patient encounter
- Currency: The data is current and up to date
- Definition: all data elements are clearly defined
- Granularity: The data is at the appropriate level of detail
- Precision: The data is precise and collected in their exact form
- Relevancy: The data is relevant to the purpose it was collected
- Timeliness: Documentation is entered promptly, is up to data and available within specified and required time frames (Buttner et al. 2021)

Using the data lifecycle and adhering to the 10 data quality characteristics allow healthcare organizations to better ensure that their performance improvement decisions are based on sound and trustworthy data and provide the foundation for their data governance strategies. Performance improvement activities are dependent on quality data.

Statistical Analysis

The mean and standard deviation (*SD*) are methods of statistical analysis that are necessary to the graphic display of data. Although an in-depth discussion of these techniques can be found in any elementary statistics text (such as White 2021), a brief review is provided here before the discussion of graphic display.

The **mean (*M*)**, also known as the average of a distribution of numerical values, is the average value in a range of values, calculated by summing the values and dividing the total by the number of values in the range. The values may be discrete or continuous in nature. If the data are discrete (or count), the mean should be rounded to the nearest whole value; if the data are continuous, whole numbers or numbers with decimal fractions can be reported.

To calculate the mean, the various observed values are first added together. There may be repetitions of specific values, all of which are included. Then, the sum is divided by the number of observations made. For example, 15 observations of a person's systolic blood pressure revealed the following data set:

| 122 | 124 | 116 | 115 | 120 | 128 | 126 | 122 | 121 | 121 | 124 | 120 | 117 | 116 | 121 |

Note that there are three 121 readings and two 122 readings in the set. All are summed. The sum of those observations is 1,813, which is then divided by the number of observations made (15). This equals 120.86666, which should be rounded to a whole number because systolic blood pressure is commonly expressed as a whole number. The reported mean (average) systolic measurement is 121.

The **median** is usually derived without calculation. The observed values are placed in ascending or descending order; the value that is in the very middle of the set is taken as the median. An odd number of observations is necessary for there to be a value in the middle. In the following data set, the values are rearranged in ascending order as follows:

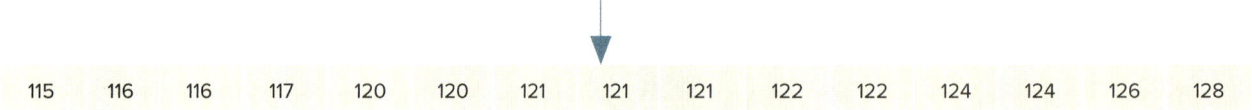

| 115 | 116 | 116 | 117 | 120 | 120 | 121 | 121 | 121 | 122 | 122 | 124 | 124 | 126 | 128 |

Note again that the repeated values are retained. The middle value is 121, as indicated by the arrow. Thus, 121 is the median. If, however, there were an even number of values, the middle would fall between the two values at places 7 and 8 in the row.

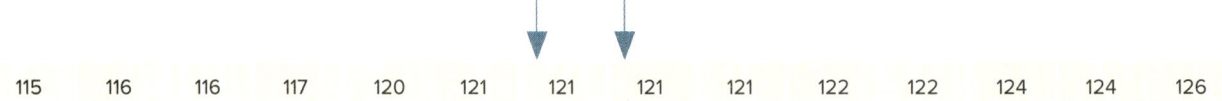

| 115 | 116 | 116 | 117 | 120 | 121 | 121 | 121 | 121 | 122 | 122 | 124 | 124 | 126 |

The values in places 7 and 8 are added together and divided by 2: 121 + 121 = 242, which divided by 2 = 121. If the values in places 7 and 8 were 122 and 125, adding them together would equal 247, which divided by 2 would equal 123.5, which should be rounded to 124 because systolic blood pressure is expressed in whole numbers.

It is sometimes better to use a median value in displaying some graphic representations of data, particularly if there is a lot of variation in the observed values or if they are skewed to one side. **Skewing** means that there are a lot of very high or very low values in the observations that distort the calculated mean and may shift the distribution one direction or the other. Because the median is not calculated, if the data set is greatly distorted by the extreme values, it can help to define a truer picture of the middle of the set.

The **standard deviation (SD)** is a complex analysis technique used in developing control charts for the display of some PI data. (See the discussion of control charts later in this chapter.) The *SD* is most easily calculated using the statistical analysis feature of a spreadsheet application. To do so, enter and highlight the column of data and select the *SD* function from the menu bar's "*fx*" button. Alternatively, choose a cell to contain the *SD*, type = STDEV(), then record the range inside the parentheses.

Although the *SD* is easily calculated using a spreadsheet application, what this statistic reveals about a data set is more difficult to understand. When a PI team begins observing a continuous measure, the observations are plotted along the *x*- and *y*-axes with very little clustering, or no discernible pattern or trend. The first nine values from the systolic blood pressure data set above can be graphed as in figure 5.8 on an *x-y* axis, where the *x*-axis is the value of the measure and the *y*-axis is the absolute frequency of that value in the set.

Figure 5.8. Spread of data in initial observations of a continuous measure

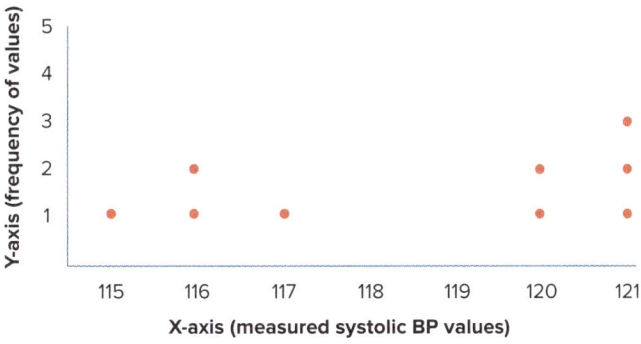

Here we see 115 with an absolute frequency of 1, 116 with an absolute frequency of 2, 117 with an absolute frequency of 1, and so on. However, as the measure is observed again and again, the observed values begin to congregate more often around the mean, as in figure 5.9.

Figure 5.9. Spread of data in later observations of a continuous measure

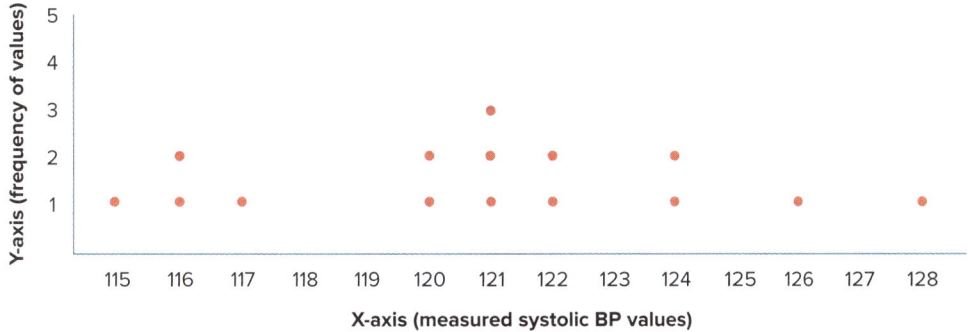

As the number of observations increases into the hundreds or thousands, a graph similar to figure 5.10 begins to form, the typical bell-shaped curve of what is called a **normal distribution**. Almost all measures, when graphed, take on this bell-shaped or "normal" appearance as the number of observations increases.

Figure 5.10. A normal distribution

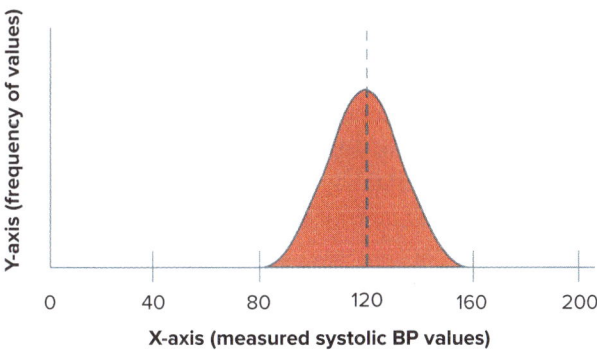

At the center or vertex of the normal distribution is the calculated mean. For the small data set in our example, 121 was calculated as the mean of the observed blood pressures. Many people know that the commonly accepted "normal" or mean value for systolic blood pressure is 120, so that calculation is relatively close. It has the greatest absolute frequency in this data set as denoted by the apex of the curve residing at that 121 value. As we examine the absolute frequencies of the measured values of the data set to the left and right sides of the mean, we see them decrease until there are no observations below 80 or above 160 in relatively "normally" functioning human beings.

For the purposes of control chart construction, the *SD* can be defined by the percentage of the frequencies contained beneath various portions of the normal distribution. Approximately 68 percent of the observations occur in the interval under the curve from −1 *SD* from the mean to +1 *SD* from the mean. (See figure 5.11.)

Figure 5.11. One standard deviation from the mean

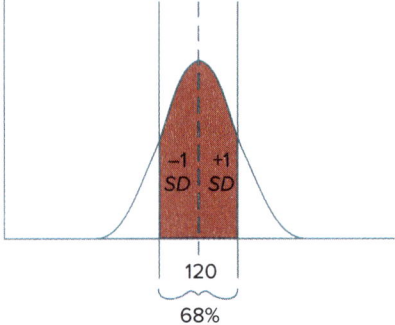

Approximately 95 percent of the observations occur in the interval under the curve from −2 *SD* from the mean to +2 *SD* from the mean. (See figure 5.12.)

Figure 5.12. Two standard deviations from the mean

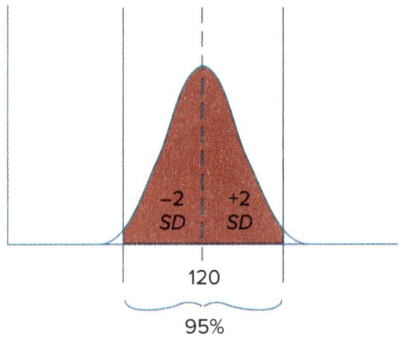

Finally, approximately 99 percent of the observations fall in the interval under the curve from −3 *SD* from the mean to +3 *SD* from the mean.

The *SD* is a useful statistic for PI in healthcare. It helps define the interval in which 95 percent of the observations should be made. Any observation that occurs outside the interval defined by +/−2 *SD* from the mean can be identified as a variant. If many observations fall outside the +/−2 *SD* interval, the process under examination could be "out of control" and contributing negatively to the provision of healthcare services.

Both Microsoft Excel and SPSS (Statistical Packages for the Social Sciences) may be used to perform data analysis and create graphs to display data. This may include the mean, median, and standard deviation, but they are also used to perform in-depth analysis such as correlation, t-test, Chi square, z scores, and many others. Review any statistical text (such as White 2021) for more information on these other statistical tests. Microsoft Excel instructions (Microsoft 365 2023a) and SPSS instructions (IBM n.d.) provide details on how to use these programs.

Artificial Intelligence

Artificial intelligence (AI) uses machine learning, but also has the ability to adapt and has cognitive-type abilities similar to those of human intelligence. AI continues to learn, adapt and change its behavior and output based on this learning. This tool has the ability to quickly assimilate large amounts of data that would have been a time-consuming and tedious task for a human. The full scope of opportunity and application of AI has yet to be realized. Although the potential for this technology is promising and could have positive impact on the healthcare system and patient outcomes, the full ramifications of this technology and its application in healthcare is yet to be determined. Healthcare organizations will need to develop policies and procedures on how this technology will be used and incorporated into their workflow (Solomonides et al. 2022). One of many possible concerns for quality managers related to the use of AI is that organizations need to ensure that their providers are making the decisions regarding patient care and not relying solely on technology to dictate care. Healthcare organizations are taking a thoughtful approach to ensure that ethical, privacy, risk, and security considerations are being addressed before implementing new products, processes, and technologies related to AI.

Predictive Analytics

Predictive analytics takes the products of statistical analysis and utilizes them in a way that provides organizations the ability to predict future events. Predictive analytics uses machine learning and historical data to help guide decision making. This process identifies patterns in the data that have been previously determined to be potential risks both in outcome and cost. Through this process, organizations are able to identify certain predictive elements in the data that have shown in the past to be key indicators of specific diseases, risk of illness, or complications. Numerous intuitive patient management systems (such as clinical decision support systems and reimbursement systems) use predictive analytics technology to support patient care, decision making, and preventable readmissions. This technology analyzes large amounts of data from disparate, structured, and unstructured data sources to identify trends that will alter patient care, treatment, and medical decision making in real-time situations.

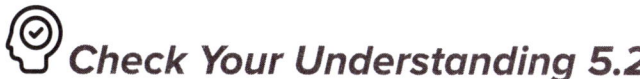

Check Your Understanding 5.2

1. Review this figure:

   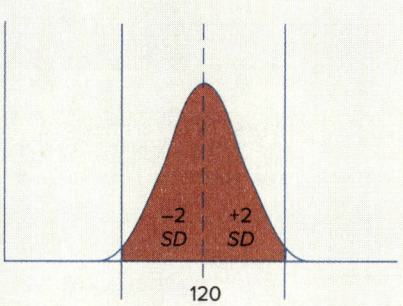

   Approximately what percent of observations occur in the interval under the curve from –2 *SD* from the mean to +2 *SD* from the mean?
   a. 50 percent
   b. 80 percent
   c. 95 percent
   d. 100 percent

2. The extent to which healthcare data are reliable and the same across the entire patient encounter is known as data:
   a. Accuracy
   b. Comprehensiveness
   c. Precision
   d. Consistency

QI Toolbox Techniques

The display tools most commonly used in PI activities include bar graphs, histograms, Pareto charts, pie charts, pivot tables, line charts, and control charts.

Once the data have been collected, the PI team should sort the data and identify any significant findings. Charts and graphs of the data make it easier to identify trends and significant relationships. Graphs can be used to compare data sets from different years or over time to visually illustrate a trend in the data or a change in performance.

The PI measures reported to a board of directors often highlight variances in data using graphs, tables, or charts. For example, in a bar graph (see figure 5.3), a change in the height of a bar indicates an increase or decrease in the data represented by the bar. The PI team would then have to determine whether this increase or decrease was a significant change in the performance of the related process.

When constructing charts, graphs, and tables, the team must provide explanatory labels and titles. Data display should be simple and accurate. Team members must report all the data, even when the data appear to have positive or negative implications for the organization. Sometimes what appears to be a negative trend may actually turn out to be a positive trend after the team fully analyzes the data. (See AHIMA 2022 for additional information.)

Spreadsheet software is helpful in creating graphs and charts. For example, using Microsoft Excel, the PI team simply needs to enter their data into the software and decide which type of graph is appropriate for the type of data. This is done by highlighting the data and selecting "Insert" and the graph or chart type. The software will then display the graph or chart. The PI team member can then add the chart title, axis labels, and any other labeling desired. Spreadsheet software instructions provide more details (Microsoft Support 2023b).

Bar Graphs

A **bar graph** (see figure 5.3) is used to display discrete categories, such as the gender of respondents or the type of health insurance respondents have. Such categories are shown on the horizontal (x) axis of the graph. The vertical (y) axis shows the number or frequency of responses. The vertical scale always begins with zero. Most spreadsheet software can be used to create a bar graph from a given data set.

Histograms

A **histogram** is a bar graph that displays data proportionally (see figure 5.5). Histograms are used to identify problems or changes in a system or process. They are based on raw data and absolute frequencies, which determine how the graphs will be structured. Unlike a Pareto chart (described in the following section), a histogram keeps the data in the order of the scale against which they were obtained. The horizontal axis measures intervals of continuous data, such as time or money. The scale is grouped into intervals appropriate to the nature of the data. For example, time might be grouped into intervals of six hours and money into groups of $5,000. The vertical axis shows the absolute frequency of occurrence in each of the interval categories. Because of its visual impact, a histogram is more effective for displaying data than a check sheet of raw data, particularly when the frequencies are large. A histogram should be used for continuous data (rather than a pie chart).

Histograms have the following characteristics:

- Display large amounts of continuous data that are difficult to interpret in lists or other nongraphic forms
- Show the relative frequency of occurrence of the various data categories indirectly using the height of the bars
- Demonstrate the distribution of the absolute frequencies of the data in the grouped intervals

The first step in creating a histogram is to gather the data. The data can be collected on check sheets or gathered from department logs or by querying computer programs and systems. A histogram should be used in situations in which numerical observations can be collected; for example, cost in dollars for a surgical procedure. Once the data have been gathered, the team can group the data into a series of intervals or categories. A check sheet can be used to count how many times a data point appears in each interval grouping. For example, the cost of a surgical procedure on each patient might be grouped into the following intervals: $0 to $24,999; $25,000 to $49,999; $50,000 to $74,999; and $75,000 to $99,999.

To analyze a histogram, look for things that seem suspicious or strange. The team should review the various interpretations and write down observations.

The histogram in figure 5.5 shows data related to the number of patients and their total charges. The horizontal axis lists the revenue per stay by dollar amounts, and the vertical axis shows the interval groupings indicating the number of patients.

Pareto Charts

A **Pareto chart** is a type of bar graph that uses data to determine priorities in problem solving. The Pareto principle states that 80 percent of costs or problems are caused by 20 percent of the patients or staff (Juran 2019). Pareto charts are useful in the following situations:

- When analyzing data about the frequency of problems or causes in a process
- When there are many problems or causes and you want to focus on the most significant
- When analyzing broad causes by looking at their specific components
- When communicating with others about your data (ASQ 2023a)

Using a Pareto chart can help the PI team focus on problems and their causes and demonstrate which are most responsible for the problem. Follow these steps to construct a Pareto chart:

1. Use a check sheet or database query to collect the required data. Figure 5.13 shows the top 10 major diagnostic categories (MDCs) by total charges. A check sheet is used to collect cases by MDC and to total the hospital charges for that MDC.

2. Arrange the data in order, from the category with the greatest frequency to the category with the lowest frequency. In figure 5.13, the data are arranged from the MDC with the highest charges to the MDC with the lowest charges.

3. Calculate the totals for each category. Figure 5.13 lists MDC 10 first, with charges totaling approximately $2,500,500; then MDC 06, with charges totaling $2,500,000; MDC 04, with charges of $2,300,000; and so forth to MDC 18, with charges totaling approximately $300,000.

4. Compute the cumulative percentage. This is accomplished by calculating the percentage of the total for each category and then adding the percentage for the greatest frequency to the percentage for the next greatest frequency, and so on. Using the example in figure 5.13, the charges for MDC 10 ($2,500,500) represent 18.7 percent of all charges listed, while the charges for MDC 06 ($2,500,000) represent 18.7 percent of all charges listed. The cumulative percentage is obtained by adding the percentages together—MDC 10's 18.7 percent plus MDC 06's 18.7 percent equals 37.4 percent. This cumulative percentage is then calculated for all categories until 100 percent is obtained.

5. Spreadsheet software can easily create a Pareto chart.

Figure 5.13. Example of a Pareto chart

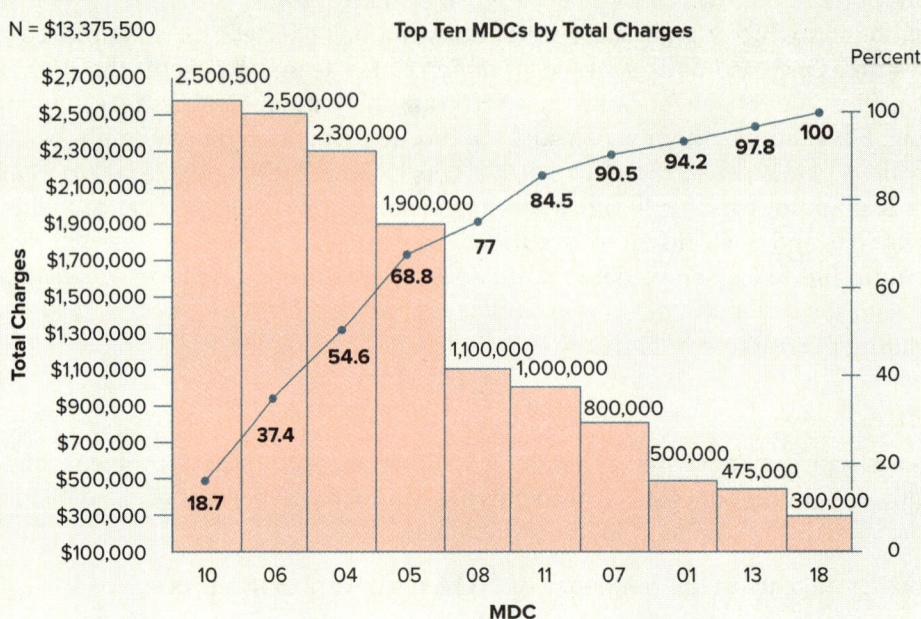

Pie Charts

A **pie chart** (see figure 5.4) is used to show the relationship of each part to the whole and reveals how each part contributes to the total product or process. The 360 degrees of the circle (pie) represent the total, or 100 percent. The pie is divided into "slices" proportionate to each component's percentage of the whole. To create a pie chart, first determine the percentages for each data element of the total population, and then draw the slice accordingly. Spreadsheet programs can automatically create pie charts from a given data set (see instructions in the Line Charts section later in this chapter).

Pivot Tables

In Microsoft Excel, a **pivot table** can be used to summarize large amounts of data according to categories for decision making. Table 5.2 is an example of a pivot table totaling hip replacement procedures by ICD-10-PCS code according to gender. Microsoft provides detailed instructions on how to create pivot tables in Excel (Microsoft Support 2023c).

Table 5.2. Example of a pivot table

Count of Hip Replacement Procedures First Quarter			
ICD-10-PCS Code	Male	Female	Total
0SR9039	5	3	8
0SR90J9	10	15	25
0SRB039	4	7	11
0SRB0J9	13	8	21
Total	32	33	65

Line Charts

A **line chart** is a simple plotted chart of data that shows the progress of a process over time. By analyzing the chart, the PI team can identify trends, shifts, or changes in a process over time. The chart tracks the time frame on the horizontal axis and the measurement (the number of occurrences or the actual measure of a parameter) on the vertical axis. The data are gathered from sources specific to the process that has been evaluated. Each set of data (measurement or number of occurrences and time frame) must be related.

A line chart can be created by completing the following steps:

1. Select a time frame.
2. Identify the data to be tracked.
3. Use a check sheet to collect frequency data or query a database or other system to collect measurement data.
4. Figure 5.6 is an example of a line chart. Let's walk through the process steps in Excel used to create this chart. First, the data points are entered into the spreadsheet. This includes one column for the dates and a second column indicating the number of charts analyzed for the corresponding date. Then, the data in both columns is highlighted using the cursor. Next, the Insert tab is used to select the type of chart—in this case, a line chart. The software will display the chart on the screen. The axis labels are added using the chart tools tab on the menu bar at the top of the screen. The layout option is selected, then the axis titles option is used to add the x-axis title and the y-axis title. The chart tools feature is used to select the layout icon and then the chart title can be added; drop-down menu options are used to define the title location. To add the data values on the chart, the data labels icon under the chart tools layout option is selected; the values should appear on the chart. The chart can then be copied and pasted into a report or other document (Microsoft 365 2023a).

To analyze the chart, the team should look for peaks and valleys that indicate possible problems with the process. Periodically redoing the line charts for a process helps the team monitor changes over time. A line chart is a good way to display trends in the data. For example, a line chart could be displayed on a large graph that could be updated each month. When the team evaluates the results, it should look for seasonal peaks and valleys. For example, summer vacation times may show a change in a chart that plots staff productivity.

Control Charts

A **control chart** can be used to measure key processes over time. Using a control chart focuses attention on any variation in the process and helps the PI team determine whether that variation is normal or a result of special circumstances. Normal variation also may be called *common cause variation*, or the expected variance in a process, because the process will not or cannot be performed in exactly the same manner each and every time. When a special circumstance or unexpected event occurs in the process, this will result in what is called *special cause variation*. It is this special cause variation that the PI team needs to investigate.

The specific statistical calculations used to determine the upper and lower limits of a control chart depend on the type of data collected. The calculations used for statistical process control are the data mean (the median of the range between data points) and the *SD* (ASQ 2023b). The appearance of the control chart is like turning the classic bell curve on its left tail and running it horizontally left to right as the time on the x-axis goes by. (See figure 5.14.)

Figure 5.14. Example of a control chart

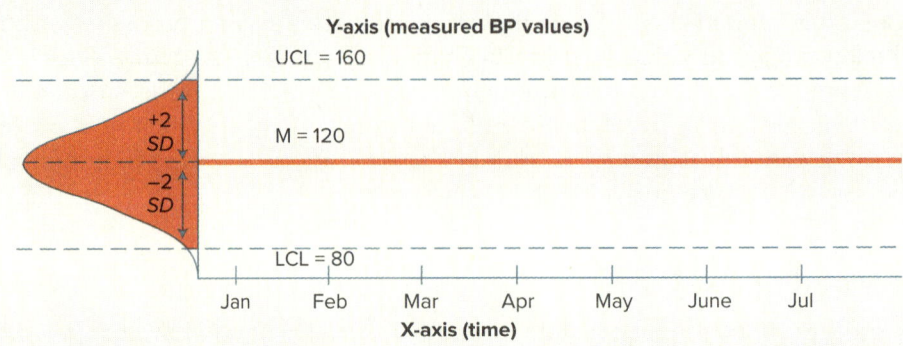

The upper and lower control limits are always +/–2 SD from the mean. As each successive month of data is added to the chart, the SDs are recalculated and may fluctuate in value. As the process is tightened up and improved over time, the SD should become smaller and smaller as variation is driven out of the process. If the SD expands, the process becomes less controlled, taking on variation and most likely less quality. The latest calculated SD is always used in the current display of the chart. Data points that lie outside the upper or lower control limits may signal special cause variation that should be examined.

A control chart can be created by completing the following steps:

1. Determine which process and what data to measure.
2. Collect about 20 observations of the measure.
3. Calculate the mean and SD for the data set. Various spreadsheet software programs can be used to make these calculations. The mean (average) becomes the centerline for the control chart.
4. Calculate an upper control limit (UCL) and a lower control limit (LCL). The upper control limit is usually represented by a dashed line 2 SDs above the mean, and the lower control limit is usually 2 SDs below the mean.

The resulting control chart becomes the standard against which the team can compare all future data for the process. For example, figure 5.14 displays systolic blood pressure measurements for a patient. The mean is calculated at 120, and the standard deviation is calculated at 20. The UCL is 2 SDs above the mean, or 160. The LCL is 2 SDs below the mean, or 80.

Scatter Diagram

A **scatter diagram** (also called a scatter plot) is used to show the relationship or association between two variables (White 2021, 54). For example, figure 5.15 shows a scatter diagram that displays the relationship between the average minutes a patient spends with their provider and the provider's average patient satisfaction scores on a scale of 1–5, with 5 being the highest score. This scatter diagram shows a positive relationship between these two variables in that the patient satisfaction score increases when the patient spends more time with their provider.

Figure 5.15. Example of a scatter diagram

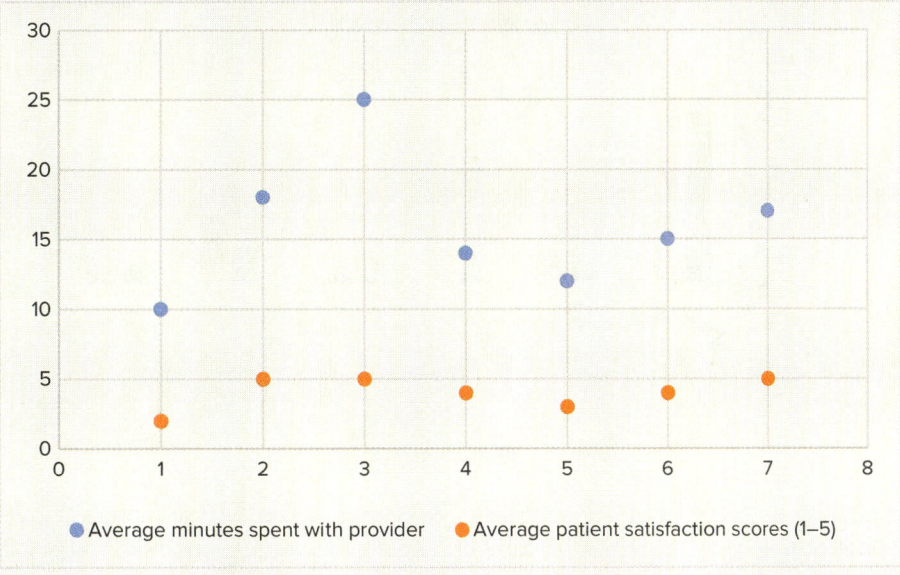

Real-Life Example

Table 5.3 shows a portion of a patient profile for one hospital in the years 2020 and 2025. When the 2020 data are compared with the 2025 data in a bar graph (see figure 5.16), we see that the hospital's customer base has experienced a significant increase in the number of patients identifying Asian as their race/ethnicity. The hospital must look at how this increase affects its processes. For example, what changes might be required in the dietary area? What staffing changes might be required to accommodate patients who have religious and cultural differences? How will the organization ensure patient rights and safety in light of potential language barriers to effective communication?

Table 5.3. Data set for bar graph

Profile of Hospital Patients			
2020		2025	
Race/Ethnicity	Discharges	Race/Ethnicity	Discharges
White	6,254	White	6,874
Black	1,859	Black	1,763
Hispanic	4,251	Hispanic	3,954
Native American	254	Native American	301
Asian	1,352	Asian	2,514
Other/Unknown	750	Other/Unknown	594

Figure 5.16. Bar graph comparison of patient profile data

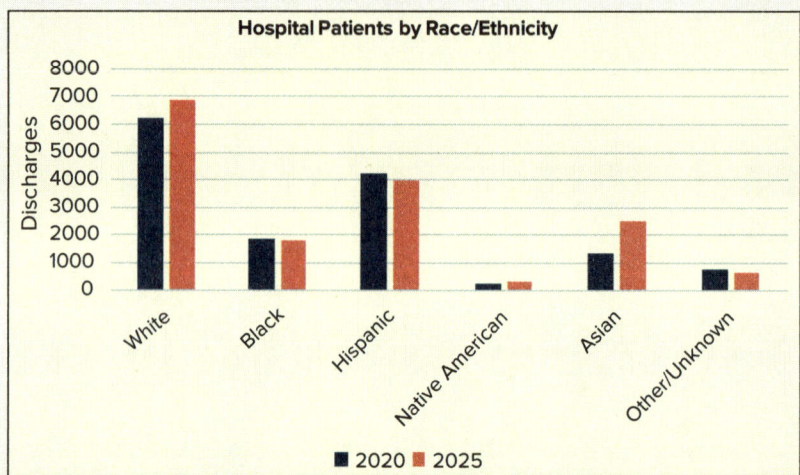

Table 5.4 shows another set of data from the hospital's patient profile. The two pie charts in figure 5.17, which were created from the data, show that over five years the number of emergency admissions increased by 24 percentage points and the number of urgent admissions decreased by 12 percentage points. This information indicates that either the admissions are being categorized incorrectly or the incidence of trauma is increasing. The facility may need to look at its emergency department capacity and procedures or consider changes to its admission criteria.

Table 5.4. Data set for pie chart

Profile of Hospital Patients			
2020		2025	
Admission Type	Discharges	Admission Type	Discharges
Emergency	2,163	Emergency	5,987
Urgent	4,325	Urgent	2,478
Elective	5,784	Elective	4,458
Newborn	1,659	Newborn	1,342
Delivery	1,478	Delivery	1,270

Figure 5.17. Pie chart comparison of patient profile data

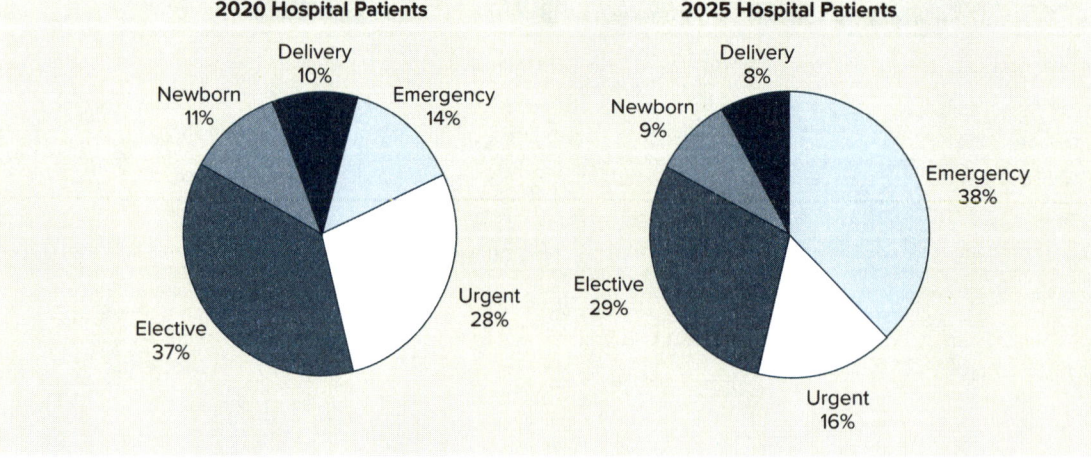

Check Your Understanding 5.3

1. If you want to plot data that displays the percentage of overall employee satisfaction by department in a healthcare clinic, which type of data display tool should be used?
   a. Pie chart
   b. Histogram
   c. Bar graph
   d. Line chart

2. A PI team wants to display the patient types that have the most coding errors in relationship to coder years of service. The desire of the PI team is to display how a coder's years of service relate to the number and type of coding errors. The type of chart best suited for this is a:
   a. Bar graph
   b. Pareto chart
   c. Pie chart
   d. Line graph

Case Study

Table 5.5 is an example of a dashboard report showing the health information department performance standards of the six hospitals within Western Healthcare System for the month of March. The data presented represent the key indicators of performance for each hospital's HI department. These data are used by the corporate HI director to evaluate the performance of each hospital and across the corporation. Western Healthcare System has established a benchmark standard for each of these key performance metrics; this is found in table 5.5 at the bottom of the report, labeled "Best Practice Standard." Each hospital within the corporation submits its monthly data to the corporate HI director.

Case Study Questions

1. If you were the corporate HI director for Western Healthcare System, what would be your overall evaluation of the dashboard report for the month of March? Specifically, based on the trends you are seeing in the data, which hospitals are not meeting several of the best practice standards?

2. Based on your answer to question 1, what additional data would you request? What additional analysis would you perform?

3. Are there trends in any metrics across the corporation that are concerning? If so, which metrics? Why are they of concern?

4. Select three data elements from table 5.5 and create an appropriate graph to represent those data, along with the corresponding best practice standard for that data element. Keep in mind the type of data in the table and choose the best graphic display tool for those data.

Table 5.5. Data set for case study

Western Healthcare System
Health Information Corporate Dashboard
March, 20XX

	Scan Days			Outpatient (OP)	Index Days				Quality Review of Scanning/Indexing Process (days)			Analysis Days			Delinquency Rate
	IP	SDS	ED		IP	SDS	ED	OP	IP	SDS	ED	IP	SDS	ED	
Community Region															
Facilities															
Hospital A	2.0	2.0	2.0	1.0	2.0	1.0	1.0	2.0	11.0	11.0	3.0	3.0	3.0	2.0	5%
Hospital B	1.0	0.5	1.0	2.0	2.0	1.0	2.0	2.0	1.0	1.0	1.0	1.0	2.0	1.0	0%
Hospital C	0.0	1.0	2.0	1.0	3.0	0.0	2.0	0.0	0.0	0.0	0.0	1.0	3.0	1.0	8%
Urban Region															
Facilities															
Hospital D	2.0	3.0	1.0	1.0	0.0	1.0	0.0	1.0	55.0	45.0	0.0	4.0	1.0	0.0	12%
Hospital E	0.0	1.0	2.0	3.0	1.0	2.0	1.0	2.0	130.0	130.0	120.0	2.0	32.0	30.0	23%
Hospital F	1.0	2.0	3.0	1.0	2.0	0.0	2.0	2.0	145.0	45.0	32.0	3.0	7.0	4.0	18%
Corporate Average	1.00	1.58	1.83	1.50	1.67	0.83	1.33	1.50	57.00	38.67	26.00	2.33	8.00	6.33	11%
Best Practice Standard	2.0	2.0	1.0	2.0	1.0	1.0	1.0	1.0	1.0	1.0	1.0	2.0	2.0	1.0	<15%

Review Questions

1. In the following data set the absolute frequency for 99/min is:

Date and Time	Pulse Rate Recorded
Jan. 5, 8:00 a.m.	100/min
Jan. 5, 12:00 noon	102/min
Jan. 5, 4:00 p.m.	99/min
Jan. 5, 8:00 p.m.	99/min
Jan. 5, 12:00 midnight	102/min
Jan. 6, 4:00 a.m.	98/min
Jan. 6, 8:00 a.m.	99/min

   a. 1
   b. 2
   c. 3
   d. 4

2. Using the data set from question 1, the relative frequency for 102/min would be _____.
   a. 42.9
   b. 28.6
   c. 14.3
   d. 57.1

3. Which type of chart is used to focus attention on any variation in the process and helps the team to determine whether that variation is normal or a result of special circumstances?
   a. Pareto chart
   b. Pie chart
   c. Control chart
   d. Line chart

4. Which type of data display tool is used to display data proportionally and to identify problems or changes in a system or process?
   a. Bar graph
   b. Histogram
   c. Pie chart
   d. Line chart

5. Which type of data display tool is used to show the relationship or association between two variables?
   a. Control chart
   b. Scatter diagram
   c. Pie chart
   d. Bar graph

References

AHIMA. 2022. "Data Presentation and Visualization." In *Introduction to Data Analytics Toolkit*. Chicago: AHIMA.
ASQ (American Society for Quality). 2023a. "What is a Pareto Chart?" https://asq.org/quality-resources/pareto.
ASQ (American Society for Quality). 2023b. "Control Chart." https://asq.org/quality-resources/control-chart.
Buttner, P., M. Meyer, R. Mikaelian, N. Miller, and B. Ruhnau-Gee. 2021. "Healthcare Data Governance." https://journal.ahima.org/page/practice-brief-healthcare-data-governance-14.

IBM. n.d. "IBM SPSS Software." Accessed December 19, 2023. https://www.ibm.com/spss.

Juran. 2019. "Pareto Principle (80/20 Rule) & Pareto Analysis Guide." https://www.juran.com/blog/a-guide-to-the-pareto-principle-80-20-rule-pareto-analysis/.

Microsoft 365. 2023a. "Microsoft Excel." https://www.microsoft.com/en-us/microsoft-365/excel?ef_id=_k_Cj0KCQiAm4WsBhCiARIsAEJIEzV2GtPw10xN3nJwnV9L6ct2k5ryawPSEgoZY3HSXYJUqAvq9dRv59AaAlPfEALw_wcB_k_&OCID=AIDcmm474qp8el_SEM__k_Cj0KCQiAm4WsBhCiARIsAEJIEzV2GtPw10xN3nJwnV9L6ct2k5ryawPSEgoZY3HSXYJUqAvq9dRv59AaAlPfEALw_wcB_k_&gad_source=1&gclid=Cj0KCQiAm4WsBhCiARIsAEJIEzV2GtPw10xN3nJwnV9L6ct2k5ryawPSEgoZY3HSXYJUqAvq9dRv59AaAlPfEALw_wcB.

Microsoft Support. 2023b. "Create a chart from start to finish." https://support.microsoft.com/en-us/office/create-a-chart-from-start-to-finish-0baf399e-dd61-4e18-8a73-b3fd5d5680c2.

Microsoft Support. 2023c. "Create a PivotTable to analyze worksheet data." https://support.microsoft.com/en-au/office/create-a-pivottable-to-analyze-worksheet-data-a9a84538-bfe9-40a9-a8e9-f99134456576.

Solomonides, A., A., E. Koski, S. M. Atabaki, S. Weinberg, J. D. McGreevey, J. L. Kannry, C. Petersen, and C. U. Lehmann. 2022. Defining AMIA's artificial intelligence principles. *Journal of the American Medical Informatics Association* 29(4):585–591, https://doi.org/10.1093/jamia/ocac006

White, S. 2021. *A Practical Approach to Analyzing Healthcare Data*, 4th ed. Chicago: AHIMA.

Resources

CMS (Center for Medicare and Medicaid Services). 2024. "2024 ICD-10-CM." https://www.cms.gov/medicare/coding-billing/icd-10-codes/2024-icd-10-cm

CMS (Center for Medicare and Medicaid Services). 2024. "2024 ICD-10-PCS." https://www.cms.gov/medicare/coding-billing/icd-10-codes/2024-icd-10-pcs

CHAI (Coalition for Health AI). 2023. "Blueprint for Trustworthy AI Implementation Guidance and Assurance for Healthcare." https://www.coalitionforhealthai.org/papers/blueprint-for-trustworthy-ai_V1.0.pdf

Hulsen, T., S. S. Jamuar, A. R. Moody, J. H. Karnes, O. Varga, S. Hedensted, R. Spreafico, D. A. Hafler, and E. F. McKinney. 2019. From big data to precision medicine. *Frontiers in Medicine* 6: 34.

Masick, K. and E. Bouillon. 2020. *Storytelling with Data in Healthcare*. New York: Routledge.

Shilo, S., H. Rossman, and E. Segal. 2020. Axes of a revolution: challenges and promises of big data in healthcare. *Nature Medicine* 26(1): 29–38.

Sullivan, L. M. 2023. *Essentials of Biostatistics in Public Health*, 4th ed. Essential Public Health Series. Burlington, MA: Jones & Bartlett Learning.

White, S. 2020. "Healthcare Data Analytics: Impact of sampling." Chapter 16 in *Health Information Management: Concepts, Principles, and Practice*, 6th ed., edited by P.K. Oachs and A.L. Watters. Chicago: AHIMA.

Communicating Performance Improvement Activities and Recommendations

Learning Objectives

- Apply communication tools such as meeting minutes, quarterly reports, and presentations in performance improvement processes
- Design a performance improvement presentation, ensuring that all key elements are included
- Critique a performance improvement presentation

Key Terms

CRAF method
Electronic presentations
Minutes
Quarterly report
Report cards
Storytelling

The effective communication of information about the activities of performance improvement (PI) teams is vital to the PI process in healthcare organizations. All PI activities should be reported using the committee or meeting structure defined by the healthcare organization. This structure may include medical staff standing committees, PI team workgroups, and/or department meetings.

The Performance Improvement and Patient Safety Council is an example of a standing committee in most healthcare organizations that is responsible for coordinating and reporting PI and safety activities. This council receives committee reports of PI activities and in turn, reports significant findings to the leaders of the organization—typically, the executive committee and board of directors.

Evidence of PI activity is required by various regulatory and accreditation agencies. Such organizations require that PI activities take place within every healthcare organization, and they look for PI compliance during the survey process.

Common methods of communicating PI activities include minutes, quarterly reports, and storytelling. This chapter focuses on these three basic communication tools. Figure 6.1 shows the flow of information from the chartered PI teams to the Performance Improvement and Patient Safety Council, regardless of the reporting method.

Figure 6.1. Flow of information from chartered PI teams to the Performance Improvement and Patient Safety Council

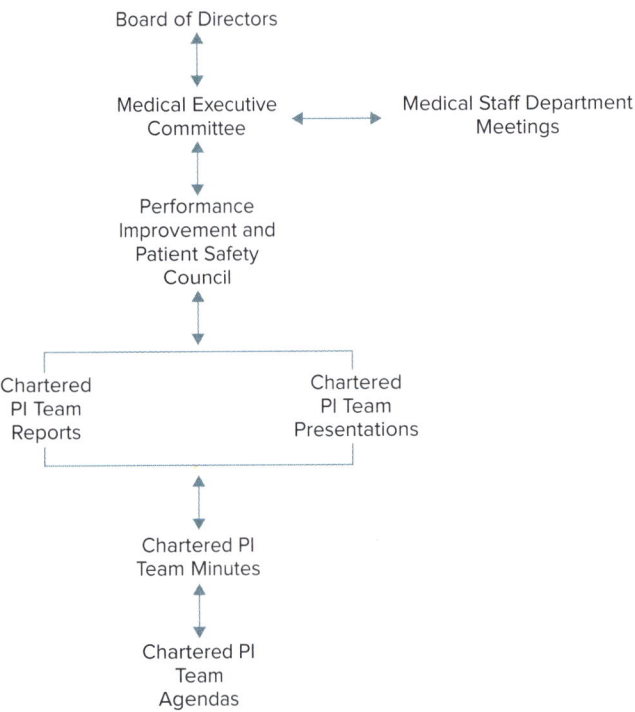

Minutes

It is important that the PI committee or team keep track of its progress and activities. Documentation of these activities is often recorded in the form of minutes. **Minutes** are the written record of key events in a formal meeting and are typically reviewed and approved by the group at the next meeting.

Organizations should select the methods they will use to set agendas for their meetings and allocate meeting times for action items and discussions. The responsibility for distributing agendas for upcoming meetings and minutes from past meetings should be discussed and assigned. The role of recorder should be assigned to an individual trained in the process of documenting minutes.

Many different formats can be used to record meeting minutes. One that is particularly helpful for PI documentation is the **CRAF method**. (See figure 6.2 for an example.) CRAF stands for the following categories of recordable information:

- **C**onclusions of group discussion
- **R**ecommendations made by the committee or team
- **A**ctions that the committee, team, or individual members decide to take
- **F**ollow-up activity

By using the CRAF format, the recorder can avoid getting distracted from the discussion. The format allows the recorder to focus only on necessary documentation.

The *Conclusions* section should document the results of the discussion and any decisions the group makes about future actions. The recorder should be sure to clarify the conclusions at the end of a discussion if there is any ambiguity.

The *Recommendations* section should capture the team's plan for putting its decision into effect, with justification points if necessary. The approach to solving the problem at hand should be listed as a recommendation.

In the *Actions* section, the recorder documents the *actions* planned for the various process steps. In figure 6.2, this section documents the person assigned to accomplish specific activities during the next work period. Activities between meetings might include gathering data, talking with people involved in and responsible for the process being examined, or doing a literature search.

The *Follow-up* section documents whether the actions were accomplished and whether the group is ready to make decisions and recommendations for future activities. Assessing and documenting progress ensures that the PI team is following the process plan appropriately and conducting sufficient analysis of previous actions.

Figure 6.2. Sample minutes from a PI meeting

Committee Name: Employee Satisfaction Survey Uptown Clinic
Attendees: Clinic Manager, Human Resource Manager, Practice Directors, Front-End Supervisor, Lab Supervisor, Radiology Supervisor, Clinical Staff Manager
Date: January 15th
Recorder: Jose Nunez
Leader: Sue Jones
Facilitator: Sandra Yu
Approval:
Beginning/Ending Time: 10:05 am – 11:20 am

Conclusions	Recommendations	Actions	Follow-up
Reviewed and finalized employee survey tool	Changes made to the survey: - Add a Likert scale (1-5) to improve the detail of employee answers - Add questions about employee engagement and growth - Add an open-ended question at the end of survey for qualitative feedback	- Human Resource Manager to update survey per recommendations by 1/20 - Human Resource Manager to ensure that survey is uploaded to the clinic survey management tool	Consensus reached on survey tool questions and administration of the survey

Figure 6.2. Sample minutes from a PI meeting (*Continued*)

Analyze survey results during meeting next month.	Review the survey data for any trends or common themes.		
Subcommittee work on developing an action plan related to the survey findings.	Document and report all meeting decisions/actions.	Subcommittee work completed on trends or common themes	Assignment complete
Survey results reviewed by entire team	Recommendations for employee engagement and growth initiatives	Plan for implementation created by 3/1	Implementation plan
Evaluate the meeting Adjourn			

Quarterly Report

In addition to documenting meeting activities, the committee or team must provide regular reports to the organization's Performance Improvement and Patient Safety Council. The frequency of reporting is usually based on the committee or team meeting schedule. At a minimum, quarterly reports should be submitted to the council. The **quarterly report** is based on the documented meeting minutes and should include information about PI activities, such as summaries of data collection, conclusions, and recommendations. (See the sample reporting form in figure 6.3.)

Figure 6.3. Example of a quarterly report

Committee Name: Employee Satisfaction Survey Uptown Clinic Date: January 15th Recorder: Jose Nunez Leader: Sue Jones Facilitator: Sandra Yu	
Opportunity Statement	Supervisors have noted a lack of employee engagement.
Performance Measures	Survey employees to assess levels of satisfaction, engagement, and perception of growth opportunities within the clinic.
Sample	All clinic employees
Summary of Progress to Date	Survey will be administered over the next month using the clinic survey management tool. Employees will be reminded to complete the survey through email notifications. Data will be analyzed, and recommendations will be made. PI team will wrap up its activities by the end of February.
Conclusions	Not applicable at this time
Recommendations	In progress
Reported to: Performance Improvement and Patient Safety Council Date: March 1st Reported by: Sue Jones	

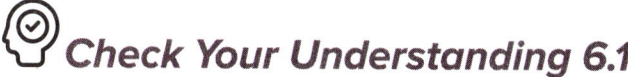

Check Your Understanding 6.1

1. Javier is serving in the role of the recorder on the PI team. One of his responsibilities is to document the key items from the meetings. This record is referred to as the:
   a. Presentation
   b. Minutes
   c. Report
   d. Follow-up report

2. PI teams must report their progress and activities to the organization's PI and Patient Safety Council. At a minimum, how often must this report be submitted?
   a. Weekly
   b. Monthly
   c. Quarterly
   d. Annually

Storytelling

It is important to share the results of PI activities. One method of doing this is **storytelling**. Storytelling is a report format that explains the PI purpose, process undertaken, analysis, and results of team activities in an easily understood manner by anyone interested (Ishikawa 1990, 254–255).

In the early 1980s, Kaoru Ishikawa called attention to the importance of communicating the PI process in a structured manner to support learning and organization-wide PI (Ishikawa 1990, 255). Since the technique was introduced, elaborate rules outlining the process have been developed. Leaders in continuous quality improvement and total quality management continue to emphasize the importance of these rules.

Storytelling remains an effective tool for healthcare organizations to facilitate PI activities by "Telling people the reality of what's going on and giving them hope by providing them with the vision. Understand deeply and describe simply, honor the past, lay out the mandate for change, and provide a rigorous and optimistic vision for the future. Put your thoughts down on paper and, if practical, do it with your team. Share what you come up with to test and improve it. And remember that your customers are resources, too… add their voices to your story" (Frei and Morriss 2023, 12–13). Key elements in successful storytelling include:

- Organization
- Structure
- Timeliness
- Frequency
- Connection
- Celebration
- Feedback

Methods of Storytelling

Storytelling has always been a powerful method of teaching and learning. Methods of storytelling include oral presentations, poster presentations, and other types of **electronic presentations**. A poster presentation is created electronically as a single slide using presentation software such as Microsoft PowerPoint or Prezi. Electronic presentation software has significantly streamlined storytelling because such software provides standard formatting and key symbols to display the PI tools. Both of these presentation techniques are used to summarize the PI team's activities. The decision to create a single-slide presentation versus a full electronic presentation with multiple slides depends on the setting or situation in which the team's results are being presented. For example, if the results are presented in a training session, a multiple-slide presentation may be the best option. If the results are being presented as a snapshot in a common area of the facility, a single-slide presentation may be better.

These storytelling methods can help teams explain their work to those who may not be familiar with the PI process. The purpose of these presentations is to summarize an entire PI project in a graphic format. The team uses words, pictures, and graphs to tell the story of the project in a way that permits the target audience to understand the team's thought process and its specific applications of PI tools. Presentations also demonstrate a growing knowledge of customer needs and the understanding of gathered statistical data. Healthcare organizations use various types of presentations because they are valuable teaching tools for customers and staff. In addition, prominent display of a presentation recognizes the accomplishments and participation of the organization's employees. Presentations force the storytelling to be far more succinct and focused, and when posted in a public place, they are available to a wider audience. They communicate PI activities to the entire organization and also recognize individual contributions to the process. The basic presentation content for PI team activities is listed in figure 6.4.

Figure 6.4. Sample presentation content

Presentation Title		
• Mission statement • Vision statement • Team members • Customers • Customer requirements	• Key team activities in process steps • Flowcharts • Cause-and-effect (fishbone) diagram • Benchmarks	• Data gathered and analyzed (baseline and during PI activities) • Gantt chart • Measurement/evaluation • Future plans and goals

Once a PI project is complete, the organization may decide to communicate the outcome to its communities of interest, such as patients, medical staff, or employers in the region. Organizations that have improved their services often want to publicize this fact.

Several approaches can be used to communicate information on PIs. For example, some large healthcare corporations routinely present performance data on their websites to show customers and other stakeholders how they are progressing with important performance measures.

Many healthcare organizations also publish information about care quality initiatives in their annual reports. Such reports are excellent vehicles for communicating performance information, emphasizing an organization's mission within its community, and communicating ongoing efforts to provide the community with the best healthcare possible.

Benefits of Storytelling

Just as storytelling is common in daily life throughout the world, it is also common in healthcare organizations. One unit or hospital can learn from the PI processes conducted in another unit or hospital, but only if their story is shared with others. Telling the story of a quality improvement initiative may be helpful to engage others in quality improvement work throughout the organization. Examples of how individuals can benefit from the storytelling process include the following:

- Team accomplishments are documented over an extended period of time in an organized and succinct way

- PI teamwork is presented in an engaging manner

- Employees are informed of important quality issues that have been addressed within the organization in a manner that draws their attention to the potential impact and creates mindfulness going forward

- Staff members continue to recognize the importance of quality patient care
- PI team members and employees of the organization have a forum to be recognized for their exceptional work on quality issues

QI Toolbox Technique: Report Cards

Report cards provide a summary of performance and outcomes related to healthcare services, facilities, and/or providers. These report cards consist of a document or system designed to offer a transparent and easily understandable evaluation of various aspects of healthcare delivery. The goal is to help patients, providers, and other stakeholders make informed decisions about healthcare quality and choose the most appropriate care options. These report cards are publicly available, through either online platforms or other means, to promote transparency and accountability in the healthcare system. Patients can use this information to make informed decisions about their healthcare providers, and healthcare organizations can use it to identify areas for improvement and showcase their strengths. Report cards play a role in fostering a culture of continuous quality improvement within the healthcare industry. For example, https://www.medicare.gov/care-compare/ allows users to find and compare different types of Medicare providers (e.g., physicians, hospitals, nursing homes, home health services).

Check Your Understanding 6.2

1. Consumers and other healthcare stakeholders use report cards for which of the following reasons?
    a. To access a detailed medical history for patients
    b. To assess the financial performance of healthcare providers
    c. To offer a transparent evaluation of healthcare quality and outcomes
    d. To determine eligibility for health insurance coverage

2. List the reasons why an organization would require all PI teams to develop an electronic presentation to communicate the details of performance improvement activities.

Real-Life Example

Figure 6.5 shows an example of a PI team's presentation of their documentation improvement project. The PI project focused on provider timeliness of documentation to meet regulatory and accrediting body compliance. The PI team developed mission and vision statements and identified the customers and their requirements for this process. The team used baseline data for documentation that showed the average time taken to complete clinical documentation across all departments in the hospital was approximately 48 hours. The team surveyed providers and staff to assess functionality and workflow with the EHR documentation process. The PI team developed interventions to address the issues discovered from the survey results and created an implementation plan for improvement. The team collected post intervention data in order to evaluate the effectiveness of the implementation plan and interventions. Specific data and information is found in the figure. The post intervention data showed a 30 percent improvement from the baseline. This presentation was presented to the Performance Improvement and Patient Safety Council and the findings were also reported to the Medical Executive Committee and the Board of Directors.

Figure 6.5. Example of a PI poster presentation

Improving Documentation Timeliness PI Team Presentation
Community Hospital

PI Team Mission
Hospital HIM Department is committed to providing quality patient care through complete, accurate, and timely EHR documentation.

PI Team Vision
To ensure EHR documentation meets hospital standards and regulations.

PI Team Members
HIM Manager, HIM Analysts, Compliance Officer, Chief of Medical Staff, EHR Quality Assurance Specialist

Customers
Providers, Patients, Hospital Staff, Payers, Accrediting bodies

Customer Expectations
Timely EHR documentation for all patient care encounters.

Baseline Assessment Data

Average Documentation Completion Time (Before Interventions):
Before interventions, the average time taken to complete clinical documentation across all departments in the hospital was approximately 48 hours.

Department Documentation Completion Time (Before Interventions) [bar chart]

Root Cause Analysis Data

Survey Results
- 72% of healthcare providers reported that they found the EHR system challenging to use efficiently.
- 64% of healthcare providers mentioned that they faced competing priorities and excessive workload that hindered timely documentation.
- 52% of healthcare providers expressed frustration with the lack of automated reminders for documentation deadlines.

EHR System Logs:
Identified instances of system lag and performance issues during peak usage times, leading to delays in documentation.

Intervention Implementation Data

EHR Training Program:
- Conducted a series of EHR training sessions for healthcare providers, and post-training assessments showed a significant improvement in their proficiency.
- 85% of surveyed healthcare providers reported increased confidence in using the EHR after training.

Workflow Redesign:
- Redesigned documentation workflows resulted in a 20% reduction in steps required to complete documentation.
- Implementation of standardized templates for common documentation tasks reduced the time needed for data entry.

EHR Alerts and Reminders:
- Implemented automated alerts and reminders for documentation deadlines.
- 70% of healthcare providers reported that the reminders had a positive impact on their documentation timeliness.

Documentation Champions:
- Appointed documentation champions in key departments to advocate for timely documentation.
- Champions reported a 40% reduction in documentation delays within their respective departments.

Measurement and Evaluation Data

Average Documentation Completion Time (After Interventions):
- After interventions, the average time taken to complete clinical documentation reduced to approximately 33 hours, a 30% improvement from the baseline.

Department Documentation Completion Time (After Interventions) [bar chart]

Survey Results (Post-Interventions):
- 90% of healthcare providers reported improved usability of the EHR system.
- 80% of healthcare providers noted reduced workload-related barriers to timely documentation.
- 65% of healthcare providers expressed satisfaction with the implementation of reminders and alerts.

Case Study

 Using the following criteria, critique the PI team presentation shown in figure 6.5.

Case Study Questions

1. Is the presentation pleasing to look at? Is the text easy to read?
2. Is the presentation set up logically?
3. Are the steps in the process clearly defined and communicated?
4. Does the presentation display data in an easily comprehended manner?
5. Does the presentation data support the team's implementation plan?
6. Are the team's recommendations based on the data the team collected? Are the recommendations sound?

Review Questions

1. Justify the value of storytelling in quality and performance improvement activities.
2. The CRAF method is used for recording PI team minutes. The acronym CRAF stands for what categories of information?
3. John was complaining to Sue about the quality council's requirement to create a digital presentation to display their PI team's latest project. Sue reminded John of the reasons why this task is necessary. Defend Sue's response and explain her reasons based on what you have learned about storytelling from the chapter.
4. LeeAnn experienced a fall in her home that required her to have a hip replacement. After her hospitalization it was determined that she would need rehabilitation services, and her family feels that she is unsafe living alone. LeeAnn's children would like to find the best nursing facility that would be able to provide rehabilitation services and then continued residential care. What is the most reliable resource LeeAnn's family could use to determine the best facility in their area?
   a. Consult neighbors to determine if they know of a good nursing facility.
   b. Access the information on the hospital compare website.
   c. Review an online report card that provides information on the nursing homes in their area.
   d. Call the local city government offices to ask about nursing homes in their area.
5. Explain why healthcare organizations must report the results of their PI activities to both internal and external entities.

References

Frei, F. X. and A. Morriss. 2023. Storytelling that drives bold change. *Harvard Business Review* 101(6):62–71.

Ishikawa, K. 1990. *Introduction to Quality Control*. Tokyo, Japan: 3A Corporation.

Medicare.gov. n.d. "Find and Compare Providers Near You." Accessed June 25, 2024. https://www.medicare.gov/care-compare/.

Resources

Masick, K. and E. Bouillon. 2020. *Storytelling with Data in Healthcare*. New York: Routledge.

Richards, D., K. Strain, L. Hawthornthwaite, I. Jordan, and C. Fancott. 2023. Storytelling at board meetings: a case study of co-developing recommendations. *Patient Experience Journal* 10(1): 173–180.

Robertson, C., G. Clegg, and J. Huntley, eds. 2023. *Storytelling in Medicine: How Narrative Can Improve Practice*, 2nd ed. Boca Raton, FL: CRC Press.

Williams, B. E., A. S. Williams, and K. M. Williams. 2021. Learning from others: A low-cost-high-impact risk/opportunity identification technique. *Journal of Healthcare Risk Management : The Journal of the American Society for Healthcare Risk Management* 40(3): 35–41.

PART II
Continuous Monitoring and Improvement Functions

Measuring Customer Satisfaction

7

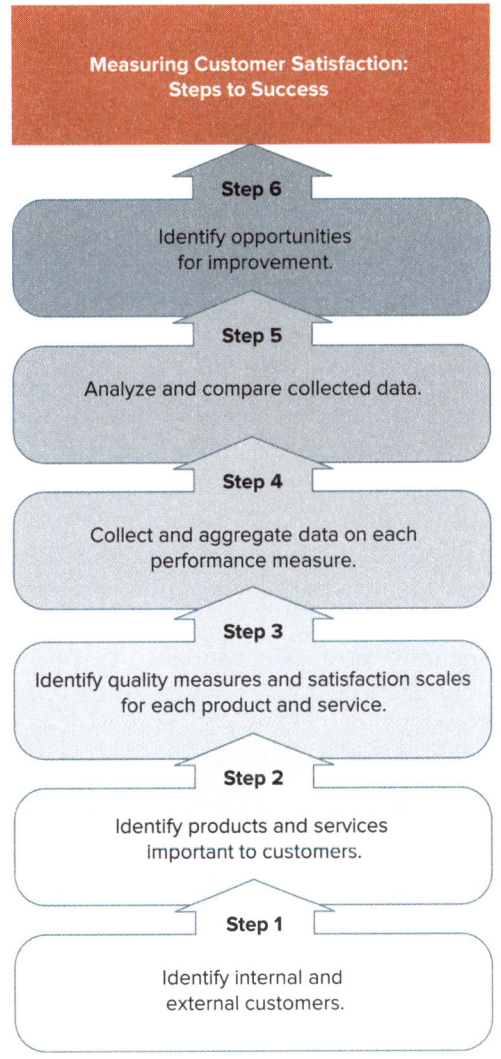

Learning Objectives

- Identify the differences between internal and external customers
- Explain why customers' perspectives are important to the performance improvement process
- Select the characteristics that make surveys and interviews effective
- Critique a survey or interview format

Key Terms

Customers
Direct observation
Expectations
External customers
Funneling
Institutional review board
Internal customers
Interviews
Operational definition
Survey tools

Researching and defining performance expectations includes an investigation of what the **customers** of an organizational process expect from that process. Because there are many types of organizational processes, there are also many types of customers. Their **expectations**, characteristics that customers want to be evident in a healthcare product, service, or outcome, must be identified and incorporated into the design or redesign of an effective process.

Customers receive a product or service as a result of an organizational process. Just as we can identify the customers of a clothing store or an auto dealership, we can also identify the customers of a healthcare process. For example, when a nurse inserts a catheter into an artery to administer medication, the patient is receiving a service from the nurse. When a pharmacist dispenses a medication to a patient, the patient is receiving a product from the pharmacist. The health information professional is a customer of the patient registrar because the health information professional relies on the patient registrar to collect accurate demographic information to properly identify the patient in the electronic health record (EHR) and assign the correct health record number.

Identifying the patient, client, or long-term care resident as a customer seems straightforward, but customers can be identified for all kinds of healthcare processes. The families and friends of patients are the customers of volunteer services when they ask for a patient's room number. Emergency department providers are the customers of central supply services when they request sterile suturing trays to close a patient's laceration. Surgeons are the customers of the pathology laboratory when they request frozen-section examination of tissue in the operating room during resection of a breast lesion.

Types of Customers

Customers can be placed in one of two categories: internal customers or external customers. Within the healthcare organization setting, **internal customers** are individuals within the organization who receive products or services from an organizational unit or department. In the preceding examples, surgeons are the internal customers of the pathology laboratory, and emergency department providers are the internal customers of central supply services.

External customers are individuals from outside the organization who receive products or services from within the organization. In the preceding examples, patients and their family members and friends are external customers. Other external customers may include regulatory agencies, accreditation bodies, payers, and public health agencies.

When determining the customers of a process, the organizational frame of reference must be taken into consideration. Sometimes the frame of reference modifies the customer type, as shown in figure 7.1.

Figure 7.1. Examples of the internal and external customers of a pathology laboratory

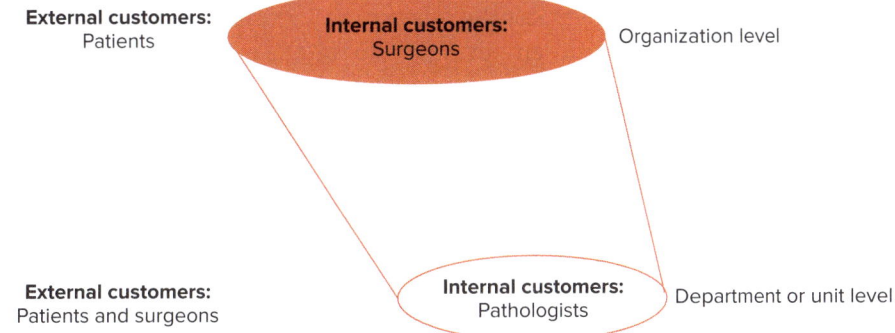

Figure 7.2 depicts an overhead view of the customers from figure 7.1. The large oval represents Western States University Hospital as a whole organization. Patients are external customers because their frame of reference comes totally from outside the organization. When considering the organization as a whole, surgeons are identified as internal customers because they are members of an organizational unit—the medical staff.

Figure 7.2. Organizational level: Patients as external customers and providers as internal customers of Western States University Hospital

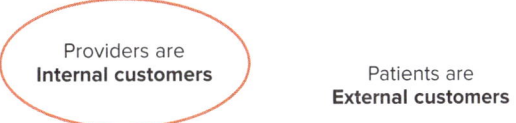

Context: Western States University Hospital as a whole organization

If the frame of reference is at the departmental level, as depicted in figure 7.3, surgeons would be identified as the external customers of pathology lab processes. The pathologists would be identified as the internal customers of the laboratory technicians who process the specimens.

Figure 7.3. Departmental level: Surgeons as external customers and pathologists as internal customers of Western States University Hospital's pathology laboratory

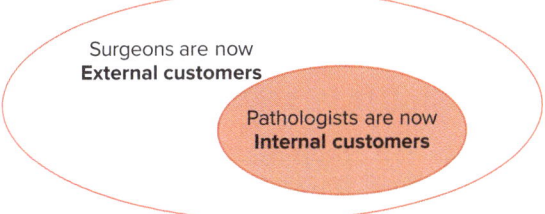

Context: Pathology services as a department of Western States University Hospital

It is important to recognize that internal and external customers must be identified in relation to the organizational process under consideration. Each process has a unique set of customers whose needs and expectations must be recognized.

The opinions of internal and external customers regarding the effectiveness of a healthcare process should be of primary importance to healthcare organizations. No one is a better judge of products and services than the customer. In addition, a dissatisfied customer is said to tell 10 times more people about a negative experience than the satisfied customer is to relate a positive experience.

There are several ways for an organization to obtain information about customer perceptions of its products and services. Organizations can ask internal customers for their feedback through a survey or informal conversations. Many internal customers never get the opportunity to express their expectations in a positive context. Often, the only time a department member hears about the expectations of internal customers is when a process has been mismanaged or has resulted in a negative outcome. Giving internal customers the opportunity to provide feedback increases their overall satisfaction. It would be important for the financial services department to provide feedback to the patient registration department on their customer expectations of the registration process. For example, the patient registration process is critical for accurate billing to occur. The registrar must capture the accurate patient type and payer information at the time of registration. In this example, the financial services (billing) is the internal customer of patient registration and expects accurate information to perform claims processing.

With external customers, particularly patients, identifying expectations about service quality is more complicated. Patients' expectations are multifaceted and often based on the condition for which the patient is being treated. Assessments of patient expectations must be undertaken judiciously.

Administrative subjects, such as parking, hours of operation, room decor, and so forth, can be assessed using an anonymous patient satisfaction survey. Clinical subject matter pertaining to the patient's condition and medical and nursing treatment may need to be assessed from the viewpoint of the clinicians involved in the patient's care and the outcomes achieved through that care.

Patient expectations about subjective topics, such as pain management, are completely different from one patient to the next. Another highly subjective area that influences patient satisfaction is the patient's return to an acceptable quality of life after treatment. Because patient expectations and results of treatment both vary based on the patient's condition and response to treatment, patients may have unrealistic expectations. For example, a patient undergoing physical therapy while recovering from a stroke may never be able to walk like they did prior to the stroke but can make progress toward achieving an acceptable gait. In this example, it would be important for providers to explain to the patient that this is the best possible outcome for them; by doing so, they are managing the patient's unrealistic expectation of a full recovery. One of the most important factors that influence patients' assessments of their care is how they are treated by caregivers and whether they feel that their concerns are addressed and their questions are answered.

Healthcare organizations collected data on patient satisfaction for many years, but there was a lack of standardization of this process. The Hospital Consumer Assessment of Healthcare Providers and Systems (HCAHPS) survey was initiated in 2006 to provide a consistent format and process for gathering patient satisfaction data and perspectives on hospital care. The HCAHPS survey has allowed valid comparisons to be made across hospitals locally, regionally, and nationally. This methodology has been expanded to include other healthcare settings and services. The HCAHPS survey includes three broad goals:

- Collect consistent data on patients' perspectives of their care that allow for comparison between hospitals
- Publicly report survey data to incentivize hospitals to improve their quality of care
- Enhance accountability for care provided (HCAHPS 2023a).

Although the HCAHPS survey consists of a core set of questions, hospitals may also add customized questions to reflect their organization and services lines. These additional questions are not publicly reported, but hospitals can use the additional data to support improvements in internal customer service and quality-related activities.

HCAHPS provides an approved vendor list of companies that assist healthcare organizations in completing their patient satisfaction surveys. (See table 7.1.) Most of these surveys also provide organizations with important benchmarking feedback, which measures their customers' satisfaction against that of similar organizations.

Table 7.1. Sample vendors of patient satisfaction surveys

Vendor Name/Contact Information	Product Description
Press Ganey Associates, Inc. http://www.pressganey.com	Specializes in patient satisfaction measurement Produces reports that detail hospital-wide performance and compare individual units, noting satisfaction trends and national benchmarking statistics for HCAHPS compliance Offers online access to completed surveys Produces special reports that contain detailed demographic analyses of individual hospital data and national comparative data
Sullivan Luallin Group http://www.sullivanluallingroup.com	Produces standard and customized patient satisfaction surveys Produces web-based surveys of internal physicians, managers, and staff members Produces patient assessments to provide feedback from the patient's view Provides coaching consultations for human resources improvement
Professional Research Consultants, Inc. http://www.prcexcellence.com	Uses proven methodology for patient satisfaction assessment Incorporates patient satisfaction and expectation assessments with outcomes research Provides statistically valid measurement of perceptions of "quality" with open-ended response capabilities

Source: Adapted from HCAHPS 2023b.

Check Your Understanding 7.1

1. The patient registration department has developed a performance improvement (PI) team to investigate a recent increase in registration errors. These errors can have an impact on the health record number assignment and insurance billing issues. As this team developed their list of all of the customers of the registration process, the health information management (HIM) department was identified as a customer. Whichat type of customer is the health information professional?
   a. External customer
   b. Experienced customer
   c. Internal customer
   d. Investment customer

2. The next step in the PI process for the patient registration PI team is to identify customer expectations for each of their customers of the registration process. List some possible customer expectations of the HI department regarding the registration process performed by the patient registration department.

3. How are HCAHPS surveys used to ensure the performance of hospitals?
   a. To assess patient satisfaction and gather feedback on various aspects of the hospital experience
   b. Solely for marketing purposes to attract new patients
   c. To track the financial performance of the hospital
   d. Only as a benchmark for comparing hospitals in the region

Monitoring and Improving Customer Satisfaction: Steps to Success

To monitor and improve customer satisfaction, an organization must know the following:

- Exactly who its customers are
- What its customers want and value
- What improvements could be made to better meet customer needs

Step 1: Identify Internal and External Customers

Assessing whether a process meets customer expectations is difficult when some customers have not yet been identified. To identify customers, the PI team should list everyone who takes away a product or a service from the process. (See figure 7.4.)

Figure 7.4. Monitoring and improving customer satisfaction

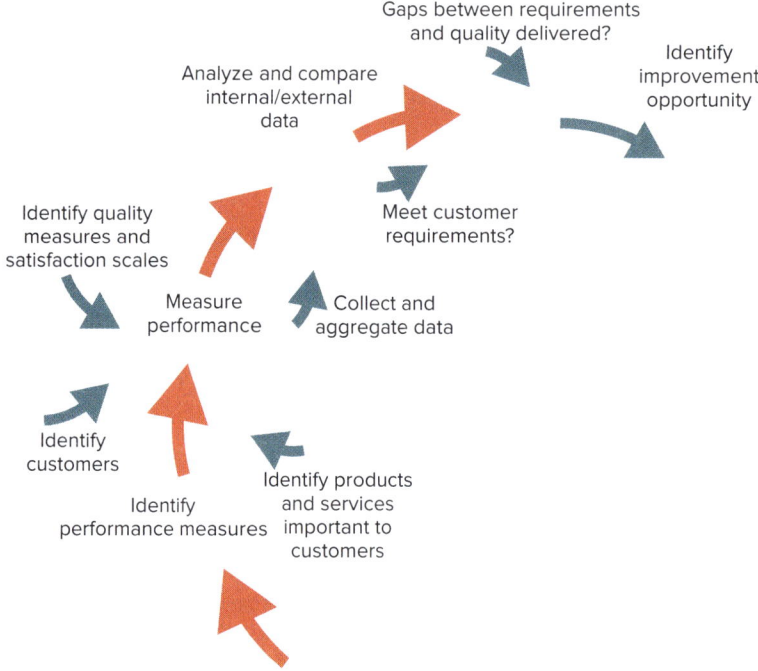

Step 2: Identify Products and Services Important to Customers

The PI team should develop a list of the products and services used by internal and external customers. However, not every product is tangible—it is not always seen and evaluated as an object in the environment, such as facilities, equipment, and supplies. Intangible products include things such as information collected in a database. This information may be used by many customers but would rarely be printed out on paper (a tangible form). Services are actions taken by organization staff to assist, care for, or do work for someone.

Outcomes of care are not necessarily tangible, either. To report outcomes of care, the recipient of the care service needs some established means of describing the outcome, or clinical staff may have to use healthcare monitoring instruments to determine improvements in the patient's condition. For example, heart monitoring equipment might need to be used to determine whether a drug has had the appropriate effect on a patient's arrhythmia.

Another aspect of quality that customers may emphasize in their evaluations of healthcare performance is reliability. *Reliability* in this context is the level at which an organization can provide an offered product or service when requested and as advertised. For example, a hospital may advertise that patients visiting its emergency department will be seen by a staff member within 15 minutes. To be deemed reliable by customers, that 15-minute goal must be met when they come to the emergency department.

Responsiveness refers to how an organization's staff responds to unanticipated service needs. This includes staff willingness to continuously monitor both the patient's condition and their satisfaction with services. Caregivers must be responsive when patients request help and provide services in a timely manner. For example, a patient needing assistance to get to the bathroom or use a bedpan will perceive the caregiver's responsiveness to be high if the call button is answered quickly.

The healthcare PI term *assurance* describes the knowledge and courtesy of the staff members who provide the goods and services. This aspect of care quality generates customer trust and confidence in both the individuals providing the products and services and the products and services themselves. For example, when a patient selects a provider, assurance is a key consideration. If new patients do not trust the provider's judgment, they will probably question the outcome of all visits or find another provider.

Empathy can be defined in this context as the staff's willingness to relate to customers as fellow human beings who have feelings and emotions. This can be a particularly important aspect in healthcare settings because when people are ill, they frequently have emotional reactions to the illness. When major illness strikes, or when fragile individuals such as children or older adults are involved, the emotional response can be intense. Healthcare customers expect staff and providers to understand these kinds of feelings and help them cope with trying situations.

Features are the aspects of healthcare services that distinguish one organization from another or that add particular value in the customer's evaluation of an organization. For example, an organization may have a track record of providing exceptionally successful heart disease treatment with few negative outcomes while employing the latest in diagnostic imaging and therapeutic modalities. Another example is a facility that has upgraded its services by adding a number of new birthing centers.

Finally, *perceived quality* is another important aspect of healthcare service. This consists of the organization's reputation for the quality of its products and services and the consumer reaction to these products and services based on their experiences with the organization.

It may or may not be important to look at the quality of a healthcare product or service from all of these aspects. In the process of planning the PI activities for a period of time, leadership must be willing to prioritize the impact of the possible projects on the organization's performance, the number and scope of projects that realistically can be undertaken given available resources, and the necessity of making the improvement at this particular time. Once a process or service is identified for improvement, the PI team must determine which aspects are relevant to the process or service under examination and then complete the cycle of measurement and improvement regarding each aspect.

Step 3: Identify Quality Measures and Satisfaction Scales for Each Product and Service

For each quality aspect of a product or service, performance measures must be identified. For example, if a PI team was assessing a patient's experience at a provider's office for a medical appointment, waiting time would be a relevant performance measure. After the team identified waiting time as a performance measure, the team would need to develop a satisfaction scale. The PI team would need to decide whether to measure waiting time in minutes or hours.

The HCAHPS survey can be used by organizations to identify their performance on quality measures and their level of patient satisfaction. The HCAHPS questionnaire is provided to a sample of discharged hospital patients. Vendors aggregate and analyze results of completed surveys. The vendor then reports the results to the Centers for Medicare and Medicaid Services (CMS). The following is a list of topics that this survey addresses:

- Quality of interactions with nurses in terms of courtesy and respect
- Quality of nurses' ability to listen to the patient
- Ability of nurses to explain relevant aspects of care to the patient
- Call button response times and attitudes
- Quality of interactions with providers in terms of courtesy and respect
- Quality of providers' ability to listen to the patient
- Ability of providers to explain relevant aspects of care to the patient
- Cleanliness and quietness of the care environment

- Quality of assistance with ambulation and elimination activities
- Education of patient about medications administered in hospital
- Planning for postdischarge assistance and continuing care
- Overall rating of the hospital (HCAHPS 2023c)

Step 4: Collect and Aggregate Data on Each Performance Measure

Next, the PI team should determine the best methods for collecting data on each performance measure being assessed. In assessments of customer satisfaction, the principal methods of data collection are survey tools, interviews, and direct observation:

- A **survey tool** is a research instrument used to gather data and information from respondents in a uniform manner through the administration of a predefined and structured set of questions and possible responses. The construction of an effective survey tool requires a significant investment of time.

- **Interviews** consist of a series of open-ended questions, which are posed to individuals in person or by telephone, to collect information about their experiences with the organization or unit. It is easier to aggregate data from a survey than information from an interview because surveys are usually composed of structured responses. By contrast, the responses to interview questions must be analyzed to identify common themes and perceptions.

- **Direct observation** is a data collection method in which the researchers conduct the observation themselves, spending time in the environment they are observing and recording these observations (Fix et al. 2022).

The healthcare organization's **institutional review board** (IRB) should preapprove the use of any data-gathering tool. IRB approval is mandated by federal regulations on the use of human subjects in biomedical and health services research. Although policies and procedures vary across organizations, PI teams using such data-gathering methodologies should recognize their responsibility to obtain IRB approval to maintain the highest research standards respecting their human subjects even when the IRB committee may deem the investigation or study to be exempt.

If the organization has no IRB, then either the quality council or the committee involved in the approval of PI projects should review the use of all tools. A statement such as "Your completion and return of this survey implies your consent to use your feedback for quality improvement purposes" should be prominent in the survey introduction to inform respondents that their responses will be used individually and collectively. If patient or client responses will be identified as specifically belonging to them by name or associated with information gathered from their health records, organizations may want to include approval from privacy officers or privacy boards to ensure compliance with current privacy laws and regulations.

Step 5: Analyze and Compare Collected Data

The PI committee should compare aggregate satisfaction ratings on performance measures with previous trends within the organization or with satisfaction levels achieved by other organizations. Such comparisons may be conducted using patient satisfaction data collected within the enterprise or satisfaction ratings published by state departments of health, national accreditation agencies, or other national organizations specializing in healthcare quality assessment. The HCAHPS survey is released to the public domain, making it available for use by hospitals and others. HCAHPS and its benchmarking database can be accessed on its website (see the Resources list at the end of this chapter) or via the Medicare.gov/care-compare website. (The vendors of patient satisfaction surveys listed in table 7.1 can also provide national data.) An organization's published performance data based on national or regional benchmarking criteria are often referred to as a "report card," providing the public with information on the quality of care provided by the organization.

Step 6: Identify Opportunities for Improvement

Finally, the committee should develop a list of areas that need improvement based on its comparisons with aggregate satisfaction ratings on quality measures. PI teams should be implemented to define appropriate performance expectations and design or redesign processes.

Check Your Understanding 7.2

1. Community Hospital advertises that all patients will receive phlebotomy services in their laboratory within 20 minutes or less. The hospital collected data over the past year and determined that they were meeting this expectation 96 percent of the time. In this situation, which aspect of quality is Community Hospital meeting?
   a. Responsiveness
   b. Reliability
   c. Assurance
   d. Empathy

2. A PI team wants to collect data from its customers in a uniform manner so the data can be tabulated easily. Some members suggest that the team should interview these customers to get at the heart of the issues quicker. Madison counters this suggestion because she feels that they will get more variations in their answers using this data collection format. Which data collection tool should the PI team use instead of interviews to collect their data using a predefined and structured set of questions?
   a. Interview
   b. Process measure
   c. QI toolbox
   d. Survey tool

QI Toolbox Techniques

Surveys and interviews are two data collection techniques commonly used to measure customer satisfaction. As mentioned earlier in this chapter, direct observation of behavior can be used as well, but behavior is difficult to analyze because it often changes when people realize that they are being observed. However, all three methods can be used to measure outcomes and processes. A discussion of some design considerations for surveys and interviews follows.

Survey Design

Surveys may be administered in many formats and via communication methods that include mailed paper surveys, telephone surveys, and emailed or text-message electronic surveys. The administration method will vary based on organizational preference, the survey vendor, and available tools.

When designing a survey, the PI team must define the goal of the survey in clear and precise terms, keeping the purpose and audience of the survey in mind. The team must carefully consider the questions asked on the survey and must have a reason to include every item. It should avoid asking for information that is interesting but not necessary for measuring process capabilities.

Survey items should be arranged from general to specific in an effort to engage the respondent in the survey process. General questions that are easily answered are an effective way to begin the survey. For example, demographic data should be followed by process-specific questions. It is helpful to identify the broad categories of necessary information and then determine their order. After the survey respondent has been asked general questions about the subject and has developed a comfort level with the survey subject, the survey questions can then move into more emotionally charged or sensitive information questions. For example, if providers are surveyed about the quality of the EHR system, the first question should not ask whether they are happy with the EHR system. The initial questions should ask how much they use the system, what types of applications they use, and so on. The next set of questions can be used to determine their level of satisfaction with the system.

After the team has determined the broad categories of information it needs, it should think about individual questions or items. Item format and content should be consistent throughout the survey to ensure clarity. Format similar questions in the same way, and use the simplest sentence structure possible to facilitate reliable responses. In addition, using a response format such as a single blank line or check box prior to the possible responses streamlines the appearance of the survey for respondents. (See figure 7.5.)

Figure 7.5. Example of inconsistent and consistent survey question format

Inconsistent Format	Consistent Format
What is your ZIP code? _____	Check which ZIP code you live in:
	___ 84065
Sex (circle one): Male Female	___ 84070
	___ 84092
	___ 84094
	___ Other (specify): _____
	What is your sex?
	___ Male
	___ Female

The survey should be written at the reading level of the respondents. Generally, surveys intended for public distribution would be written to the average reading level. The average reader in the US reads at the sixth-grade level, so vocabulary should be simple, rather than sophisticated medical or technical terminology that the average person would not understand. Surveys intended for providers would be written at a higher reading level. In addition, sensitivity to diverse patient mix should be considered when developing any survey instruments. Furthermore, the items should be written in an objective manner so that they do not imply that any particular response is either desired or correct. Figure 7.6 provides an example of poor wording; medical terms are used for healthcare services rather than simple statements that the respondent would understand. Figure 7.6 also provides an example of simpler wording that is appropriate for the general public.

Figure 7.6. Example of poor wording and appropriate wording of survey items

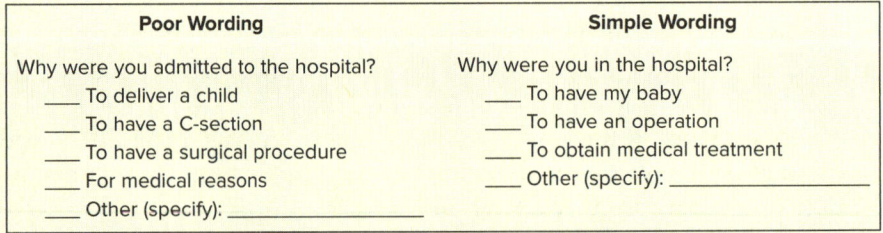

Poor Wording	Simple Wording
Why were you admitted to the hospital?	Why were you in the hospital?
___ To deliver a child	___ To have my baby
___ To have a C-section	___ To have an operation
___ To have a surgical procedure	___ To obtain medical treatment
___ For medical reasons	___ Other (specify): _____
___ Other (specify): _____	

Surveys may incorporate a variety of question types. Open-ended questions allow respondents to construct an answer in their own words that may qualify their responses in a more detailed format. However, responses to open-ended questions are difficult to score, and response data are difficult to aggregate because there is no defined scale of responses. Therefore, responses may show no clear connection or pattern.

Open-ended questions should be used only at the end of the survey, and they should not be used to elicit information that could be more easily collected in a structured format. (See figure 7.7.) Placing open-ended questions at the beginning of a survey may discourage respondents from participating in the survey. If open-ended questions are placed after short-answer or structured-format questions, respondents may be more invested in the survey and complete the open-ended questions. When the researcher wants specific information about a particular area of investigation, the items must be worded precisely so that comparable data can be collected.

Figure 7.7. Example of an open-ended question and a more structured question

Open-Ended Question	More Structured Question
How has your coronary artery disease affected your lifestyle?	Now that you have heart disease, are you exercising: ____ More than before ____ Same as before ____ Less than before ____ Not at all, before or now

The use of structured questions on a survey limits the number of possible responses and thus standardizes the data collected. Care should be taken to include all possible responses to each question. Respondents must be able to select their answers from the choices provided. One method of ensuring this is to include a choice of "Other (specify)" so that respondents can record an answer when the desired answer is not among the choices offered. Even then, it is important in survey construction to provide all of the possible answers to minimize the number of free-text responses. When items include categories of responses, the categories must be mutually exclusive, meaning that categories should not overlap. (See figure 7.8.)

Figure 7.8. Example of overlapping (poor) and distinct (good) response choices

Poor Question Construction	Good Question Construction
What is your present age? ____ 0–17 ____ 17–35 ____ 35–45 ____ 45–60 ____ 60–75	What is your present age? ____ 20 or younger ____ 21–30 ____ 31–40 ____ 41–50 ____ 51–60 ____ 61–70 ____ 71 or older

Another important issue in survey design involves the use of words and phrases that are known to both the PI team and the respondent. Careful word choice reduces ambiguity and can improve data collection. This clarity of terminology is called an **operational definition** (Vogt 2007, 114). (See figure 7.9.)

Figure 7.9. Example of unclear and clear terminology

Unclear Terminology	Clear Terminology
Have you received treatment in the ambulatory surgery unit? ____ Yes ____ No ____ Don't know	Have you had surgery at this hospital for which you came to the hospital in the morning and left after surgery in the afternoon or evening? ____ Yes ____ No

Interview Design

Interviews can provide important insight into quality issues in healthcare. Interviews may be unstructured or structured. In an unstructured interview, the sequence of questions is not planned in advance. Instead, the interview is conducted in a friendly, conversational manner. This type of interview is helpful when the interviewer is trying to uncover preliminary problems that may need in-depth analysis and investigation.

By contrast, a predetermined list of questions is used in a structured interview. The team knows exactly what information is needed, and the interviewer must know and understand the purpose and goal of each question so that a meaningful response can be recognized.

During the interview process, the interviewer must establish rapport with the respondent. Without this trust, respondents may not reveal their true opinions. Some techniques to keep in mind during the interview process include funneling, using unbiased questions, and clarifying responses.

Funneling is the process of moving questions from a broad theme to a narrow theme in an unstructured interview. This technique helps the interviewer establish trust with the respondent and address the pertinent quality issues. For example, if a supervisor in central supply wanted to discuss service to the emergency department with the nursing coordinator from that unit, the following series of questions might be used. The questions become more specific as the interview proceeds:

Question: Overall, how do you rate our service to the department?
Response: In general, I think your department is doing a better-than-average job.
Question: A better-than-average job? Where have you experienced problems?
Response: There have been problems at times getting cath packs when we need them.
Question: Cath packs. Any particular shift?
Response: Definitely in the late afternoons of the day shift.

The interviewer must state each question in a clear and somewhat benign manner so that bias is not introduced. If a specific word or phrase were overemphasized, it might elicit a different response than if all the words were spoken in the same tone. The interviewer should restate each response for clarification. This ensures the correct interpretation of each response.

Sometimes the interviewer may choose to use closed-ended questions, with all of the possible responses specified. In such cases, the interviewer must examine each question carefully to ensure that the wording and delivery do not bias the response. Similar to the survey formatting discussed earlier in this section, questions should begin with broader issues and work toward more specific areas of concern to garner greater participation by the interviewee.

Check Your Understanding 7.3

1. Bob is collecting information from patients about their experience with the reception staff at Dr. Reddy's office. Bob calls each patient and asks questions in no particular order in a friendly, conversational manner. Which type of interview is Bob conducting?
   a. Structured interview
   b. Unstructured interview
   c. Planned interview
   d. Unplanned interview

2. Gabriella has a developed a survey to assess the employee satisfaction of the cafeteria. Which following would be the most appropriate question to start this survey?
   a. How likely are to use cafeteria during your shift?
   b. How often do you feel the food quality is less than par when you use the cafeteria?
   c. When you use the cafeteria is it always clean and neat?
   d. Is the cafeteria staff always pleasant and friendly when you use the cafeteria?

Real-Life Example

The director of quality and service excellence for a large US healthcare organization is working with one of the organization's smaller facilities, an acute-care hospital with 80 beds. She created a patient satisfaction survey to evaluate the food service quality at the facility. The survey was to be emailed to patients after they were discharged from the hospital.

One part of the survey asked for patient feedback on inpatient food services, including the following items:

- Taste of the food
- Temperature of the food
- Appearance of the food
- Variety of menu items
- Overall satisfaction with the food

The quality of food services was rated on a five-point scale, ranging from "very satisfied" to "very dissatisfied."

After administering the survey for several months, it was noted that only 10 percent to 30 percent of patient ratings of food services fell within the "very satisfied" category.

The percentage of responses in the "very satisfied" category was considered a reflection of the loyalty of a facility's customers. Customers who ranked food service as less than "very satisfied" may or may not return to the facility for care in the future. In a highly competitive environment, developing market loyalty is extremely important to the survival of a facility.

Historically, institutional food does not get rave reviews. Upon review of the literature for institutional nutrition services, the investigators found that the research noted that assessment of food quality is highly subjective. Everyone has their own ideas about what is high quality. The fact that the respondents are hospitalized further complicates the assessment because illnesses and medications often significantly affect taste sensation. Institutional food services have traditionally received lower satisfaction ratings compared to other hospital departments. Yet, despite this precedent, administration and management of the food services department decided to see if they could improve ratings in this area.

Using PI methodology, the PI team developed an entirely new approach to menu selection for inpatients. The team focused on lunch and dinner, leaving breakfast as it was, providing the usual standard breakfast items. The directors had read about a few hospitals that use a method similar to hotel room service. They contacted a hospital that had implemented such a program and invited the staff to give a presentation about the pros and cons of the program. Following the presentation, the team did additional research to locate other facilities that used the system and identified the system's successes and challenges. It became apparent that every facility needed its own process for designing this service. The service features needed to be based on the specific organization's patient population, staffing, equipment, and financial resources. The pilot hospital assembled a multidisciplinary team to identify possible issues that could arise with such a change. The food services team needed the support of the administration, staff, ancillary staff, and especially nursing.

The program was implemented as planned. Patients on regular diets had a three-and-a-half-hour window during which they could order from a menu similar to a hotel room-service menu. Patients on therapeutic diets were visited by the dietitian, who helped them develop appropriate diets for their medical conditions.

Over the following months, the ratio of "very satisfied" ratings increased from 10 percent to 30 percent to more than 50 percent. The ratio of ratings in the "satisfied" and "very satisfied" responses rose to more than 80 percent. Annual projected costs in food services decreased thanks to a decrease in the amount of wasted food. Patients could now eat what they wanted, when they wanted it, and they were more likely to eat all of it.

Long term, the system has worked extremely well. Food services staff members who were initially skeptical would not go back to the old way of doing things. Patient satisfaction scores have remained high. There is less food waste, and the nursing staff keeps all liquid diet products on the units so that patients have access to them whenever they want them. Nursing staff also knows when patients are moving from a liquid diet to a solid diet, and they can help their patients order appropriate food.

The food services department at the hospital has become a revenue-generating unit because the room-service menu has been expanded to serve visitors. Families are thrilled to be able to have meals with the patients, and they are willing to pay for the meals. This service has recently been expanded to the hospital staff. The hospital cafeteria is closed on weekends, and the staff can call for room service at any time. They love it, and the program has improved employee satisfaction as well.

A copy of a patient satisfaction survey is provided in figure 7.10.

Figure 7.10A. Example of a patient satisfaction survey

Patient Satisfaction Survey

Answer only the questions that apply to your stay in the hospital.

Select one of the responses provided for the following questions.

1. Was this the first time you came to this hospital for inpatient care?
   ○ Yes   ○ No
2. Would you recommend this hospital to a friend or family member who needed inpatient care?
   ○ Yes   ○ No
3. Where were you admitted into the hospital?
   ○ Registration Area   ○ Emergency Department   ○ Other
4. How long did you wait before you were taken to your room?
   ○ Less than 20 minutes   ○ 21 to 30 minutes   ○ 31 to 60 minutes   ○ More than 1 hour
5. Did you have surgery while you were hospitalized?
   ○ Yes   ○ No
6. Were you in an intensive care unit at any time during your stay?
   ○ Yes   ○ No

7. Courtesy and friendliness of the registration staff   ○ ○ ○ ○ ○
8. How well the registration staff answered your questions   ○ ○ ○ ○ ○
9. Amount of time needed to complete the registration process   ○ ○ ○ ○ ○
10. Overall satisfaction with registration procedures   ○ ○ ○ ○ ○

Nursing Staff

11. Caring and concern of the nurses who cared for you   ○ ○ ○ ○ ○
12. Skill of the nurses who cared for you   ○ ○ ○ ○ ○
13. Time it took for nurses to respond to your calls   ○ ○ ○ ○ ○
14. Willingness of your nurses to listen to your concerns   ○ ○ ○ ○ ○
15. Amount of time your nurses spent with you   ○ ○ ○ ○ ○
16. Overall satisfaction with nursing staff   ○ ○ ○ ○ ○

Figure 7.10B. Example of a patient satisfaction survey (*Continued*)

Medical Staff	Very Dissatisfied	Somewhat Dissatisfied	Neutral	Somewhat Satisfied	Very Satisfied
17. Caring and concern of the doctors who cared for you	○	○	○	○	○
18. Availability of your doctors	○	○	○	○	○
19. Ways your doctors worked together and with your nurses	○	○	○	○	○
20. Information your doctors provided about your condition	○	○	○	○	○
21. Amount of time your doctors spent with you	○	○	○	○	○
22. Overall satisfaction with medical staff	○	○	○	○	○
Housekeeping Services					
23. Cleanliness of your room	○	○	○	○	○
24. Overall cleanliness of the hospital	○	○	○	○	○
25. Overall satisfaction with housekeeping services	○	○	○	○	○
Food Services					
26. Taste of the food	○	○	○	○	○
27. Temperature of the food	○	○	○	○	○
28. Appearance of the food	○	○	○	○	○
29. Variety of menu items	○	○	○	○	○
30. Overall satisfaction with food services	○	○	○	○	○
Other Hospital Services					
31. Overall satisfaction with x-ray services	○	○	○	○	○
32. Overall satisfaction with respiratory therapy services	○	○	○	○	○
33. Overall satisfaction with rehabilitation services	○	○	○	○	○
34. Overall satisfaction with emergency department services	○	○	○	○	○
35. Overall satisfaction with the care and services you received	○	○	○	○	○

36. What did we do really well? (Please be specific.) _____
_____
_____

37. What do we need to improve? (Please be specific.) _____
_____
_____

REMEMBER: ALL OF YOUR RESPONSES ARE CONFIDENTIAL.
THANK YOU FOR PARTICIPATING.

Case Study

Using the http://medicare.gov/care-compare website, select "nursing homes including rehab services" to compare three nursing homes in your area. Select the three nursing homes you want to compare. Once the data is populated, select two data points from each section (overview, health inspections, staffing, quality measures, fire safety inspections and emergency preparedness, and penalties), and create a report on your findings that would inform a consumer about the overall quality of these three nursing homes. This report should be detailed enough to allow the consumer to make an informed choice between the three facilities.

Review Questions

1. Dr. Gallegos is filing for board certification in gastroenterology and has requested a report of all of the endoscopic procedures she performed last year from the health information (HI) department manager. Is Dr. Gallegos considered a customer of the HI department? If so, is she an internal or external customer? Explain your reasoning.

2. An important strategy in survey design involves the use of terms, phrases, and words that are known to both the PI team and respondents. This clarity of terminology is called _____.
   a. assurance
   b. responsiveness
   c. operational definition
   d. direct observation

3. The three broad goals of the HCAHPS survey are: (1) to collect consistent data on patients' perspectives of their care that allow for comparison between hospitals, (2) to publicly report survey data to incentivize hospitals to improve their quality of care, and (3) to enhance accountability for care provided. A department director was complaining about the time it takes to review and analyze the results of the HCAHPS survey, and questioning the value to the organization. Construct a defense for how and why the organization can benefit from participating in the HCAHPS survey and what the organization can learn from the results of the survey.

4. Joan is choosing to have her surgery at University Hospital over the other options in her area. Joan makes this choice because of the hospital's reputation and past patient experiences of her family and friends. The aspect of quality that this example illustrates is:
   a. Reliability
   b. Assurance
   c. Features
   d. Perceived quality

5. Which of the following are considered external customers of a hospital?
   a. Hospital administrators and staff
   b. Clinical and nonclinical departments within the hospital
   c. Healthcare providers within the hospital
   d. Insurance companies providing coverage

References

Fix G.M., B. Kim, M. Ruben, and M.B. McCullough. 2022. Direct observation methods: A practical guide for health researchers. *PEC Innovation* 1:100036, https://doi.org/10.1016/j.pecinn.2022.100036. PMID: 36406296; PMCID: PMC9670254.

HCAHPS (Hospital Consumer Assessment of Healthcare Providers and Systems). 2023a. "HCAHPS Background." https://www.hcahpsonline.org/#Background.

HCAHPS (Hospital Consumer Assessment of Healthcare Providers and Systems). 2023b. "HCAHPS Approved Survey Vendors as July 6, 2023." https://www.hcahpsonline.org/en/approved-vendor-list/.

HCAHPS (Hospital Consumer Assessment of Healthcare Providers and Systems). 2023c. "HCAHPS Survey." https://www.hcahpsonline.org/en/survey-instruments/.

Vogt, W. P. 2007. *Quantitative Research Methods for Professionals*. Boston: Pearson.

Resources

AHRQ (Agency for Healthcare Research and Quality). n.d. "CAHPS Hospital Survey." Accessed December 13, 2023.

Medicare.gov. n.d. "Find & Compare Providers Near You." Accessed December 13, 2023. https://www.medicare.gov/care-compare/.

Refining the Continuum of Care

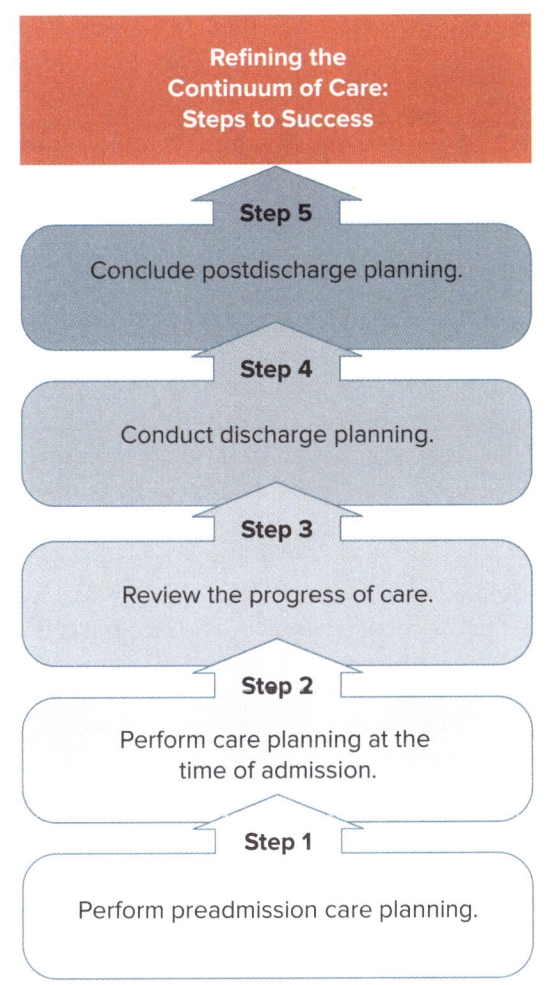

Learning Objectives

- Analyze how processes are used to optimize the continuum of care
- Plan for a balanced continuum of care in a community healthcare setting
- Identify the steps in the case management function
- Compare the steps in the case management function
- Assess how paying for value has influenced quality of care in the US healthcare system

Key Terms

Case management
Continuum of care
Critical pathway
Gantt chart
Indicator
Intensity of service
Ratio
Severity of illness
Utilization review (UR)

American consumers are demanding more extensive and complete healthcare services in the hope of improving the quality and longevity of their lives. Third-party payers, both private and governmental, are trying to ensure profits, minimize costs, and address healthcare fraud. Public and private purchasers, such as businesses buying health insurance for their employees, are looking for comprehensive coverage at affordable premium rates.

The mission of healthcare organizations is to make a positive contribution to the health of their communities by providing safe, cost-effective, and ethical treatment. The increasing nature of litigation in healthcare, coupled with the increased cost of malpractice insurance, places an additional financial burden on healthcare organizations. In the US, these conflicting objectives and values have led to a variety of attempts to control the healthcare market, none of which has been entirely successful. PI monitoring of the utilization of healthcare services began in many facilities when efforts to control costs and ensure quality were initiated.

The goal of this chapter is to provide a basic understanding of the US healthcare system's history, successes, and failures to enhance understanding of the issues surrounding the concept of the continuum of care. **Continuum of care** can be defined as the totality of healthcare services provided to a patient and their family in all settings, from the least to the most extensive. The emphasis is on treating individual patients at the level of care required by their course of treatment. Figure 8.1 shows various types of treatment settings available along the continuum of care.

Figure 8.1. The continuum of care

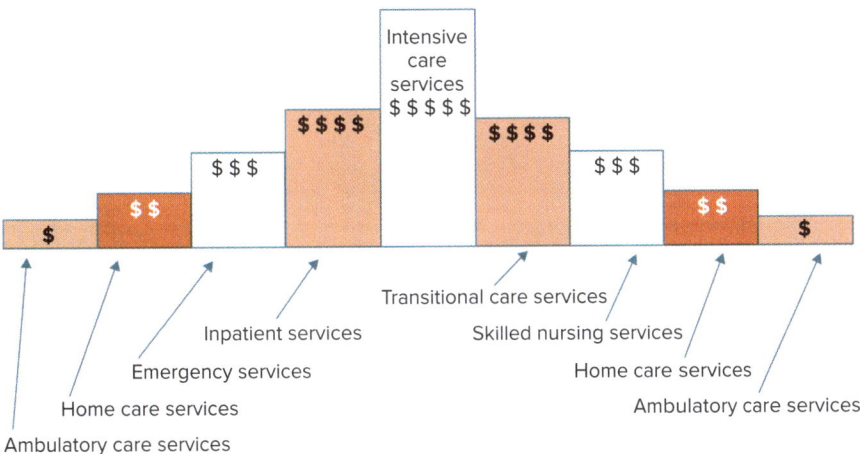

Healthcare in the US

In discussions of healthcare in the US, there are many typical viewpoints on topics including public and private regulation, healthcare economics, and the human desire to benefit personally and collectively.

Over time, attempts have been made to balance the competing needs and expectations of consumers, providers, and payers. At different times, each group has dominated the marketplace, though none has been on top for long. The products of this competition have included health services organizations, advanced technology, private health insurance plans, the broadest range of the most effective pharmaceuticals available, government payers, preferred provider arrangements, and health maintenance organizations.

While learning about healthcare quality and performance improvement (PI), it is also important to review the economic and policy issues inherent in US approaches to delivering healthcare.

The overall goal of the US healthcare system is to achieve equilibrium between health and spending, as illustrated in figure 8.2. As the figure shows, a finite level of optimal collective health can be realized in US society. Although many factors influence collective health, the system today seeks to identify the optimal level of spending that will achieve the optimal level of collective health. Expenditures are funded by a combination of public and private resources, including public health agencies, Medicare, Medicaid, insurance, and private payers. But there comes a point where more spending does not mean more collective health.

In figure 8.2, the shaded triangle that represents total spending extends above the line that represents optimal health. This representation acknowledges the realization that all the healthcare spending a society could possibly do would not necessarily achieve the goal of optimal collective health. At some point for every patient within the healthcare system, no additional health benefit would be achieved by further spending. Any additional expenditure would, in effect, be wasted. The money could have been used for another patient who might still have benefited. Because millions of Americans never approach the optimal health condition, that waste is considered intolerable. The continuum of care system seeks to provide benefits up to the point of optimal health for each individual, thereby realizing optimal health collectively.

Figure 8.2. Optimal spending for optimal health

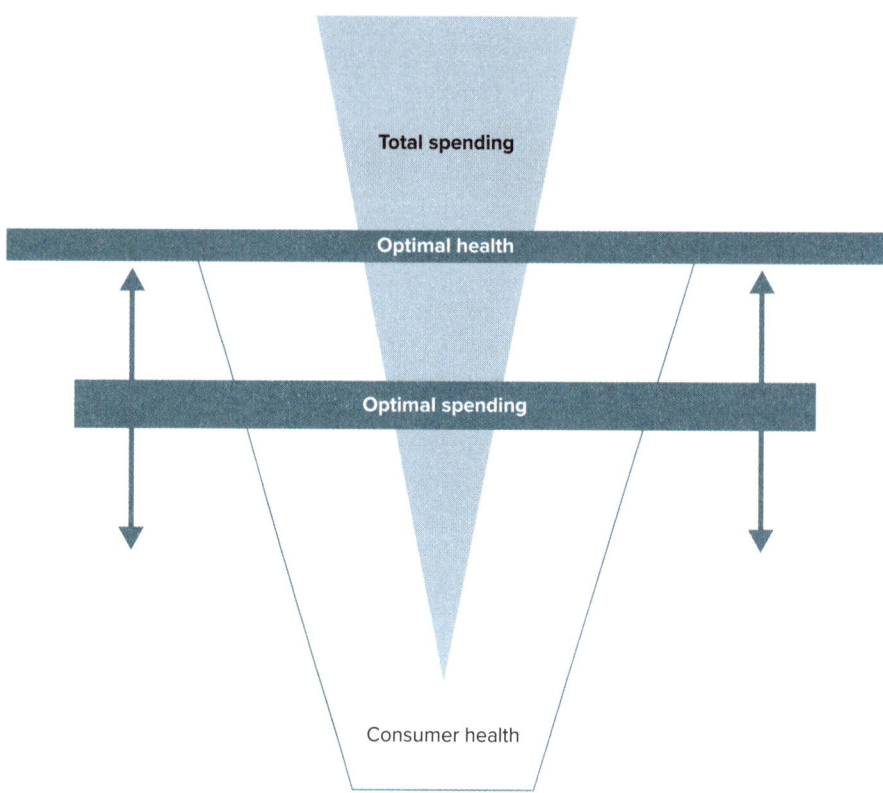

For example, Mr. Carl Goldberg is an 80-year-old white male who has, in recent years, developed a heart condition known as chronic ventricular fibrillation. The condition is manageable with medication, but patients often continue to experience occasional periods of the arrhythmia (irregular heart rhythm) even when taking their medication as prescribed. Mr. Goldberg experiences such arrhythmias. Each time the fibrillation begins, he feels weak and unwell, his face flushes, and he can feel his heart fluttering in his chest. He is afraid that he is going to die. Immediately, he calls to his wife to take him to the emergency department of his local hospital. By the time the couple drives to the hospital and Mr. Goldberg is checked by a provider, the fibrillation has subsided, and his heart has returned to a normal sinus rhythm. The emergency department provider on duty examines him, performs an EKG, and draws blood for analysis, The results indicate no cardiac event has occurred. Each time the arrhythmia occurs, the symptoms could be those of a heart attack, but they are not. Mr. Goldberg should contact his provider at the recurrence of his symptoms for direction and advice before going to the emergency department. Additionally, chronic disease management has evolved to include home monitoring of conditions in an effort to treat at the lowest cost source. This home tracking might include a monitoring device to record his heart rate.

This patient's visits to the emergency department accomplish nothing, but no one is prepared to tell him not to go when he experiences arrhythmias, especially in light of the litigious nature of US society. Yet emergency visits are among the most expensive types of ambulatory care. Every time Mr. Goldberg visits the emergency department needlessly, he wastes resources that could have been used by someone for whom the emergency visit would have been more helpful. His use of healthcare services is not optimal, either for him or for society.

Regulatory approaches seek to control expenditures on individuals such as Mr. Goldberg in the hope that more resources will be available for those who can still benefit. In the mid-1960s, Medicare regulations mandated **utilization review (UR)**, the process of determining whether the medical care provided to a specific patient is necessary according to preestablished objective screening criteria at time frames specified in the organization's utilization management plan. The system required provider committees to review the practice patterns of their colleagues at institutions receiving Medicare dollars. The difference between those who could afford good healthcare coverage and those who could not was very wide. As a result, directives were issued to the effect that organizations receiving federal Medicaid and Medicare funds must provide the same care to all patients without differentiation based on their ability to pay.

In the 1970s, Medicaid programs in most states trained their own reviewers to visit hospitals and make sure that Medicaid patients met set criteria for hospitalization and were staying in the hospital only as long as absolutely necessary. In the mid-1980s, the prospective payment system was implemented for Medicare and Medicaid patients. Under this system, standardized payments are made to hospitals according to the diagnosis-related group (DRG) into which a patient falls. In the 1990s, the private and public sectors wrestled with the sometimes unfortunate decisions of managed care officials. These efforts have attempted to accomplish a balance between health benefits and health spending.

The issue remains important in the administration of healthcare organizations today. Services are to be accorded to, and expenditures made for, individuals who can still benefit. Organizations must be able to demonstrate that rational decisions were made about a patient's care and that those decisions were in the patient's and society's collective best interests. Healthcare organizations must also be able to demonstrate that the services provided to the patient were safe and appropriate to the patient's physical and quality-of-life needs across the continuum of care.

The continuum of care consists of all the possible settings in which patients may receive care. (See figure 8.1.) Currently, care is delivered in patients' homes, providers' offices, clinics, hospitals, long-term care facilities, and residential care facilities. Each of these care settings provides a more or less complex set of services, all of which depend on the identified needs of the patient during the initial assessment. In addition, each patient's needs may change, depending on the time that the needs are identified: prior to hospital admission, during the admitting process, during the hospital stay, during the discharge process, or during any immediate subsequent care episode. The expectation of public and private regulatory agencies is that patients' needs will be identified, prioritized, and provided for in the setting most appropriate to their requirements for care.

Understanding that the patient-centered approach to care that is common today (see table 8.1) has evolved from a very unilateral, authoritarian system of care (see figure 8.3) is an important starting point. In the past, medicine was practiced as an art, with most information for treatments based on the individual provider's skill and knowledge. Most patients expected their providers to tell them what to do regarding their health. A provider was seen either as a separate, individual provider who treated only one aspect of a patient's illness or as the family practitioner who treated everything. For example, a surgeon practiced only surgery, and patients with other health issues were referred to another provider for care of those issues. Providers ordered the tests they felt were necessary for treatment, and patients did not question providers' diagnoses or whether a test was required. There was little review of whether tests and care were necessary and little supervision or assessment of how one provider initiated and treated a patient compared with how another provider might have treated the same patient for the same illness. Best-practice standards were not a common approach to care. Sometimes, patient care and hospitalization were provided on the basis of the patient's ability to pay. Some providers and clinics provided free care for indigent patients, but this was at their own discretion.

Table 8.1. Healthcare staff roles in patient-centered approach to care

	Patient Registration	MD or DO	RN	Licensed Clinical Social Worker	Treatment Team	Discharge Planner/UR	Educator
Prescreen	x	x				x	
Registration	x	x	x			x	
Assessment		x	x	x			
Care/treatment		x	x	x	x	x	x
Patient teaching			x	x			x
Discharge		x	x	x	x	x	x
Follow-up		x					

Figure 8.3. Authoritarian approach to care

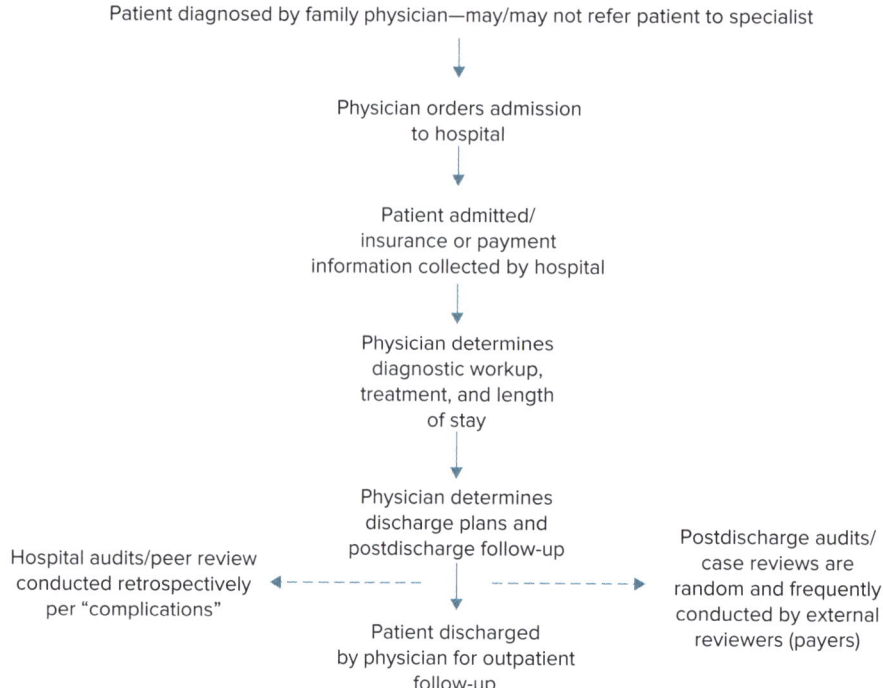

Each individual provider maintained health records on each patient, and providers had to make formal requests to get patient information from another treating provider. Transfer of information was not always reliable and was often a cumbersome and lengthy process that required a written request to be mailed and the requested information then returned by mail. The concept of a seamless patient health record entered the picture in the 21st century, just as the pace of healthcare and the complexities in providing total care necessitated better communication among treating providers and entities.

As treatments and technologies developed, the cost of research and knowledge-based care began to rise. As the cost of treatment rose, insurance companies experienced higher payouts for treatments and interventions that were sometimes duplicated and not always best for the patient. For example, at one point, it was routine practice for OB/GYN providers to remove both the ovaries and the uterus during a hysterectomy to prevent future problems. It was later discovered that women seemed to fare better hormonally when healthy ovaries were allowed to remain after surgery. Research demonstrated the importance of maintaining ovaries in young women who were not menopausal as a protection against early onset of menopause. Insurance companies then stepped in to state that they would no longer reimburse providers for the additional surgery unless there was clear indication of a need to remove the ovaries.

The increased awareness of duplication of services increased the drive to determine the medical necessity for treatments and care. Purchasers and payers of healthcare services began to demand a more comprehensive approach to care—one that decreased costs and improved the quality of care provided. Along with this demand came standards intended to ensure that the services provided were timely, cost-efficient, and appropriate to the patient's medical condition. As patients were stuck with medical bills that insurance companies refused to pay and providers were unwilling to write off because services were deemed "not medically necessary," new processes were developed to address these concerns. Insurance companies and healthcare organizations developed a role for case managers who worked with providers and hospital employees to ensure that the care ordered was appropriate to the diagnosis and that it was a payable covered item under the patient's insurance policy. Thus, the continuum of care model was developed to meet the needs of patients, providers, and payers. A review system was put into place to address medical necessity issues and fraudulent billing practices that occurred as a result of the treatment restrictions placed on providers. Millions of dollars continue to be lost due to fraud each year.

One product of these changes was the establishment of health maintenance organizations (HMOs), a type of managed care health insurance plan in the 1980s. These organizations provided their members with many levels of care at reduced costs through a network of healthcare providers contracted by the HMO. Members of HMO plans were rewarded with lower premiums for utilizing only those services provided by the HMO's network of providers, hospitals, and pharmacies. These organizations strove to keep all patient care within their own continuum of services. Since the HMO functioned as both insurer and provider, it offered many different services at substantial savings because of the ability to contract for them to meet the needs of its substantial number of members.

The health of the community and the US population as a whole has become an increased topic of focus with the passage of the Affordable Care Act (ACA) of 2010. Additional attention was placed on providing more preventive care. Healthcare services have been traditionally targeted at patients with illnesses rather than focused on preventing people from getting sick in the first place. A provision of the ACA is that health insurance companies must cover recommended preventive services to their beneficiaries. Furthermore, the ACA has urged healthcare organizations and providers to align their networks in an effort to better coordinate patient care and deliver care more efficiently. These networks are encouraged to create an accountable care organization (ACO) that is responsible for the health of its entire patient population. The ACO will direct resources to healthy patients and patients with illnesses in an effort to increase the overall health of the community.

Shift to Paying for Value

In an effort to align payment to quality of care, the Centers for Medicare and Medicaid Services (CMS) developed its first pay-for-performance (P4P) initiatives in 2005. Providers under this arrangement are rewarded for meeting preestablished targets for delivery of healthcare services that improve quality and efficiency. This was a fundamental change from fee-for-service payment. CMS collaborated with many public and private organizations, including the National Quality Forum, the National Committee for Quality Assurance (NCQA), the American Medical Association (AMA), and the Joint Commission, in an effort to improve quality of care while containing and decreasing the cost of care. The following subsections discuss these programs.

Medicare's Hospital Value-Based Purchasing Program

As part of the move to pay for value, CMS developed their value-based purchasing (VBP) program as part of the Affordable Care Act of 2010. This program began in fiscal year 2013 and incentivized acute-care hospitals to provide better quality of care to Medicare patients. VBP supports the CMS three-part aim: better care for individuals, better health for populations, and lower costs. Hospitals are no longer paid solely based on the volume of services they provide but also on the quality of care and how well the hospital adheres to best-practice standards. This VBP program includes four domains: safety, clinical outcomes, efficiency and cost reduction, and person and community engagement (see figure 8.4). Each domain includes a variety of measures that must be reported to CMS regularly (see figure 8.5).

Figure 8.4. Medicare VBP domains and weights for fiscal year 2025

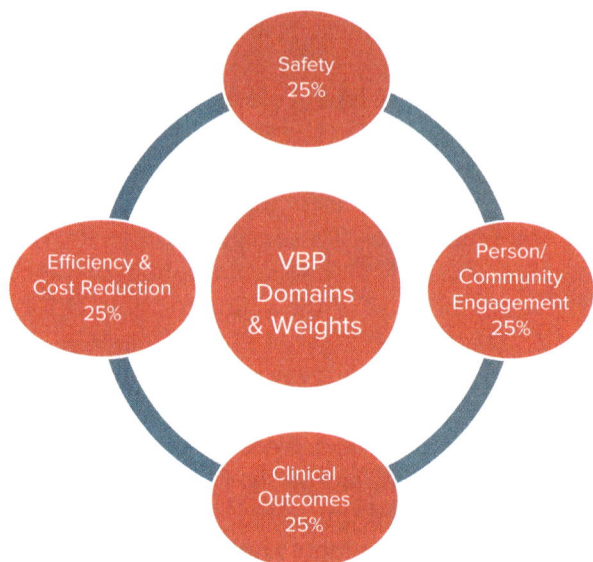

Source: Adapted from CMS 2023a.

Figure 8.5. Examples of hospital VBP program measures

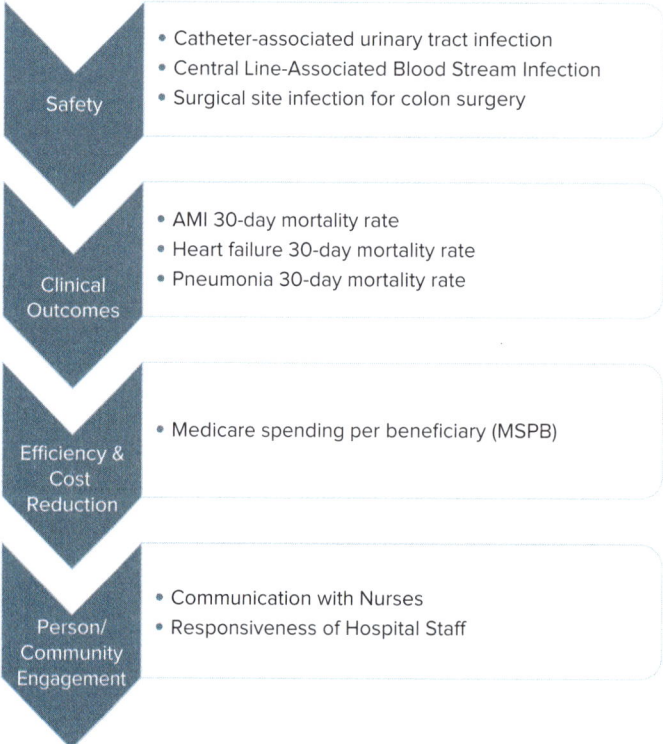

Source: Adapted from CMS 2023b.

The VBP program uses reported data to establish threshold values. Hospitals are rated based on the achievement and improvement for each of these measures against the threshold values. When a hospital does not meet the calculated score, it will result in a payment reduction (CMS 2023b).

Hospital Outpatient Quality Reporting Program

CMS's Hospital Outpatient Quality Reporting (Hospital OQR) program requires hospitals to report standardized measures of care to receive the full update to their outpatient prospective payment system (OPPS) payment rate. Participating hospitals agree that CMS may publicly report their data. Hospitals that do not participate or fail to meet the requirements may receive a 2 percent reduction of their OPPS payment rate (CMS n.d.a). These measures are listed in figure 8.6.

Figure 8.6. Outpatient quality reporting measures

- OP-8   MRI lumbar spine for low back pain
- OP-10   Abdomen CT—use of contrast material
- OP-13   Cardiac imaging for preoperative risk assessment for noncardiac low-risk surgery
- OP-18   Median time from emergency department (ED) arrival to ED departure for discharged ED patients
- OP-22   ED Patient left without being seen
- OP-23   Head CT or MRI scan results for acute ischemic stroke or hemorrhagic stroke patients who received head CT or MRI scan interpretation within 45 minutes of arrival
- OP-29   Appropriate follow-up interval for normal colonoscopy in average-risk patients
- OP-31   Cataracts—improvement in patient's visual function within 90 days following cataract surgery
- OP-32   Facility 7-day risk-standardized hospital visit rate after outpatient colonoscopy
- OP-35   Admissions and ED visits for patients receiving outpatient chemotherapy
- OP-36   Hospital visits after hospital outpatient surgery
- OP-37   Outpatient and Ambulatory Surgery (OAS) CAHPS Survey
- OP-38   COVID-19 vaccination coverage among healthcare personnel
- OP-39   Breast cancer screening recall rates
- OP-40   ST-elevation myocardial infarction (STEMI)

Source: CMS n.d.b

Physician Practice Program

The physician quality reporting system (PQRS) transitioned to the Quality Payment Program (QPP). This program was designed to reduce the paperwork burden on physicians while improving care to Medicare patients (see figure 8.7). Under the QPP, providers have two tracks to choose from based on practice size, specialty, location, or patient population: the merit-based incentive payment system (MIPS) or the advanced alternative payment model (APM). Under MIPS, provider payments are based on quality of care (a feature of the former PQRS program), promoting interoperability (a feature of the former Meaningful Use program for electronic health record technology), improvement activities, and cost (CMS n.d.c). The advanced alternative payment models are designed to incentivize providers who give high-quality and high-value care to their patients.

Figure 8.7. Quality Payment Program

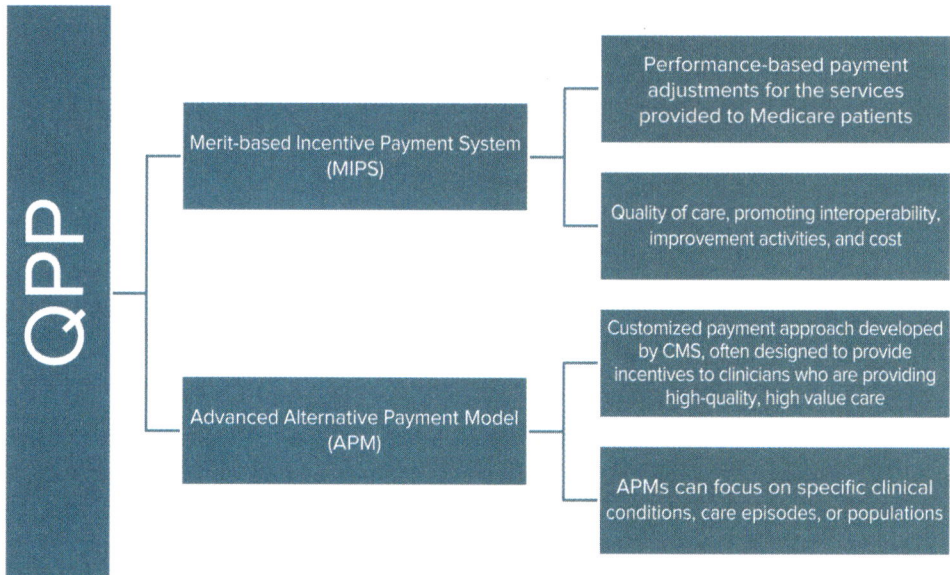

Source: CMS n.d.c

Ambulatory Surgical Center Quality Reporting Program

As with other pay-for-performance programs, the ambulatory surgical center quality reporting (ASCQR) program promotes higher quality through quality-of-care measurement, quality improvement, and information transparency through public reporting. Ambulatory surgical centers (ASCs) must meet administrative, data collection, and data submission requirements to receive the full payment update. ASCs that do not meet these requirements, including allowing the data to be publicly reported, are subject to a 2 percent reduction to any payment update for the year (CMS n.d.d). See figure 8.8 for a list of the ASC quality measures.

Figure 8.8. ASC quality measures

ASC-1	Patient burn
ASC-2	Patient fall
ASC-3	Wrong site, wrong side, wrong patient, wrong procedure, wrong implant
ASC-4	All-cause hospital transfer/admission
ASC-9	Endoscopy/polyp surveillance—appropriate follow-up interval for normal colonoscopy in average-risk patients
ASC-11	Cataracts—improvement in patient's visual function within 90 days following cataract surgery
ASC-12	Facility 7-day risk-standardized hospital visit rate after outpatient colonoscopy
ASC-13	Normothermia
ASC-14	Unplanned anterior vitrectomy
ASC-17	Hospital visits after orthopedic ASC procedures
ASC-18	Hospital visits after urology ASC procedures
ASC-19	Facility- 7-day hospital visits after general surgery procedures
ASC-20	COVID-19 vaccination coverage among healthcare personnel

Source: CMS n.d.e

Other Medicare Value-Based Programs

CMS has developed additional value-based programs for other healthcare settings. These programs include the end-stage renal disease (ESRD) quality incentive program (QIP), the inpatient psychiatric facility quality reporting (IPFQR) program, the PPS-exempt cancer hospital quality reporting (PCHQR) program, the skilled nursing facility value-based purchasing (SNF VBP) program and the home health value-based purchasing (HHVBP) model. Details on these programs may be found on the CMS website.

Hospital Readmission Reduction Program

The hospital readmission reduction program (HRRP) lowers payments to inpatient prospective payment system hospitals with too many readmissions. This program is designed to improve care coordination and postdischarge planning. CMS calculates an excess readmission ratio (ERR) for hospitals, which is the ratio of predicted-to-expected readmissions. This ERR is determined for each of the following conditions and procedures:

- Acute myocardial infarction
- Chronic obstructive pulmonary disease
- Heart failure
- Pneumonia
- Coronary artery bypass graft surgery
- Elective primary total hip arthroplasty or total knee arthroplasty

Any readmissions to any acute-care hospital for any condition is factored into the readmission rate (CMS 2023c).

 Check Your Understanding 8.1

1. Which of the following is an example of the hospital value-based purchasing program measure for clinical outcomes?
   a. Surgical site infection
   b. HCAHPS survey results
   c. Heart failure 30-day mortality rate
   d. Catheter-associated urinary tract infection

2. A 68-year-old female, Keilani was recently discharged from the hospital after been treated for pneumonia. She began experiencing reoccurring symptoms and was sent back to the emergency department. After evaluation, Keilani was taken back to the medical floor of the hospital for further care. The hospital will receive lower reimbursement for Keilani's care based on which of the following programs:
   a. Medicare's hospital value-based purchasing
   b. Physician practice quality payment
   c. Ambulatory surgical center quality reporting
   d. Hospital readmission reduction

Refining the Continuum of Care: Steps to Success

The principal process by which organizations optimize the continuum of care for their patients is **case management**. Case managers review the condition of patients to identify each patient's care needs and to integrate patient data with the patient's course of treatment. The subsections that follow outline common steps in the case management process.

The case manager in many organizations matches the patient's course with a predetermined optimal course (also known as an integrated care map, **critical pathway**, or practice guideline) for the patient's condition. This pathway is a multidisciplinary outline of anticipated care within an appropriate time frame to aid a patient in moving progressively through a clinical experience that ends in a positive outcome.

The case manager identifies, in conjunction with the treatment team, actions to be taken when the patient's care is not proceeding optimally. UR is an integral part of case management. As part of this UR process, the case manager reviews for medical necessity and appropriateness. This UR process helps to improve patient outcomes and lower healthcare spending, while still providing appropriate care to patients at the appropriate time (Giardino and Wadhwa 2023). Managed care plans use case management to define when a patient may have a procedure or to stipulate a particular course of treatment that the payer believes will be equally effective but less costly than another option.

URAC, formerly known as the Utilization Review Accreditation Commission, was formed in the late 1980s to address the lack of uniform standards for UR services. This organization promotes quality and accountability of healthcare organizations through accreditation, education, and measurement programs. URAC supplies the healthcare industry with standards to evaluate an organization's processes and programs for utilization review (URAC 2023).

Step 1: Perform Preadmission Care Planning

Preadmission care planning is initiated when the patient's provider contacts a healthcare organization such as a hospital or nursing facility to schedule an episode of care service. The case manager reviews the patient's projected needs with the provider. Admission criteria are established on the basis of a suggested diagnosis. The case manager also may contact the patient directly to obtain further information.

The hospital case manager may contact the patient's payer to confirm that all necessary preadmission authorizations have been obtained, that admission criteria have been met, and that the payer will pay for the patient's services. This process is called *preauthorization*. As part of preauthorization, the payer's representative will have compared the planned services with the payer's criteria of care for the patient's diagnosis. Some payers will pay 80 percent to 100 percent for care provided by facilities and providers in their preferred provider network. Patients who opt to go to an out-of-network facility or provider usually have to pay a higher share of the cost than those who receive services at in-network facilities. Some insurance plans allow the patient to choose to receive services at any facility and from any provider, but these plans usually have a lower reimbursement rate, and the cost to the patient is higher.

Step 2: Perform Care Planning at the Time of Admission

When the patient is admitted to the hospital, the case manager will review all the information gathered by the clinicians assigned to the case to confirm that the patient meets the admission criteria for an admitting diagnosis. The case manager will confirm that the patient requires services that can be performed at the facility. If it is determined that the facility cannot perform the services needed, the case manager will arrange for the patient to be transferred to another facility.

Figure 8.9. Sample Gantt chart format in an excerpt of a critical pathway

Western University Regional Medical Center
Department of Nursing
Case Management Plan

Diagnosis: Idiopathic pediatric scoliosis, with surgery, without complications   **Unit:** 9 East   **DRG:** 215

Average Length of Stay: 7 days   **Usual OR Day (admission day = 1):** 2

Clinical Milestones:

	Prior to Admission	Day 1	Day 2	Day 3	Day 4	Day 5	Day 6	Day 7	Day 8	Day 9	Day 10	Day 11	Day 12
Self-donation of blood	X												
Chest x-ray, chem panel	X												
Labs, EKG, blood type & crossmatch	X												
PM admission		X											
H&P		X											
Care planning		X											
Surgery			X										
Surgical ICU			X										
Catheter removed				X									
Patient sits up in bed					X								
Transfer to surgical floor					X								
Physical therapy					X	X	X						
Patient walks down corridor						X							
Patient education for self-care								X					
Patient receives meds and instructions for follow-up care										X			
Outpatient physical therapy scheduled						X							
Patient discharged to home								X					

Health Outcomes:

Diagnosis	Outcome (The patient . . .)	Day–Visit	Intermediate Goal (The patient . . .)	Day–Visit	Process (The nurse . . .)	Day–Visit	Process (The physician . . .)
Fluid-electrolyte imbalance: third space shifting secondary to large volume loss and replacement	Has stable vital signs consistent with baseline at admission	5–6 4–14	Is afebrile	4	Takes vital signs every 2 hours	PTA	Arranges for self-donation of blood before surgery
		4–6	Maintains urine output over 1 cc/kg/hr while catheterized	4	Measures and records urine output every hour	1	Assesses patient's cardiac status on admission
						1	Orders lab workup
	Has a baseline normal voiding pattern	6–8	Voids 8 hours after Foley is discontinued				
		4–14	Maintains specific gravity under .1020	4	Monitors specific gravity		
	Has no edema	8–9	Returns to baseline skin turgor	4–8	Balances IV and oral intake to achieve maintenance fluid requirements		

If the facility uses care-mapping methodology, the case manager will assign the case to the appropriate critical pathway (see figure 8.9) and verify that all services stipulated in the critical pathway have been initiated.

Step 3: Review the Progress of Care

The case manager periodically reviews the patient's progress throughout the entire episode of care. When a critical pathway is being used, the case manager will reintegrate care data (such as vital signs, response to treatment, and lab results) each time the case is reviewed and compare the patient's progress with the pathway. When variations from expected progress occur, the case manager coordinates interventions among the clinicians and therapists assigned to the case to move the patient along the path.

From the beginning of the episode of care, the case manager continuously monitors the patient's acuity level and requirements for services. At the same time, they plan—in conjunction with the patient, the patient's family, and the clinical team—for the services the patient will need after discharge. The case manager will arrange for the patient to be transferred to another facility or nursing unit to meet the patient's care needs. Ultimately, the goal is to maintain the least costly level of care possible for the patient based on assessed needs.

Step 4: Conduct Discharge Planning

Discharge planning is an integral part of the clinical team's decision-making regarding length of stay, services rendered, and provision of benefits. As the patient's requirements for care decrease and the patient moves toward discharge, the case manager undertakes final discharge planning. In this step, the patient's continued care after discharge is planned. Many times, family members and significant others are an active part of this process because they will often assist with care after discharge. Postdischarge medications are prescribed, and therapies are scheduled. A detailed list of current medications is shared with providers in the next step of the continuum. Arrangements to transfer the patient to a subacute facility are made when necessary. Effective discharge planning often begins at the time of admission to ensure that the patient will be prepared to leave the facility as scheduled.

Step 5: Conclude Postdischarge Planning

Once the patient has been discharged, the case manager shares information about the patient's course of treatment with the clinicians who will continue to care for the patient. At this point, the case management function is returned to the patient's provider and office staff. Some healthcare organizations follow up with patients after discharge to ensure that the transition has gone smoothly and that the patient is receiving all required services.

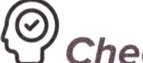

Check Your Understanding 8.2

1. Upon receiving a call from Kathy's provider to schedule a hysterectomy, the hospital case manager contacts Kathy's insurance company to get their approval for the procedure. This is an example of which step in the case management process?
   a. Preadmission care planning
   b. Care planning at time of admission
   c. Review the progress of care
   d. Discharge planning

2. Maddie was admitted to the hospital after she fell and fractured her right hip. She will need rehabilitation services after leaving the hospital. The hospital case manager assisted with her placement at Sunnyville Rehab Center. Which case management step is being performed to plan for continued care after hospital services end?
   a. Preadmission care planning
   b. Care planning at time of admission
   c. Review the progress of care
   d. Discharge planning

QI Toolbox Techniques

 Indicators (criteria) and Gantt charts are often used in assessments of continuum of care issues.

Indicators

An **indicator**, also called a criterion, is a performance measure that enables healthcare organizations to monitor a process to determine whether it is meeting requirements. The criteria may be established and implemented internally, externally, or generically.

Internal criteria are usually developed by an interdisciplinary team made up of providers, nurses, and other clinical staff to monitor specific processes within the organization. External criteria are created by an organization outside the healthcare facility. Insurance companies, peer review organizations, CMS, and other regulatory agencies develop healthcare criteria.

Generic criteria have been developed by many of the same agencies for use across the continuum of care and in various regions of the country. The term *generic* implies that the criteria are applicable across many organizations and with many different kinds of patients.

One of the most common applications of generic criteria measures is in admission certification. Admission criteria are used to establish that each patient requires care at the level at which they have been admitted. Usually, admission criteria in acute-care settings have two categories: intensity of service and severity of illness. For a patient to meet the admission criteria, they must meet a clinical measure in both categories. **Intensity of service** refers to the type of services or care the patient requires. **Severity of illness** refers to how sick the patient is or what level of care the patient requires, such as intensive care or general medical care. (See the list of admission criteria in the following case study.)

Each indicator, written in the form of a **ratio**, is used as a tool for monitoring care and service. All ratios are listed as a percentage when reported. An indicator for the number of admissions that meet set admission criteria might be the following ratio:

$$\frac{\text{Number of admissions meeting criteria}}{\text{Total number of admissions}}$$

A target or goal set by a healthcare facility might be, "Admission criteria met 99 percent of the time." Meeting such high expectations is very important to healthcare organizations because care rendered to patients who do not meet admission criteria is generally not reimbursed.

Monitoring these indicators allows the organization's leadership to identify cases in which a patient did not receive the best care. The indicators also identify excessive numbers of cases in which this was true, thus providing an opportunity for improvement in organizational processes.

An example of hospital standard measures (indicators) used by one community hospital is provided in table 8.2. These indicators were used to provide standardized reporting. (See the discussion on standardized reporting in chapter 17.) The formula for each criterion is given, along with the benchmark the organization wants to meet, how often the indicator is measured, which organizational unit is responsible for the measure, the source of data used to compute the measure, and where the results are reported.

Table 8.2A. Examples of hospital standard measures

Measure of Process	Type Out/Proc	Measured Y/N	Indication/Formula	Benchmark	How Often Measured	Owner	Source of Data	Results Given to
Discrepancies—Pre-op/Post-op/Path	O	Y	# cases with discrepancy / # of pathology cases	0%	Quarterly	OR	OR data sheet	QC, Med Exec & the Board
Complications of post-procedure care	P	Y	# pts w/complications / # patients operated on	0%	Quarterly	OR	OR data sheet	QC, Med Exec & the Board
Preparing and dispensing: Dispensing errors	O	Y	# dispensing errors / # inpatient days	0%	Quarterly	Pharmacy	Pharmacy tracking system	P&T Med Exec
Monitoring the effects on patients: Adverse drug reactions	O	Y	# ADRs / # of admissions	0%	Quarterly	Pharmacy	Incident report	P&T Med Exec
Administration: Blood hung within 20 minutes of dispensing	P	Y	# units hung within 20 minutes / # units dispensed	100%	Quarterly	Lab	Blood slips	QC & Med Exec
Monitoring effects on patients: Potential transfusion reactions	O	Y	# of true reactions / # transfusion episodes	0%	Quarterly	Lab	Transfusion reaction investigations	QC & Med Exec
Utilization management: Patients admitted to observation who should have been inpatients	P	Y	# pts not admitted as IPs who met inpatient criteria / # pts admitted	0%	Quarterly	UR	Utilization management form	QC & Med Exec
Adverse events during anesthesia	O	Y	# adverse events / # pts given anesthesia	0%	Quarterly	OR	OR data sheet	QC & Med Exec
VBAC rate	O	Y	# VBAC / # repeat C-sections	36%	Quarterly	Labor & Delivery	Obstetric report	QC & Med Exec
Joint replacements with complications	O	Y	# joint replacements with complications / # joint replacements	0%	Quarterly	OR	Patient record & surgical stats	QC & Med Exec
Notice of intent	O	Y	# for current quarter	1%	Quarterly	Risk Mgmt.	Receipt of atty letter or notice	QC & Med Exec

Table 8.2B. Examples of hospital standard measures (*Continued*)

Measure of Process	Type Out/Proc	Measured Y/N	Indication/Formula	Benchmark	How Often Measured	Owner	Source of Data	Results Given to
Patient/Family complaints—care	O	Y	# complaints / # patient days	1%	Quarterly	Risk Mgmt.	Complaint system	QC & Med Exec
Medical device reporting (manufacturer)	O	Y	# complaints / # patient days	<0.1%	Quarterly	Risk Mgmt.	Complaint system	QC & Med Exec
Patient satisfaction: Inpatient	O	Y	Percentage reported only	93%	Quarterly	QRS	Gallup results	QC, Med Exec & the Board
Completion of competency testing of employees	O	Y	# employees completing competency testing / # of employees	100%	Annually	Human Resources	Results of tests	QC, Med Exec & the Board
Hospital-acquired infection rate	O	Y	# hospital-acquired infections / # patients	<1%	Quarterly	Infection Control	Culture reports & Pt records	QRIC Committee
Surgical wound infection rate	O	Y	# post-op infections / # surgeries	0.8%	Monthly/ Quarterly	Infection Control	Culture reports & Pt records	QRIC Committee
Medical record delinquency: Overall	O	Y	# charts 21 days delinquent / # discharges for month	<50%	Quarterly	HIM	Record report	QC, Med Exec & the Board
Suspensions	O	Y	# suspensions / # physicians	0%	Quarterly	HIM	Record report	QC, Med Exec & the Board

Gantt Charts

A **Gantt chart** is a project management tool used to schedule important activities. Gantt charts divide a horizontal scale into days, weeks, or months and a vertical scale into project activities or tasks.

Gantt charts are used in clinical process improvement to depict clinical guidelines or critical pathways in the treatment of common medical conditions. The tool provides a visual method for showing the simultaneous and interdependent treatments for a clinical condition that are most likely to result in the best possible outcome. Figure 8.9 is an example of a Gantt chart. The chart depicts the clinical guidelines used for cases of idiopathic pediatric scoliosis at a large medical center.

Check Your Understanding 8.3

1. An indicator that refers to how sick the patient is or what level of care the patient requires is assessing the _____ of the patient.
   a. Intensity of service
   b. Ratio
   c. Severity of illness
   d. Critical pathway

2. For a large PI project, Joe would like to diagram all of the required important steps in the process, their dependency, interaction, and schedule requirements. What would you recommend Joe use to do this?
   a. Affinity diagram
   b. Pareto chart
   c. Gantt chart
   d. Control chart

Real-Life Example

Information collected in the form of valid and reliable data is the starting point for management of the continuum of care. Established criteria for care and clinical paths are crucial to the quality of patient care. Such guidelines, coupled with the clinical expertise of the case manager, can make the process of case management more effective.

At one hospital, care guidelines used internal and external criteria for the process of utilization review and case management. It also used feedback provided by third-party payers.

The quality leadership had noted through data collection that the process of admission, treatment, and discharge planning was not well coordinated among the associated caregivers and the business operations of the organization. Key issues included the following:

- Patients were admitted to the hospital for diagnosis and treatment in cases in which the patients could have received appropriate care in a less-intensive care setting.
- Hospital stays were continued after symptoms and treatment had reached a point at which the patient could have received appropriate care in a less-intensive care setting.
- Families were not involved in decisions regarding discharge placement options or care plans. Home health agencies, skilled nursing care facilities, and hospices were not being contacted early enough in the patient's stay to facilitate postdischarge transition to other levels of care.
- Insurance carriers and Medicare were denying payment because services had not been preauthorized and had been rendered after discharge criteria had been met and documented.
- Health records contained inadequate documentation of medical conditions, interventions, and outcomes.

At first, hospital utilization and quality department personnel organized themselves to better communicate the needs, problems, and obstacles associated with establishing an effective case management system. However, it quickly became apparent that they alone could not make the kinds of differences necessary to improve the ailing system.

A PI team was formed. The team included a representative from the registration department, business office and financial counselors, the admissions nurse, the operating room scheduler, the operating room manager, a representative from outpatient services, representatives from the nursing units, discharge planners, the utilization review or case managers, and the director of the utilization or quality department.

The team discovered that it had not included all individuals and departments that were closely associated with the process. The team realized that it also needed representatives and participants from providers' offices. The team members invited key office personnel to participate on the team.

The newly composed team spent several weeks working on team building. Leading this group of people to form a cohesive team was a difficult task. Accusations and feelings of failure ensued. But eventually, an important breakthrough occurred. After repeated reinforcement of the concept that improving this process would benefit all departments, the team was able to break down departmental barriers, focus on its common mission and goals, and get to work.

Team members found more purpose and pleasure in their work and felt more powerful and less frustrated. The team collected and analyzed the information and reported it to those persons who could directly make a difference. The medical staff was educated regarding the problems and proposed solutions that could help develop an effective case management model. Other office personnel and service departments were included to complete the circle of participants.

The team's achievements included the following:

- Critical information was shared about postdischarge planning (such as treatment plans and care goals) and financial information (including benefits, limits, out-of-pocket expenses, and deductibles).
- Primary care providers were included in the decision-making process and were given information that benefited not only patients and their families but also the providers' practices and the hospital.
- Coordination of services was improved, and access to specialists and special services was provided in a timely manner, including options for alternative care placement and the wise use of financial resources. Often, with completed care plans, the payers were willing to pay for services that would complete the healing process and avoid readmission or duplicate extended care and testing.
- The number and dollar amounts of payment denials decreased. The organization's fiscal situation improved, thus allowing staff to purchase equipment and expand services.
- The quality of health documentation improved. Some forms and the flow of some medical information were changed.
- Having a proven method of case management served as an asset in subsequent contracting with new providers and payers.
- Departments, personnel within the organization, and provider offices became more unified. The team approach served as a catalyst for change within the organization. Individuals realized that they could make a difference and that they had the ideas and power to make change happen. The PI activity strengthened the employees' commitment to the mission and vision of the organization.

Case Study

A large integrated health system's chronic disease management program is currently facing challenges in providing seamless and comprehensive care to patients with long-term health conditions. Within this organization's integrated care model, patients often experience fragmented care. The lack of coordinated care has led to suboptimal health outcomes and increased healthcare costs, which is placing an undue burden on emergency services within the system. Patients are also voicing concerns about their experiences within the system and patient satisfaction scores are trending downward. Many patients feel that they have little control over their healthcare decisions and are often not educated on treatment options. Patients and their families are often tasked with determining the next steps for care after discharge from the hospital. Case management and utilization review teams within the system's hospitals lack processes to effectively manage these processes for patients. Although the system has an enterprise-wide EHR system in place, the tools to manage and coordinate chronic care have not been used to their full potential.

Case Study Questions

1. Using information in the Refining the Continuum of Care: Steps to Success section in this chapter, provide a framework that could be used by case management teams at the hospitals in this integrated health system.
2. How does the organization's current lack of care coordination directly impact the overall care and health of the patients it serves?
3. Provide examples of how a more robust use of the organization's EHR system could help case management teams better manage these processes.

Review Questions

1. Compare and contrast two of CMS's value-based purchasing programs.
2. Caitlin's provider suspects that she has cholecystitis and has ordered a gallbladder ultrasound to be performed. The staff at the provider's office contacts her health insurance company to determine benefits and coverage for this procedure prior to scheduling the cholecystectomy. What is this process called?
    a. Utilization management
    b. Explanation of benefits
    c. Payment adjudication
    d. Preauthorization
3. Which of Medicare's value-based purchasing programs includes measures related to median time from emergency department (ED) arrival to emergency department departure for discharged ED patients?
    a. Hospital value-based purchasing program
    b. Physician quality reporting system
    c. Ambulatory surgical center quality reporting program
    d. Hospital outpatient quality reporting program

4. If a patient comes into the emergency department with left-sided hemiparesis that started within the last three hours, which admission criterion would be used to justify admitting this patient as an inpatient?
   a. Intensity of service
   b. Indicator
   c. Severity of illness
   d. Standard of care

5. Which organization was formed in the late 1980s to address the lack of uniform standards for utilization review services by promoting quality and accountability of healthcare organizations through accreditation, education, and measurement programs?
   a. The Joint Commission
   b. CMS
   c. NCQA
   d. URAC

References

CMS (Centers for Medicare and Medicaid Services). n.d.a. "Hospital Outpatient Quality Reporting (OQR) Program." Accessed December 13, 2023. https://qualitynet.cms.gov/outpatient/oqr.

CMS (Centers for Medicare and Medicaid Services). n.d.b. "Outpatient Quality Reporting (OQR) Program Measures." Accessed December 13, 2023. https://qualitynet.cms.gov/outpatient/oqr/measures.

CMS (Centers for Medicare and Medicaid Services). n.d.c. "Quality Payment Program Overview." Accessed December 13, 2023. https://qpp.cms.gov/about/qpp-overview.

CMS (Centers for Medicare and Medicaid Services) n.d.d. "Ambulatory Surgical Center Quality Reporting (ASCQR) Program." Accessed December 13, 2023. https://qualitynet.cms.gov/asc/ascqr.

CMS (Centers for Medicare and Medicaid Services). n.d.e. "Ambulatory Surgical Center Quality Reporting (ASCQR) Program Measures." Accessed December 13, 2023. https://qualitynet.cms.gov/asc/ascqr/measures.

CMS (Centers for Medicare and Medicaid Services). 2023a. "Hospital Value-Based Purchasing (VBS) Program." https://qualitynet.cms.gov/inpatient/hvbp.

CMS (Centers for Medicare and Medicaid Services). 2023b. "Hospital Value-Based Purchasing (VBS) Program: Performance Standards." https://qualitynet.cms.gov/inpatient/hvbp/performance.

CMS (Centers for Medicare and Medicaid Services). 2023c. "Hospital Readmissions Reduction Program (HRRP)." https://www.cms.gov/medicare/payment/prospective-payment-systems/acute-inpatient-pps/hospital-readmissions-reduction-program-hrrp#:~a:text=The%20Hospital%20Readmissions%20Reduction%20Program,in%20turn%2C%20reduce%20avoidable%20readmissions.

Giardino, A.P. and R. Wadhwa. 2023. *Utilization Management*. In: StatPearls [Internet]. Treasure Island, FL: StatPearls Publishing. https://www.ncbi.nlm.nih.gov/books/NBK560806/.

URAC. 2023. "About URAC." https://www.urac.org/about/.

Resources

Joint Commission. 2024. *Hospital Accreditation Manual*. Oakbrook Terrace, IL: Joint Commission Resources.

Rotter T., R.B. de Jong, S.E. Lacko, et al. 2019. "Clinical Pathways as a Quality Strategy." Chapter 12 in *Improving Healthcare Quality in Europe: Characteristics, Effectiveness and Implementation of Different Strategies* [Internet], edited by R. Busse, N. Klazinga, D. Panteli, et al. Copenhagen, Denmark: European Observatory on Health Systems and Policies. https://www.ncbi.nlm.nih.gov/books/NBK549262/.

Improving the Provision of Care, Treatment, and Services

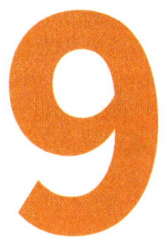

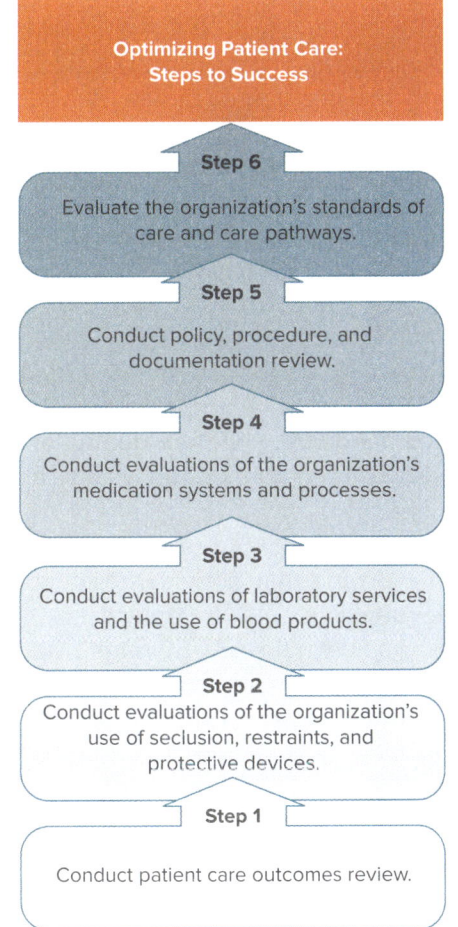

Chapter 9 Improving the Provision of Care, Treatment, and Services

Learning Objectives

- Identify four core processes or elements in the care, treatment, and services provided to patients and recognize the common means by which healthcare organizations monitor and improve the quality of these elements of care
- Explain how the National Patient Safety Goals interface with the performance improvement cycle during the patient care process
- Determine the roles that clinical practice guidelines and evidence-based medicine play in standardizing patient care
- Analyze how patient preferences impact patient-centered care and outcomes

Key Terms

Clinical guidelines
Clinical Laboratory Improvement Amendments (CLIA)
Clinical practice standards
Core processes
Evidence-based medicine

Facility quality-indicator profile
Minimum Data Set (MDS) for long-term care
Patient-centered care
Standards of care
Transfusion reaction

The preceding chapters discussed the performance improvement (PI) model, its goals, and some of the factors involved in working with PI processes. This chapter focuses on a systematic approach to PI that can ultimately benefit the patient. Patient care is a complex process that begins at any point of entry into the healthcare system and may last from one brief emergency department (ED) visit to a lifetime of frequent outpatient visits and hospitalizations for a patient with a chronic illness. Every interaction within the healthcare system provides an opportunity to improve care processes for patients and their families.

The individual medical requirements of a single patient can initiate the PI cycle. The critical factor in optimizing patient care is the organization's ability to improve patients' understanding of their health, their ability to care for themselves, their independence, and their quality of life. The goal of PI in healthcare is to design and implement systems that provide consistency and quality in all patient care processes performed to improve each individual patient's health.

With respect to the provision of care, treatment, and services, PI efforts provide a process for evaluating every service, provider, setting, and outcome that patients, residents, and clients expect in a healthcare organization. The **core processes** involved in care, treatment, and services are *assessing* patient needs; *planning* care, treatment, and services; *providing* the care, treatment, and services that the patient needs; and *coordinating* care, treatment, and services. The greatest responsibility for care lies within these processes. Activities involved in providing these four core processes include:

- Assessing and providing appropriate access to levels of care
- Providing interventions based on the plan of care developed in conjunction with the patient and significant others
- Teaching patients what they need to know about their care, treatment, and services
- Coordinating care, treatment, and services when the patient is referred, transferred, or discharged.

The Patient Care Process Cycle

In practice, the core patient care processes actually become part of a cycle that begins with the patient's initial assessment and concludes with their discharge or referral to another care provision venue. (See figure 9.1.)

Many patients have to go through this cycle several times during the duration of an illness, and the cycle may occur in one facility or across the continuum of facilities involved in the patient's care.

Figure 9.1. Patient care process cycle

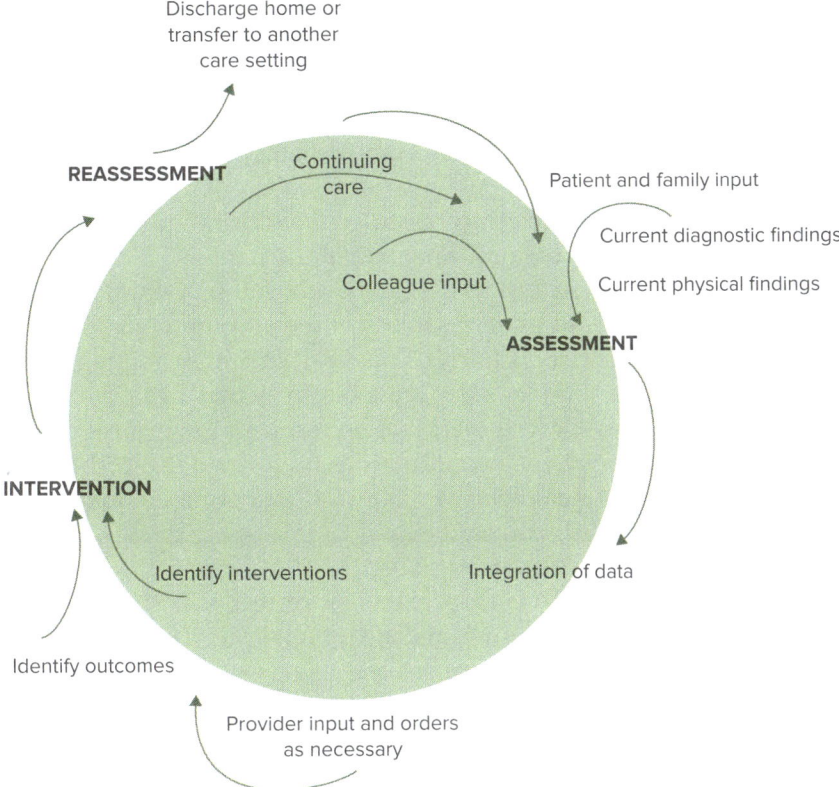

Core Process 1: Assessing the Patient's Needs

The cornerstone of good patient care is the initial assessment, which determines the patient's appropriateness for admission to the facility and the level of care to be rendered. Specific admission criteria based on defined services help determine which patients will benefit most from services the facility offers during the assessment and reassessment period. Community standards and accrediting and licensing entities require collection of the following information in the initial patient assessment for admission:

- Physical, psychological, and social assessment
- Nutrition and hydration status
- Functional status (how well an individual performs activities of daily living)
- Social, spiritual, and cultural variables that influence the patient's and family members' perceptions of their lives

In addition to physical conditions, patients are assessed for issues related to legal or correctional status, experience of abuse and neglect, alcoholism and substance use disorders, presence of pain, and emotional or behavioral disorders. The organization may refer individuals with mental illness and/or alcoholism or substance abuse disorders for care, treatment, and services as consistent with its written plan of care.

If the organization provides services for alcoholism and substance abuse disorders, a thorough assessment would be conducted. That assessment includes history of each substance use, age at onset, duration, intensity, patterns of use, consequences of use, types of previous treatments, and responses to those treatments. If the patient is receiving psychosocial services, they would also be assessed for a history of mental, emotional, and behavioral problems and co-occurrence with substance use disorders and treatment. Items typically included in this type of assessment include religious and spiritual beliefs, values and preferences, living situation, leisure and recreational activities, military service history, peer group, social factors, ethnic and cultural factors, financial status, vocational and educational background, legal history, and communication skills.

Organizational policy determines whether one of the initial assessments requires a more in-depth evaluation and whether a referral to consulting providers is necessary. All facilities have policies that outline the required information to be collected for an adequate assessment and initial treatment plan. Policies also outline who is authorized to collect this information. Family members may be a source of data collection for an initial assessment if the patient is not capable of providing coherent information.

Diagnostic testing and procedures are performed as ordered in the initial assessment period in compliance with specified time frames as defined by organizational policy.

Regulatory and licensing agencies usually also define the education, training, and experience required of team members to perform an adequate assessment. Only licensed and competent healthcare professionals are allowed to assess patients. For example, most hospital medical staff rules and regulations require a medical history and physical examination be completed by a physician within 24 hours of inpatient admission or within 30 days prior to the admission. Even if there has been a physical exam within 30 days, an updated physical to note any changes in the patient's condition needs to be done within 24 hours of admission. A registered nurse completes a nursing assessment within 24 hours of a patient's inpatient admission and determines the patient's need for nursing care on the basis of this assessment. A functional screening is also completed for each patient within 24 hours of admission.

The care team, patient, and family, if available, establish priorities for treatment. If this is done early in the course of treatment, it is classified as an initial treatment plan. This plan is usually a blueprint for a more complex plan that will follow and addresses the most emergent need of the patient. An initial problem list is also developed to reflect the most critical problems to be managed. Some treatment issues may be delayed or postponed on the basis of urgency or immediacy of care needs. For example, a patient admitted to an ED with active upper gastrointestinal bleeding and diabetes may undergo treatment for the acute bleeding first and evaluation of the diabetes later. The diabetes may be listed as a problem on the treatment plan and documented as deferred to a later time. Goals and interventions are developed by the team to address the patient's need for services and to evaluate clinical improvement. Staff are assigned to accomplish interventions for each goal, and a time frame for completion or frequency of intervention is identified.

Core Process 2: Planning Care, Treatment, and Services

If an appropriate need for admission has been determined, the establishment of an interactive care plan that is specific, individualized, and based on a thorough assessment of the patient's physical, emotional, social, cognitive, and cultural needs is the next step in the care process. In the example of the patient with diabetes being treated in the ED for gastrointestinal bleeding, the ED treatment team will begin an initial treatment plan addressing the patient's most critical needs. The treatment plan may have a goal of stabilizing his body fluid level and preventing further blood loss since this could be a life-threatening issue. The objectives for this goal would include stopping blood loss through gastric lavage with ice water, intravenous fluids to balance fluid loss, and hourly lab values to ensure blood loss is stabilized. The interventions would be listed as hourly hemoglobin and hematocrit draws, D5NS at a rate of 200 cc per hour, NPO status, and gastric lavage until bleeding ceases. Most of these immediate interventions are clinical practice guidelines or best-care standards that have been researched to provide the most expedient and lifesaving measures (Torrey 2020).

The collaborative plan of care for patients is begun at the time of admission by the interdisciplinary admitting team, the patient, and perhaps the family, and is revised as the patient's condition changes. Healthcare facility policy determines when the plan of care is due and is based on the patient's goals and the time frames, settings, and services required to meet those goals. With the use of disease-specific care plans or care paths, many of the objectives and goals will be determined on the basis of researched and established guidelines in the clinical care pathway.

Core Process 3: Providing Care, Treatment, and Services

In many healthcare settings, the clinical care pathway has become the model for the documented outline of patients' progression of treatment. A multidisciplinary team using data developed through team assessment processes initiates the clinical care pathway. The goals of the clinical care pathway are broad in scope and set the overall direction for care. The pathway defines the specific treatment and its timing and frequency. (See figure 9.2.)

Many healthcare facilities use a system of care based on established national clinical standards for treatment interventions, which have been extensively researched. Much of a patient's care is provided by a group of professionals operating as a collaborative team. A team approach is necessary in every care process, as the team will contribute significantly to improving patient care and to decreasing the number of patient care errors (McLaney et al. 2022).

Once the clinical care pathway has been developed, implementation begins. The patient's status is continuously monitored for signs of stabilization, improvement, or destabilization. Revisions of the clinical care pathway and treatment interventions are developed in response to changes in the patient's clinical status. Most care teams meet daily to evaluate patient data, interventions, and improvement. The flow of patient care is cyclical and integrated in the following way (see figure 9.1):

- Assessment to treatment planning
- Treatment planning to care or service
- Care or service to reassessment
- Coordination of care when improvement is demonstrated or reassessment when the patient is referred, transferred, or discharged

As the patient's care proceeds, some key care procedures are implemented. These procedures involve services such as laboratory, radiology, pharmacy, dietary, nursing, and physical and respiratory therapy. Each department that provides these services has licensing requirements for monitoring and data collection for quality verification. Each department must also ensure that the service provided is specific to the patient's written plan of care and accommodates the patient's cultural and religious needs.

Patients and families should be involved in this process and should be actively encouraged to take part in the ongoing cycle of planning care. The patient's strengths and limitations should be considered when developing the treatment plan and completing the goals. Clinical care pathways also need to reflect the cultural values that affect a client and their family in the care setting. For example, in some Asian countries, it is traditional to serve certain types of cold and hot foods to a newly delivered mother to ensure her health and well-being. Making dietary accommodations to meet each patient's needs can ease the transition and improve their perception of holistic, individualized care. In many instances, family members and other significant persons will be educated about the patient's treatment process and care needs and encouraged to become involved. However, adult patients need to approve of this involvement before any confidential health information is shared, in compliance with federal and state privacy laws.

Core Process 4: Coordinating Care, Treatment, and Services

The expected eventual outcome of this flow of care is an improvement in the patient's condition that allows discharge to the patient's home or a different care setting. The coordination of patient services and care is often discussed among care team members. There is a defined process in the healthcare facility to receive

Figure 9.2. Integrated clinical care pathway

Example of an integrated care pathway for the management of adults with MRSA

Guidance for use

This ICP represents usual practice, and variations are expected as clinical staff use their own professional judgement.

ICP developed 1.2.20xx **Review date 1.2.20xx**

The main source of information for this ICP was the Hospital Infection Society (1998) Working Party Report: Revised guidelines for the control of methicillin-resistant *Staphylococcus aureus* infection. *J Hosp Infect* 1998; **39:** 253–290.

Local protocols may differ as the guidelines must be adapted to fit in with local circumstances.

Decision to treat

Following a positive result of MRSA from the pathology department, an informed decision is to be made to treat or not treat the patient. Please complete all the boxes and sign at the bottom of the page.

Outcomes:

1. Decision to treat based on site of infection and degree of risk to other patients.
2. Isolation precautions are met.

Outcome 1 achieved *yes* ☐ *no* ☐
Outcome 2 achieved *yes* ☐ *no* ☐

Management plan for treatment of adult patient colonised with MRSA

Use this page only when managing a colonised infection.

Outcomes:

1. Infection is contained to patient identified with MRSA.
2. Treatment is successful.

Outcome 1 achieved *yes* ☐ *no* ☐
Outcome 2 achieved *yes* ☐ *no* ☐

Management plan for systemic treatment of patient infected with MRSA

Use this page only when managing a systemic infection.

Outcomes:

1. Treatment successful.
2. Plasma levels, liver function tests and clinical checks are monitored.

Outcome 1 achieved *yes* ☐ *no* ☐
Outcome 2 achieved *yes* ☐ *no* ☐

Recording of variance

Variance from the planned care must be recorded, signed and dated, together with the reason why this happened and the alternative plan of care.

Decision to treat

Patient name: Hospital number:

Please remember: *Staff hands are the main route of cross-infection in wards
*Early communication is essential in minimising spread of MRSA

Site	**Colonised** (Organism is present but not causing symptoms of infection)	**Infected** (Organism is present and has resulted in signs and symptoms of infection)
Nose		
Throat		
Perineum/groin		
Skin lesion		
Burn		
Catheter urine		
Indwelling intra-vascular catheter		
Central line		
Intravenous infusion		
Tracheostomy		
Sputum		

Low risk Medical ward, general and acute elderly care, non-neonatal paediatrics	• Isolate if possible • Basic infection control measures • Full screen of index case • Topically treat **NB:** screening of other patients is not necessary
Moderate risk General surgery, urology, neonatal, gynaecology/obstetrics, dermatology	As above plus: • Screen other patients in the event of two or more cases
High risk Intensive care unit, special care baby unit, transplantation, cardiothoracic, burns, orthopaedic, trauma, vascular, regional, national/international referral centres	As above plus: • Isolate in single room • Screen other patients in the unit after one case • Treat patient topically (and systemically if necessary) • Policy of admission screening is advised

If there are **any** variances to ICP, please sign and date the reason(s) and alternative action taken

• Inform hospital hotel services
• Place isolation notice on door
• Discuss with patient
• Give written information to visitors

Isolation precautions

Hand washing following contact
Gloves when dealing with infected site(s)
Apron for close contact

Decision to treat

Colonisation: *yes* ☐ *no* ☐
Infected site: *yes* ☐ *no* ☐

Signature Date / /

Treatment of adult patient colonized with MRSA

Patient name: Hospital number:

Please remember:

- Re-emergence of resistant strains is common; these patients should always be considered as carriers
- If surgery is required, systemic prophylaxis may be necessary
- Treatment may be decided upon due to risk and vulnerability of other patients
- A carrier may become a heavy disperser of Staphylococcus if he/she develops an upper respiratory tract infection
- The throat is more likely to be infected if the patient has dentures

Management: five-day topical treatment plan

		1	2	3	4	5
Nasal	Bactroban **Nasal preparation** Apply to nose three times a day					
Axillae and groin	Hexachlorophane powder (Sterzac) apply daily					
Broken skin	Bactroban **Skin preparation** Apply to any small broken skin sites daily					
Daily bathing	Triclosan 2% Apply to wet skin					
Shampoo	Triclosan 2% Apply on days 1 and 3					

Is this the 1st ☐ or 2nd ☐ treatment?

Doctor's signature: Date:

Screening schedule	Date taken	Results due	Positive/ negative
48 hours after treatment ends (day 7)			
48 hours after 1st screen (day 9)			
48 hours after 2nd screen (day 11)			

Patient is clear only when 3rd set of swabs are negative

If any of three screens positive, start 2nd treatment cycle

If positive after 2nd treatment cycle, contact infection control team for further advice

Transfer/discharge of patients

Inform relevant people
Wear gloves and apron, and wash hands
Send curtains for cleaning
Decontaminate non-disposable equipment with detergent and water folled by weak hypochlorite solution
Allow all surfaces to dry before using equipment/room again
Place last on list for OPD or surgery

If there are **any** variances to ICP, please sign and date the reason(s) and alternative action taken

Systemic treatment of adult patient infected with MRSA

Patient name: Hospital number:

Please remember:

- Delay in initiating effective MRSA therapy is a significant mortality risk factor
- Intensive care patients have a higher risk of developing MRSA infection than medical patients
- A combined medical and surgical approach may be necessary

Drug 1	Dose	Route	Duration	Frequency	Signature and date
Monitoring					**Caution**

Drug 2	Dose	Route	Duration	Frequency	Signature and date
Monitoring					**Caution**

Side-effect	Present (date)	Drug stopped (specify)
Inflammation		
Pain		
Oedema		
Nausea/vomiting		
Diarrhoea		
Rash		
Headache		
Pruritus		

Treatment of side-effect(s)

Isolation precautions

Hand washing following contact
Gloves when dealing with infected site(s)
Apron for close contact

If there are **any** variances to ICP, please sign and date the reason(s) and alternative action taken

Systemic treatment of adult patient infected with MRSA (continued)

Vancomycin or teicoplanin, possibly combined with rifampicin, may be used for severe infections
For continuing treatment or less severe infection, a combination of rifampicin and fusidic acid may be used (if organism susceptible)
Quinupristin/dalfopristin should be reserved for unresponsive severe infections or for when IV therapy is appropriate

Drug	Dose	Route	Frequency	Guidance on dosage until levels available
Vancomycin	1,000 mg	IV, given over at least 100 mins	12-hourly	CrCl (ml/min): >50: 12-hourly 30-50: 24-hourly <30: load, then measure levels*

Monitoring

Plasma levels
Pre-dose 'trough' 5–10 mg/l checked at 48 hours
If >10 mg/l increase dose interval/perhaps omit a dose
Monitor every two days when previous level satisfactory

Renal function tests may be helpful

Clinical checks on hearing (eg, tinnitus)

*Discuss with microbiologist

Drug	Dose	Route	Frequency	Guidance on dosage until levels available
Teicoplanin	400 mg (reduced from day 4 in renal impairment)	IV	12-hourly for three doses, then daily	Reduced renal function: CrCl (ml/min): 40–60: reduce by 50% <40: reduce by 66%**

Monitoring

Plasma levels helpful in complex cases
Pre-dose ('trough') >10 mg/l
Post-dose ('peak') 20–50 mg/l

**Discuss with microbiologist if patient on renal support

Drug	Dose	Route	Frequency	Caution
Rifampicin	600–1,200 mg	Oral or IV	Daily (divided doses)	Rifampicin must always be combined with another agent active against MRSA in order to prevent emergence of resistance
Monitoring		Liver function tests		

Drug	Dose	Route	Frequency	Caution
Fusidic acid	500 mg	Oral	8-hourly	
Monitoring		Liver function tests		

or share patient information when the patient is referred to another internal or external provider of care, treatment, or services. A clear picture of the patient's requirements must be developed for the following:

- The primary care provider
- Community resources that will be involved following discharge, such as home health agencies or social workers
- Family or friends who will assist the patient at home following discharge
- Rehabilitation or long-term care settings to which the patient is transferred from a hospital

Coordinating care services includes resolving conflicts in scheduled appointments, preventing duplication of services, and ensuring that care is administered within a time frame that meets the patient's needs. Specific information must be given to the patient regarding exercise and activity levels, medication regimens, weight monitoring, sexual activity, and acceptable dietary habits, as well as what to do if their condition deteriorates following discharge. Information regarding diagnoses and procedures performed must also be transmitted to primary care providers other follow-up providers.

Check Your Understanding 9.1

1. The core care process that determines the patient's appropriateness for admission to the facility and the level of care and services to be rendered is _____.
   a. Planning care, treatment, and services
   b. Providing care, treatment, and services
   c. Coordinating care, treatment, and services
   d. Assessing the patient's needs

2. Betsy was admitted to the hospital through the emergency department with congestive heart failure. After the initial assessment was completed, it was determined that Betsy met the criteria for inpatient admission to treat her condition. Her nurse is writing a care plan based on an established protocol. In this scenario, what is the nurse using to develop Betsy's care plan?
   a. Minimum data set
   b. Quality-indicator profile
   c. Assessment standards
   d. Clinical care pathway

Optimizing Patient Care: Steps to Success

In a healthcare system, the treatment and care of a patient can be measured in many ways. Different measures can be used to identify problems, demonstrate compliance with regulations, or reflect improvement in patient care processes. However, some problems are more easily measured than others. For example, it is easier to measure the number of patients who receive a preoperative dose of antibiotics to prevent postoperative wound infection than it is to measure that intervention's effect on the occurrence of infection in a specific individual. People respond differently to medication interventions. Such differences create variation in the overall response to medication. The focus of improvement processes, therefore, must be tied to patient-specific data about the care processes provided at any given facility. Several common improvement processes are discussed in the following steps.

Step 1: Conduct Patient Care Outcomes Review

Patient care outcomes are reviewed to improve the safety and quality of care and to identify issues related to medical necessity for treatment and appropriateness of care. The intent of requiring organizations to collect performance data on their outcomes of care allows accreditation organizations, CMS, the healthcare organizations themselves, and other external entities to review and compare data trends and patterns in treatment among similar organizations to help improve patient care processes. The number of measures that providers and healthcare organizations must collect and report data continues to grow. Because of the increase in the amount of data required to be collected and reported, insurance plans, CMS, physician groups, provider organizations, and consumers joined to create the Core Quality Measures Collaborative (CQMC) in an effort to establish an agreed-upon set of quality measures. The CQMC reviews current measures for relevancy and new measures for priority and supports the following sets of core measures (Partnership for Quality Measurement n.d.):

- Accountable care organizations (ACOs), patient-centered medical homes (PCMHs), and primary care
- Behavioral health
- Cardiology
- Gastroenterology
- Human immunodeficiency virus and hepatitis C
- Medical oncology
- Neurology
- Obstetrics and gynecology
- Orthopedics
- Pediatrics

Accrediting and licensing entities expect that healthcare organizations will choose appropriate measures for the services they offer and that the data collected will be reported through the PI systems in the organization. The Joint Commission uses the performance measure data as part of its scoring mechanism for accrediting facilities (Joint Commission 2024a, APR 5–6).

Step 2: Conduct Evaluations of the Organization's Use of Seclusion, Restraints, and Protective Devices

The facility must have written behavior management policies approved by the facility's clinical leaders and an external expert that define which behavior management procedures can and cannot be used. Procedures that may physically harm a patient or place the individual at psychological risk are not allowed.

Because a restraining device may be part of the patient's written plan of care, all facility, state, and federal guidelines must be complied with and defined in the plan of care. Protective restraint devices include wrist restraints, jacket restraints, chairs with restraining tables, restraints to stabilize a patient's body during surgery, and side rails on hospital beds. Such protective restraint devices prevent the patient from injuring themselves. One example is the use of head stabilization devices for dental procedures.

The use of restraints involves an increased risk of client deaths with associated legal risks and requirements for monitoring during their use. On admission, an initial assessment of the patient's need for restraint should occur, including a discussion with the patient and their family about a least-restrictive progression of interventions prior to the possible use of restraint; this assessment and discussion should be documented.

Providers should be credentialed for the privilege of assessing and applying restraint and seclusion. Continued training and staff competency for seclusion and restraint procedures and protective devices must be documented. It is also very important to document leadership philosophy, education, and commitment to the facility-wide elimination of the use of seclusion and restraint. The primary focus of training for facilities includes staff competency in a number of de-escalation techniques and safety procedures as well as the facility philosophy about restraint and seclusion. The healthcare facility should reduce the frequency of seclusion and restraint uses through the PI process to identify opportunities to reduce the risks associated with these procedures. Accrediting bodies are particularly concerned about the use of restraint and seclusion and protective devices in long-term care and rehabilitation settings because the procedures may infringe on patients' rights and have been identified through the sentinel event alert process as high risk.

Restraint and seclusion standards are highly defined by accrediting bodies, CMS, and state licensing agencies. There is a clear distinction in the regulations about the use of restraint and seclusion for nonbehavioral health patients versus behavioral health patients. There are multiple PI monitors required for any use of restraint or seclusion in all facilities. Restraint or seclusion is limited to emergencies in which there is an imminent risk of a patient inflicting physical harm to themselves, staff, or others and in which nonphysical interventions would not be effective. Most of the monitors are directed toward patient safety, timeliness, care, dignity, and least-restrictive use.

Step 3: Conduct Evaluations of Laboratory Services and the Use of Blood Products

The organization's compliance with established standards related to the use of laboratory equipment and the handling of laboratory specimens must be monitored. Laboratory services are regulated by established protocols from the Centers for Disease Control and Prevention (CDC) and the **Clinical Laboratory Improvement Amendments (CLIA)**, the federal regulations outlining the quality assurance activities required of laboratories that provide clinical services. Equipment calibration and other parameters of laboratory values must be monitored daily.

The handling of blood and blood products for transfusions is also regulated and monitored. Measuring, assessing, and improving the ordering, typing, matching, dispensing, and administering of blood and blood products are a standard part of continuous monitoring for most clinic and hospital settings. The review process seeks to validate the need for transfusion, the use of the appropriate type of blood product, and effective procedures for blood product administration.

Two patient identifiers are used when administering medications, blood, or blood components (Joint Commission 2024b). Two identifiers must also be used when collecting blood samples and other specimens for clinical testing. In addition, one of the goals is that containers used for blood and other specimens are labeled in the presence of the patient. Following are common current implementation expectations:

1. Before a blood product transfusion is initiated, the patient is matched to the blood product, and the blood product is matched to the order using either a two-person verification process or an automated identification technology such as bar coding.
2. When using a two-person verification process, one individual conducting the identification verification must be the qualified transfusionist who will administer the blood product to the patient.
3. When using a two-person verification process, the second individual conducting the identification verification must be qualified to perform this task (Joint Commission 2024b, NPSG 2–3).

The cause of every **transfusion reaction**—the signs, symptoms, or conditions suffered by a patient as the result of the administration of an incompatible transfusion—must be investigated. Most deaths resulting from hemolytic transfusion reactions were primarily attributable to incomplete patient identification processes for blood verification. Some were a result of improper handling and processing of samples for many patients at the same time in the same location. Some risk-reduction strategies identified through the analysis of these events are in-service training on transfusion-related processes, revision of staffing models for these work areas, improved patient identification processes for blood verification, environmental redesign to accommodate fewer specimens in one location, and procedures to restrict simultaneous cross-matching of many patients.

Step 4: Conduct Evaluations of the Organization's Medication Systems and Processes

Over the last few years, several advocacy groups have noted that medication use is one of the most complex healthcare processes and is fraught with the greatest possibilities for error. This situation has made a healthcare organization's medication systems and processes one of the aspects most examined by accreditation and licensing agencies. Because of its complexity and impact on the patient care process cycle, it is acknowledged as one of the most important areas for examination with respect to PI.

Step 5: Conduct Policy, Procedure, and Documentation Review

The development of policies on standard practices in a facility should be multidisciplinary in nature and design. Most facilities operate within a standard set of policies developed by a multidisciplinary team of clinical and administrative professionals who meet regularly. Policies are updated and revised as national standards of care change. The governing board and leadership of an organization are ultimately responsible for the services provided in the facility and generally recommend changes and set time frames for the review of every policy and procedure to be followed. Some facilities operate with a separate policy and procedure committee.

A key quality and performance concern is the adequate and reliable documentation of care. Poor documentation leads to the largest number of risk management and legal situations in the industry. Accreditation and licensing agencies have standards on the documentation of patient care and expect that a sample of clinical documentation will be regularly reviewed as part of an organization's PI activities. The expectation is that all records have been authenticated and contain the necessary reports and that they appropriately document the condition and treatment of the patient. An example of this type of standard would be the timeline requirement for signing off on a verbal order from a provider to a nurse in the client record. Each licensing agency will have a directive regarding this standard, and facility policies will direct the time frame for verbal order sign-offs based on the facility and type of care provided.

Step 6: Evaluate the Organization's Standards of Care and Care Pathways

For a healthcare organization to define optimal care, it must first establish a set of clinical decisions and actions taken by clinicians and other representatives of healthcare organizations in accordance with state and federal laws, regulations, and guidelines known as **standards of care** and care policies. Some healthcare organizations have moved from a policy and procedure format to a **clinical practice standards** model. This model defines practice based on diagnosis. The flow of treatment interventions and the patient's progress are evaluated on the basis of nationally accepted standards of care for the diagnosis. As each standard is developed and approved, a baseline for performance in the healthcare setting develops. Variations from the standards of care; sentinel events; and high-risk, problem-prone activities must be examined. Action plans are then developed to improve care in areas identified through the monitoring process. A decline in performance or a lack of improvement may require further evaluation and redesign of care processes. One way to facilitate this is through comparing organization performance on the core measures with that of other organizations.

Check Your Understanding 9.2

1. Jim was admitted for hip replacement surgery, and during his procedure blood products were administered. Postoperatively, Jim developed a rash and fever. The presence of these symptoms will be investigated by the hospital as a possible:
   a. Blood verification
   b. Core measure
   c. Comorbidity
   d. Transfusion reaction

2. Which of the following issues is tied to the largest number of risk management and legal situations in the healthcare industry?
   a. Transfusion reactions
   b. Use of physical restraints
   c. Poor documentation
   d. Core measure data collection

Ongoing Developments

It is important to recognize that the PI processes discussed in the preceding section are part of a continuum of development in the evaluation of patient care. This continuum of development began, effectively, with the initiation of accreditation and standardization programs decades ago and will continue in the future. In addition, major national developments that must be monitored by healthcare administrators will eventually affect all healthcare organizations. Discussion of some of these developments follows.

Focus on Patient Safety: National Patient Safety Goals

It is significant to note that in spite of the tremendous amount of data collection that has occurred in healthcare, there continues to be a huge number of errors in care administration that occur on a daily basis in organizations across the country. The development of the Patient Safety and Quality Improvement Act of 2005 and the National Patient Safety Goals (NPSGs) have demonstrated a national focus on improving safety for patients (Joint Commission 2024b, NPSG 1–20). All healthcare organizations are mandated to examine care processes that have a potential for error that can cause injury to patients.

The 2024 NPSGs for hospitals, established by the Joint Commission at the time of publication of this text, are presented in figure 9.3. Goals for other settings such as long-term care and behavioral health facilities are similar. Safety goals are reviewed and revised each accreditation year, and some become permanent standards in the applicable accreditation manual. In previous iterations of the NPSGs, one of the goals was to prevent wrong-person, wrong-site, and wrong-procedure surgeries. This transitioned to a universal protocol by the Joint Commission, similar to the universal protocol used to prevent the spread of hospital-acquired infection. The elements of this universal protocol are listed in the "prevent mistakes in surgery" section of figure 9.3.

Figure 9.3. Joint Commission 2024 Hospital NPSGs

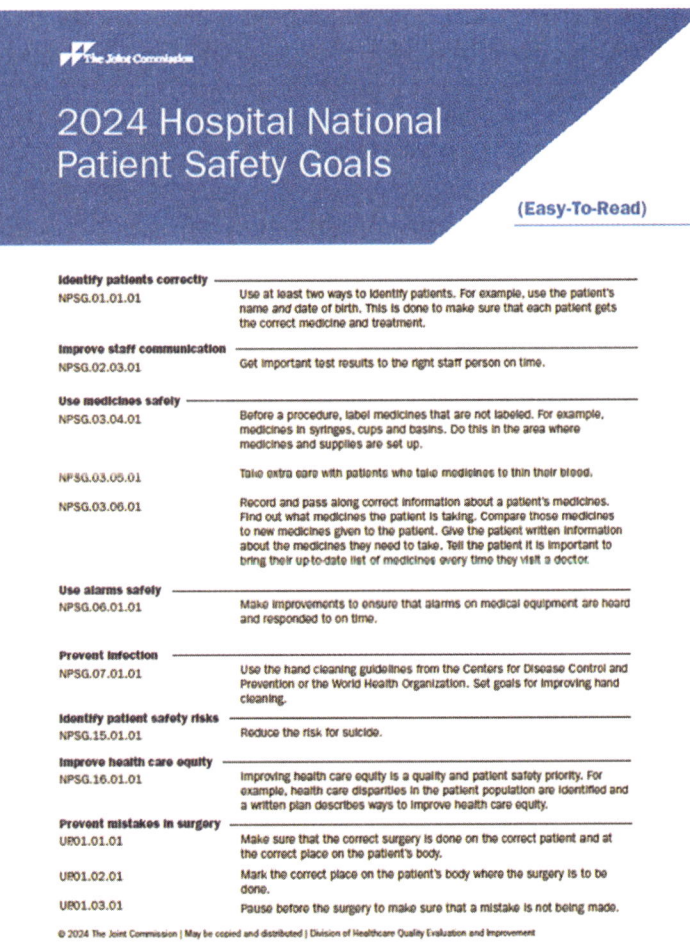

Source: Joint Commission. 2024c

National Standardization of Care Processes

The evaluation of patient care across all settings is extremely difficult. The expectation is that healthcare will be individualized because what works well for one patient may not work well for another. Some healthcare researchers, particularly those working in the federal government, have spent millions of dollars and years of research to develop **clinical guidelines**, descriptions of medical interventions for specific diagnoses in which treatment regimens and the patient's progress are evaluated on the basis of nationally accepted standards of care for each diagnosis. These guidelines attempt to standardize the care of a single condition across the entire country; however, many clinical practitioners find the guidelines difficult to implement or even contraindicated in some cases because of comorbid conditions or social ramifications in a patient's clinical presentation.

Other healthcare researchers developed the concept of **evidence-based medicine**. Evidence-based medicine attempts to identify the care processes or interventions that achieve the best outcomes in different types of medical practice. Researchers perform large population-based studies. Such studies are difficult to do without a well-developed information infrastructure to provide data for analysis.

Patient-Centered Care

The term "patient-centered care," sometimes called person-centered care, was coined by the Picker Institute, which was an organization dedicated to the perspective of patients and their families. The organization's research led to the Picker Principles of Patient-Centered Care, which was developed based on the 1993 groundbreaking book *Through the Patient's Eyes*. Researchers from Harvard Medical School, working with the Commonwealth Fund, used a variety of focus groups that included recently discharged patients, their family members, providers, and other healthcare professionals. As part of the Picker Institute research, patient surveys were developed to gain a patient's perspective (Picker 2024). These surveys were the basis of the Hospital Consumer Assessment of Healthcare Providers and Systems (HCAHPS) surveys used today .

Elements of the Patient Protection and Affordable Care Act of 2010 placed renewed emphasis on the concept of patient-centered care. Many of the central and most important processes inherent in **patient-centered care** (discussed earlier in The Patient Care Process Cycle section) emphasize respect for patient values, preferences, and expressed needs. They also place an emphasis on providers' cultural competence, information, and education regarding the patient's conditions under treatment and the modalities of treatment being utilized, access to care at levels appropriate to the patient's current progress, family involvement to the level that the patient desires, pain management, and continuity and coordination of care as the patient progresses from one level of care to another and from one type of provider to another. The concepts were emphasized for many years, but healthcare organizations across the US did not universally put them into action or make planned improvements where necessary to accomplish them. This legislation sought to encourage the development of patient-centered care principles.

Patient-centered care continues to be an increased focus for healthcare organizations, especially in discussions about quality care. Patients are routinely asked for their opinions on surveys, and the results of these surveys impact everything from publicly reported data to reimbursement. Survey results can be used by organizations to improve the care and satisfaction of patients. Patients are becoming more involved in their care, and healthcare organizations and providers must include and engage patients in their care and treatment decisions. It is important to include family members and caregivers in the process, if this is the wish of the patient.

Patient preferences are a key aspect of patient-centered care. Something as simple as asking patients the preferred name they would like to be called or if they would like the lighting dimmed in their room are small things that make a difference. Healthcare providers should also be trained to be sensitive to other cultures, languages, and when to request interpreter services. Providing patients with care at the time they need it is also a key aspect of patient preference. After-hours appointments at clinics for working professionals and telehealth options are also gaining traction.

Telehealth relies on technology to link healthcare organizations and patients from diverse geographic locations using video, text, and images as part of medical consultation and treatment. The COVID-19 pandemic accelerated the use of telehealth services, which have become more widely used. The pandemic was a catalyst that motivated healthcare payers to more readily reimburse for these services. Telehealth enables more choice for patients if their preference is to access treatment where they are located, or possibly closer to home, reducing the need to travel for care. In addition, telehealth is used by providers in rural areas to connect with specialists in larger facilities for consultation on emergent healthcare issues.

Other opportunities for organizations to provide patient-centered care arise when thinking about the timing of care. Is it necessary to wake inpatients early to have laboratory and other test results for providers' morning rounds, or is there a better time for this to occur? Can a patient's condition be monitored by a home health service instead of requiring the patient to travel to a facility, which may be challenging to do? Designing care around the patient is one way of increasing patient-centered care. As technology continues to evolve, there will be increased capacity to put patients first.

Development of organization-specific advances in the continuing deployment of patient-centered care processes will be at the forefront of accreditation and regulatory monitoring activities for the foreseeable future, even if redirection occurs with changes in the political scene at the national level.

Long-Term Care and Home Healthcare Monitoring

Another approach to monitoring care and identifying opportunities for improvement within healthcare organizations has arisen in the long-term care setting. In June 1998, the federal government mandated use of the **Minimum Data Set (MDS) for long-term care** to plan the care of long-term care residents. The MDS 3.0 version became effective in 2010. This data set structures the assessment of long-term care residents in the following areas:

- Delirium
- Cognitive loss and dementia
- Communication
- Vision function
- Activities of daily living function and rehabilitation potential
- Urinary incontinence and indwelling catheter status
- Psychosocial well-being
- Mood and behavior symptoms
- Activity-pursuit patterns
- Falls
- Disease diagnoses
- Oral and nutritional status
- Oral and dental status
- Dehydration and fluid maintenance
- Pressure ulcer
- Medication use
- Treatments and procedures
- Pain
- Return-to-community referral

The federal government requires that long-term care facilities receiving Medicare or Medicaid funding transmit patient-specific data to state departments of health for processing and use in the long-term care certification and survey review process. The certification and survey review process is carried out by state departments of health on behalf of the federal government to certify that facilities receiving Medicare or Medicaid funds are complying with federal regulations. The departments of health pay special attention to data on the occurrence of decubitus ulcers in low-risk patients (e.g., those who can ambulate, can turn over in bed, are not cognitively impaired), dehydration, and fecal impaction.

On the basis of the data gathered via the MDS, the facility is provided a **facility quality-indicator profile** that shows what proportion of the facility's residents have deficits in each area of assessment during the reporting period and, specifically, which residents have which deficits. In addition, this report includes data on recent health and fire inspection status and citations. The profile also provides data comparing the facility's current status with its preestablished comparison group. Data from the facility quality-indicator profile are also forwarded to CMS and made available to the public on the CMS care compare website.

CMS has developed and maintains data for the Outcome and Assessment Information Set (OASIS), which is used in home health agencies (CMS 2023). The OASIS lists a core of items for the comprehensive assessment of an adult home care patient. The data also help measure patient outcomes for outcome-based quality improvement.

Check Your Understanding 9.3

1. Describe the potential benefits of telehealth technologies to healthcare providers and patients in remote locations as a way to improve access to and outcomes of healthcare.

2. Diane has bilateral painful bunions, and hher right foot is so painful that she cannot walk properly. She consults her physician to seek removal of the bunion from her right foot. She does not want to have surgery on both feet at the same time as it will make the recovery too challenging. Upon waking up from her surgery Diane discovers that her left foot is bandaged and throbbing. It is soon discovered that the surgery was performed on the incorrect foot.. Evaluate how this error could have been avoided.

Real-Life Example

A typical example of an improvement effort might begin with an assessment of an overweight adolescent who is being treated for psychosis with the antipsychotic drug Zyprexa. One side effect of Zyprexa is a decrease in satiety factors in the brain, which creates a sense of hunger even when adequate food is provided. Upon assessment of the patient, based on national standards for height and weight of adolescents (body mass index [BMI]), the individual might be identified as being in a high-risk category for obesity. An evaluation of the causative factors might reveal a genetic component, a disease component, medication side effects, poor personal habits, and/or a knowledge deficit regarding healthy nutrition. A multilayered action plan would be initiated after an investigation of all aspects of the contributing factors. This plan might include a nutritional consult, a dietary regimen, a medication evaluation, and/or a psychiatric consult. At some point in the process, an activity therapist might be consulted to direct physical exercise as an intervention to increase and support muscle strengthening as the patient loses weight. This example demonstrates how the PI process may be individualized for a patient.

A system-wide PI measure could be instituted in a care setting in regard to the problem of obesity in adolescents. If providers noted significant weight increases over a brief period of time in many adolescent patients started on medications with the side effect of promoting weight gain, they might standardize their case management. Baseline evaluations of weight and height could be mandated for all patients taking this type of medication. Significant weight gains could be tracked, and interventions could be instituted for the most effective outcomes. The outcomes may result in a change in treatment that would lead providers to order dietary consults and weight monitoring for all patients taking this medication. Other preventive measures could be instituted early in treatment to avoid excessive weight gain and alleviate the patient's risk of obesity-related cardiovascular disease. The potential outcome from this PI process could lead to healthier patients who require fewer medical services in the future.

Case Study

Joan arrived at a local hospital with her father-in-law, Nigel, to seek treatment for him. Nigel was visiting Joan and her husband from Nigeria. While Nigel was at their home, Joan and her husband noticed that he has not been feeling well. He told them that he has not felt well for quite some time but did not want to worry them. His condition worsened today, and Joan decided that she would take him to the emergency room.

When they were taken to an exam room, Joan asked for an interpreter, as Nigel is a non-English speaker and Joan has limited fluency in the language he speaks. The ED physician completed his examination of Nigel, ordered several tests based on Nigel's symptoms, and left the room. After the tests were completed, Nigel and Joan were left in the room for several hours. The interpreter was no longer with them, and no member of the hospital staff came by to check on them. Joan was afraid to leave the room in case the physician would return while she was away. At one point a nurse returned to the room and began discussing the need to set up an appointment with an oncologist. She also provided information on the side effects of chemotherapy, after which she promptly left the room before Joan could ask any questions. Nigel was confused about what was said as there was no interpreter present during the conversation with the nurse. Joan was in shock realizing that her father-in-law had cancer and that she was now tasked with telling him using her limited vocabulary in his language. She proceeded to tell him that he had cancer.

Case Study Questions

1. Identify the many mistakes that were made regarding the care of this patient.
2. Explain how a patient-centered care perspective would have changed the experience of both Nigel and Joan.

Review Questions

1. List the four core processes involved in the care, treatment, and services provided to patients.
2. Select one of the NPSGs for hospitals, and construct the process improvement plan a PI team would use to improve their outcome on the NPSG goal.
3. The descriptions of medical interventions for specific diagnoses in which treatment regimens and the patient's progress are evaluated based on nationally accepted standards of care for each diagnosis is called _____.
   a. Clinical practice standards
   b. Clinical guidelines
   c. Clinical pathway
   d. Clinical standards
4. A graphic tool used to communicate established standards of patient care for specific diagnoses is called _____.
   a. Clinical practice standards
   b. Clinical guidelines
   c. Clinical care pathways
   d. Clinical standards
5. Nurse Terry prepares to administer a unit of packed red blood cells to a patient. He has verified that the patient was correctly matched to the blood product using bar-coding technology. What protocol was Terry adhering to?

References

CMS (Centers for Medicare and Medicaid Services). 2023. "Home Health Quality Reporting Program." https://www.cms.gov/medicare/quality/home-health.

Joint Commission. 2024a. "Accreditation Participation Requirements." In *Hospital Accreditation Standards*. Oakbrook Terrace, IL: Joint Commission Resources.

Joint Commission. 2024b. "National Patient Safety Goals." In *Hospital Accreditation Standards*. Oakbrook Terrace, IL: Joint Commission Resources.

Joint Commission. 2024c. "2024 Hospital National Patient Safety Goals." https://www.jointcommission.org/-/media/tjc/documents/standards/national-patient-safety-goals/2024/hap-npsg-simple-2024-v2.pdf.

McLaney, E., S. Morassaei, L. Hughes, R. Davies, M. Campbell, and L. Di Prospero. 2022. A framework for interprofessional team collaboration in a hospital setting: Advancing team competencies and behaviours. *Healthcare Management Forum* 35(2):112–117, https://doi.org/10.1177/08404704211063584.

Partnership for Quality Measurement. n.d. "Core Sets." Accessed January 8, 2024. https://p4qm.org/CQMC/core-sets.

Picker. 2024. "Our History." https://picker.org/who-we-are/our-history/

Torrey, T. Verywell Health. 2024. "Understanding Standard of Care for Patients." https://www.verywellhealth.com/standard-of-care-2615208.

Resources

Leape, L. L. 2021. *Making Healthcare Safe: The Story of the Patient Safety Movement.* New York: Springer.

Oster, C.A. and J. S. Braaten. 2021. *High Reliability Organizations: A Healthcare Handbook for Patient Safety & Quality*, 2nd ed. Indianapolis, IN: Sigma Theta Tau International.

Patient Safety and Quality Improvement Act of 2005. Public Law 109–41.

Simpson K.,W. Nham, J. Thariath, H. Schafer, M. Greenwood-Eriksen, M. D. Fetters, D. Serlin, T. Peterson, and M. Abir. 2022. How health systems facilitate patient-centered care and care coordination: A case series analysis to identify best practices. *BMC Health Services Research* 22(1):1448, https://doi.org/10.1186/s12913-022-08623-w. PMID: 36447273; PMCID: PMC9710067.

Weick, K. and K. M. Sutcliffe. 2015. *Managing the Unexpected: Sustained Performance in a Complex World*, 3rd ed. San Francisco: Jossey-Bass.

Preventing and Controlling Infectious Disease

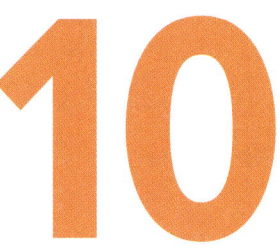

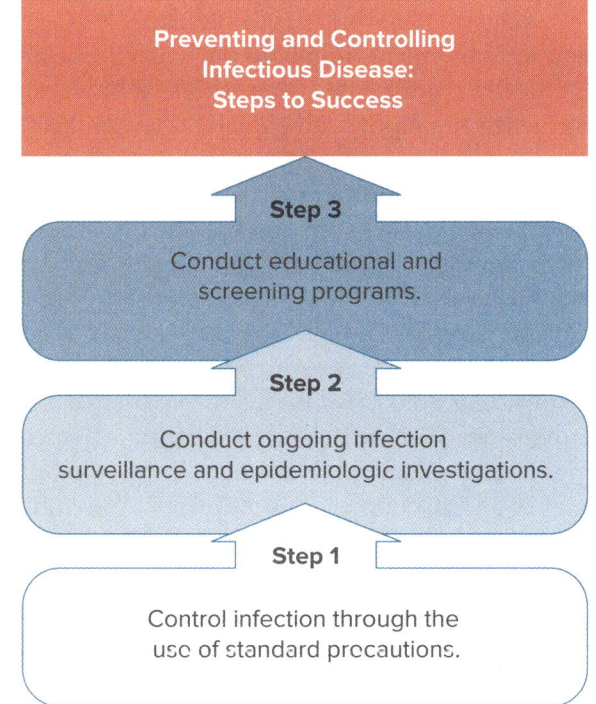

Chapter 10 Preventing and Controlling Infectious Disease

Learning Objectives

- Explain why the control of infection is so important in healthcare organizations
- Differentiate healthcare-associated infections from community-acquired infections
- Describe the various approaches that healthcare organizations use to incorporate risk-reduction strategies regarding the occurrence of infection
- Compare the governmental organizations that develop regulations in this area, and explain the regulatory approaches often taken by healthcare facilities

Key Terms

Blood-borne pathogen
Community-acquired infection
Flow charts
Healthcare-associated infection (HAI)
Icons
Multiple drug-resistant organisms (MDROs)
Standard precautions

Infectious diseases are illnesses caused by microorganisms such as viruses and bacteria that may be easy to catch and in some cases, may be deadly if not treated appropriately. Epidemics of infectious disease such as bubonic plague, tuberculosis, influenza, smallpox, and cholera have resulted in major loss of life throughout the centuries.

New diseases are still emerging today, including mutations of COVID-19, influenza (e.g., avian influenza, also called bird flu [H5N1], and swine flu [H1N1]), pneumonia, Ebola, chikungunya, severe acute respiratory syndrome (SARS), and hantavirus. Another significant problem related to the spread of infectious disease is antibiotic-resistant strains of bacteria known as multiple drug-resistant organisms. **Multiple drug-resistant organisms (MDROs)** are strains of bacteria that have become resistant to many different antibiotics.

In the US, infectious diseases inflict a heavy economic burden on the healthcare industry and on society in general. One in every 31 hospital admissions is estimated to experience one or more healthcare-associated infections (CDC 2023). A **healthcare-associated infection (HAI)** is an infection occurring in a patient in a hospital or healthcare setting in whom the infection was not present or incubating at the time of admission. HAI also describes the remainder of an infection acquired during a previous admission. HAIs added $14.9 billion to inpatient costs in 2016 (Forrester et al. 2022). Treatment of hospitalized patients with MDROs was estimated at $4.6 billion in 2017 (Nelson et al. 2021).

The discovery of pathogenic organisms such as bacteria, viruses, fungi, and parasites as the causative agents of infection has led to the development of important tools in controlling and preventing disease. Understanding microorganism replication and disease vectors (living organisms that transmit infection) has allowed scientists the opportunity to control and cure many diseases. Based on this understanding, procedures and vaccines were developed to limit the spread of infectious disease. Antibiotics were created to help limit the growth and spread of pathogenic organisms within the human body. Because of vaccinations, a much smaller portion of the world population today is affected by infectious diseases. Currently, the most effective means of stopping the spread of diseases is through education, preventive measures, and sanitation procedures.

US government agencies and professional associations such as the Centers for Disease Control and Prevention (CDC) and the Association for Professionals in Infection Control and Epidemiology (APIC) maintain national standards for disease prevention and treatment based on careful research. APIC and the American Public Health Association (APHA) are involved in training communicable disease specialists. In addition, most state licensing agencies and healthcare accrediting agencies publish standards of care for the management of infection and disease prevention within organizations. The Occupational Safety and Health Administration (OSHA) has regulations that protect the worker in the workplace from exposure to infectious materials. These regulations can be found in OSHA standard 1910.1030 (Bloodborne Pathogens). Organizations that do not comply with OSHA's basic safety standards can be fined.

Infections and infectious disease processes play a prominent role in the management of quality and performance in every healthcare facility from acute-care hospitals to community day-care program for senior citizens. Consumers who hear about HAIs in facilities may be concerned about receiving services from those facilities. Patients who acquire an infection while hospitalized may spread the word about their experience to their families, friends, neighbors, and coworkers. The infectious disease experience in healthcare facilities is of paramount importance in terms of its effect on patients' lives, costs of care, and a facility's reputation and accreditation status. If a patient is admitted for a minor procedure and dies from infection-related complications, the consequences to the facility extend beyond a bad patient outcome.

The Joint Commission has included unexpected deaths or unanticipated major loss of function from HAIs as *sentinel events*, which require review using a tool such as credible root-cause analysis. This is such an important issue that the Joint Commission established a National Patient Safety Goal (NPSG) to address the concern (Joint Commission 2024a, NPSG 10). This approach is patient-focused and evaluates systems and processes as well as disease clusters, providing a more balanced assessment of the cause of infection or death.

Because of the potential for rapid spread of infection in a healthcare setting, it is critical to have a team in place that can prevent or control the acquisition and transmission of infectious agents. This team must have the ability to move rapidly and assume its own authority to regulate care and employ resources if there is an influx of contagious patients. The governing board is required to determine and verify qualifications for an infection prevention and control (IPC) team leader (frequently a physician or epidemiologist). They must also ensure that appropriate resources are granted to the team so the goals for the IPC plan can be met. The governing board reviews IPC data on a quarterly basis and annually reviews the IPC plan and goals for the year.

The IPC team must report data to state health departments. All state health departments have a division that is required to track and record communicable diseases. When a patient is diagnosed with one of the diseases from the public health department's communicable diseases list, the IPC team must notify the public health department. (See figure 10.1 for a sample list.) The CDC provides guidelines and disease management assistance to all healthcare facilities. Most IPC plans have the CDC protocol for handwashing as the key element of training and prevention.

Preventing and managing infectious disease is an organization-wide performance issue that involves every area of the facility and affects every employee, medical staff member, patient, client, and visitor. In most facilities, a multidisciplinary approach to infection management involves the patient's provider and nursing staff, pharmacy and clinical laboratory staff, the patient's case manager, the patient, and family. The goal is to prevent infection and initiate appropriate treatment should an infection arise. A certified professional, such as an epidemiologist trained to evaluate the appropriateness of infection management measures, may be assigned to review unusual cases of infection.

Managing Infectious Disease: Steps to Success

Institutional settings are prime locations for transmission of communicable infections since they bring susceptible individuals together in one place. IPC, surveillance, and management become critical to patient safety and wellness and can be performed in a variety of ways. In some facilities, an IPC committee composed of providers, nurses, and clinical laboratory staff performs weekly reviews of the facility-wide incidence of infectious disease. In others, one individual (or a specialized department, depending on the size of the organization) with training and expertise is assigned to infection surveillance and control and is authorized by the governing board to institute any measures needed to prevent the spread of infection. In large facilities, a provider usually heads this committee. In smaller organizations, a consulting provider or epidemiologist may provide clinical oversight. The number, competency, and skill mix of the IPC staff are determined by the goals and objectives of the IPC activities. The IPC committee meets monthly to evaluate risks for infectious diseases in the facility and to establish priorities and strategies for management of the risks. The committee reviews the data collected and reports the information to the quality council. The IPC performance data are

Figure 10.1. Sample list of reportable diseases

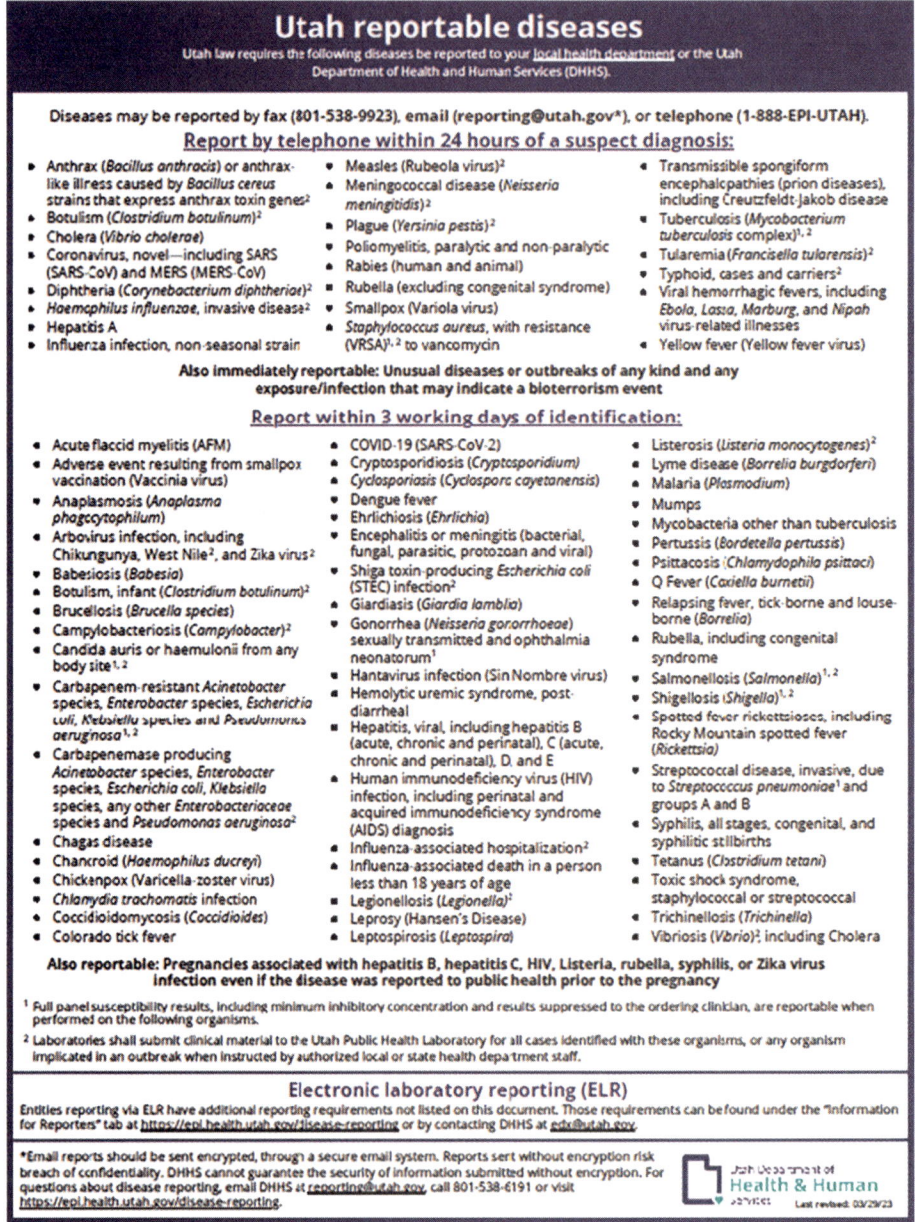

Source: Utah Department of Health 2023. Reprinted with permission.

reported on a quarterly basis to the leadership council and the governing body. Staff members involved in IPC are usually licensed, such as registered nurses, providers, epidemiologists, and pharmacists, or are certified laboratory technicians.

Data reporting for IPC usually includes data related to HAIs, community-acquired infections, antibiotic usage, culture reports, immunization data, employee illness, bloodborne pathogen exposures, and staff and patient IPC education. The goal of the reporting procedure is to identify any trends in infection and develop effective strategies to reduce the risk of infection among patients, employees, volunteers, families, and visitors.

Infection management should be based on a formal plan developed by the clinical staff and that has clearly defined goals for the prevention and control of infectious diseases in the facility. The plan should be specific to that facility's identified and prioritized risks for acquiring and transmitting infections based on geographic location, community, and population served, as well as the care, treatment, and services it provides. The goals include limiting unprotected exposure to pathogens; limiting the transmission of infections associated with procedures; and limiting the transmission of infections associated with the use of medical equipment, devices, and supplies. Another important goal is improving compliance with hand hygiene guidelines. The plan should include methods of surveillance and tracking of infections in all facility components and functions, such as medical and surgical units, dietary services, newborn nurseries, and clinical laboratories. The plan should address major communicable diseases that affect the facility's client population, such as tuberculosis, COVID-19, MDROs, community-acquired pneumonia (CAP), hepatitis B and C, and human immunodeficiency virus (HIV). In addition, the plan should outline the types of routine surveillance and procedures the organization will undertake to limit the transmission of infectious agents. This plan should be based on evidence-based national guidelines and/or expert consensus.

Step 1: Control Infection through the Use of Standard Precautions

The mandate of applying standard precautions in healthcare services has been the cornerstone of IPC since the 1980s. **Standard precautions** can be defined as the use of infection prevention and control measures to protect against possible exposure to infectious agents. The concept behind these general precautions is that every individual encountered in the healthcare setting should be treated as if they may have an active **blood-borne pathogen** disease. Blood-borne pathogens such as HIV and hepatitis B and C are transported through contact with infected body fluids such as blood, semen, and vomitus. The precautions are described as "standard" because any individual may potentially be infected or could potentially infect others. Each facility should define the employee level of risk for infection associated with their job classification and define the proper precautions needed to prevent exposure.

Transmission-based precautions are measures used to protect against exposure to a suspected or identified pathogen based on the way the pathogen is transmitted. Means of transmission of infections include direct contact, droplet, airborne, insect-borne, or any combination of these. Transmission-based precautions are used in addition to standard precautions for patients who may be infected with agents for which additional precautions are needed. Information regarding these precautions can be found on the CDC website.

Standard precautions require that caregivers be educated about proper handwashing techniques, including appropriate types of hand cleansers and proper handwashing procedure. Proper handwashing has been identified by the CDC as one of the single most important methods for preventing the spread of infection. Employees should wash their hands between patients and wear gloves when they examine patients and administer therapies. Caregivers also must wear gloves, gowns, masks, and eye protection whenever they perform procedures that disrupt the patient's skin or mucous membranes. Standard precautions assume that all patients carry infectious disease agents. Therefore, barriers are erected between patients and between patients and caregivers when blood or body fluids are involved in any way.

Step 2: Conduct Ongoing Infection Surveillance and Epidemiologic Investigations

This step incorporates substeps A through E.

A: Healthcare-Associated versus Community-Acquired Infections

Within the healthcare facility, any occurrence of infection should be evaluated to determine whether the infection was healthcare associated or community acquired. A **community-acquired infection** is an infection that was present in the patient before the patient was admitted to a healthcare facility.

Specific guidelines have been developed to determine whether an infection is healthcare associated or community acquired. For example, if a child was admitted to a hospital with a fever and within 24 hours measles developed, this disease would be considered community acquired. The incubation period for measles is between 10 and 14 days; therefore, it can be determined that the patient's exposure to the disease occurred prior to admission. However, if a patient was admitted for treatment of an intervertebral disk injury and then a urinary tract infection with fever developed several days after undergoing surgery, the infection was probably acquired while the patient was hospitalized. This infection would be classified as an HAI, especially if a urinalysis done prior to surgery did not indicate infection at that time.

Both instances of infectious disease would be tracked and reported to the Performance Improvement and Patient Safety Council and to the required state agency, but for different reasons. The measles would be tracked to document that the facility's staff took appropriate action to prevent exposure and transmission to other patients. The urinary tract infection would be tracked to document initiation of appropriate treatment interventions and to identify any presurgical measures that might be taken to prevent such infections in the future.

It is important to track HAI rates for each area of the facility that works with patients. HAI rates vary greatly depending on the nursing unit and the types of patients for whom care is provided. For example, an organization might look at central line–associated bloodstream infections in the intensive care unit (ICU). Other types of procedures commonly associated with HAIs that should be tracked include the use of indwelling urinary catheters, surgical wounds, and mechanical ventilation devices.

Other possible sources of HAIs include exposure to clinical or nonclinical staff who may carry infectious diseases, substandard surgical or postsurgical care, noncompliance with standard precautions, and improper equipment sterilization techniques. Decubitus ulcers and surgical-site infections are often associated with hospital care.

B: Surveillance of Employee Health and Illness

A different aspect of infection surveillance involves employee health and illness tracking. Employees can bring community-acquired infections into healthcare settings. Policies related to the tracking of employee absences exist for the specific purpose of preventing infection via healthcare workers. Reports of absences are tabulated and examined for any possible connection to HAI cases. Employees who are absent from work for infection-related reasons may be asked to verify their fitness for duty by bringing in a clearance from a treating physician or clinic. Accreditation organization standards generally address employee or patient exposure to infectious diseases. These standards make provisions for screening, assessment, testing, immunization, prophylaxis or treatment, or counseling for patients or staff members who have been exposed to an infectious disease in the hospital.

An additional set of standards for employees requires an influenza (flu) and COVID-19 vaccination program that offers education about the vaccines; nonvaccine control and prevention measures; and the diagnosis, transmission, and impact of influenza. There is a requirement for on-site vaccinations at sites accessible to staff and providers. Part of the performance improvement (PI) aspect of this program is that the facility must evaluate staff vaccination rates and reasons given by staff for declining vaccinations (e.g., a past adverse reaction to the vaccine, religious reasons, or fear of infection developing from the vaccine).

C: Surveillance of the Facility Vaccine Program

The key areas for surveillance are developing and implementing protocols for COVID-19, flu, and pneumococcal vaccine administration and documentation, and implementing a protocol to identify new cases of infection and ways to manage an outbreak. Each state health department must develop its own plan, and each facility's IPC plan must include how it will manage an influx of patients with infectious disease who might need isolation and intensive care.

Most healthcare facilities require employee job descriptions to carry a definition of blood-borne pathogen risk associated with the job tasks. Employees in high-risk categories are required to have hepatitis B vaccinations. Documentation of employees' blood-borne exposures and tracking of the follow-up procedures are other aspects of employee health data collection.

D: Surveillance of the Healthcare Environment

Monitoring the care environment is another aspect of infection surveillance. Facilities with on-site laboratories must meet standards for safety and IPC through a rigorous inspection process since these areas perform very high-risk procedures and deal with infectious body fluids and tissue samples. Most laboratories have to be nationally certified to provide credible services to healthcare facilities. In many facilities, specimens from patient care areas are obtained and cultured monthly to identify any pathological bacteria growing in the care environment (on door knobs, counter surfaces, computer keyboards, and such). These cultures are reported and tracked. When the presence of a significant infectious agent is identified, another specimen is cultured after the area has been cleaned to determine whether the area was sufficiently disinfected.

Many healthcare facilities have a team of providers who regularly inspect all areas in the facility for health and safety issues. The IPC team usually provides someone to assist with identifying potential areas of concern related to IPC, such as patient care rooms, laundry rooms, bathrooms, central supply areas, laboratory areas, the pharmacy, and food service areas. Results from these inspections are reported through the Infection Prevention and Control Committee along with any necessary corrective actions.

E: Surveillance of Food Preparation Areas

The cleanliness of food preparation and service areas is also tracked, and records are kept to document that all local and state regulations regarding safe food-handling procedures are being followed. The training and safety performance of food service staff is also documented. Most food preparation and service areas in facilities must be inspected and certified annually by the state department of health. Records of cleaning are documented daily.

Food temperatures and refrigerator temperatures are tracked daily, as are records of the cleaning of food preparation and service areas. Refrigerators containing medications are kept separate from refrigerators containing food.

Kitchen areas are required to record water temperatures of dishwashing machines. Food that is received must be dated and stored in rodent-proof containers, and a rotating stock is tracked to prevent food spoilage.

The IPC committee approves all substances used for cleaning in the facility. In many facilities, the IPC coordinator conducts monthly environmental rounds to look for areas of noncompliance with standards. The governing body that grants authority for IPC measures in an agency or facility may also review the results of the monthly rounds along with any actions for improvement suggested by the committee.

Step 3: Conduct Educational and Screening Programs

An effective IPC program routinely evaluates all the means of transmission of infection throughout the facility and develops educational programs that promote disease prevention. These programs include tuberculosis testing, handwashing campaigns, influenza vaccination programs, hepatitis B vaccinations for high-risk employees, sterile technique in-services, and needlestick prevention programs. Education on standard precautions is mandatory for all employees in healthcare facilities and frequently occurs before the employee is allowed access to the work environment, to ensure both the employee's and potential patients' safety.

Tracking exposures to blood-borne pathogens such as HIV is required by all states and is outlined in OSHA regulations (OSHA 2024), which require the monitoring of employees after exposure and postexposure prophylaxis treatment if indicated. HIV testing and screening for employees known to have been exposed to HIV require the informed consent of individual employees. OSHA also mandates that specific education on the risks and outcomes of testing be provided to employees by a certified HIV instructor or provider.

When state law requires the facility to report positive test results to the state department of health, the employee involved must be notified ahead of time. Many state departments of health provide programs to test, treat, and educate employees, clients, and patients regarding the HIV and AIDS disease process.

Due to the Health Insurance Portability and Accountability Act of 1996 (HIPAA) regulations, client and patient rights of protection and notification related to infectious diseases have increased. Most states require facilities to outline a tuberculosis prevention plan that involves the careful screening of employees, clients, and patients to identify those who have active tuberculosis as well as those who may have been exposed but do not have an active disease process. State licensing agencies require testing of employees as an occupational safety measure, but testing of patients and clients varies considerably from state to state. Often, the testing of patients and clients is required in long-term rehabilitative settings. The tuberculosis plan for most facilities outlines the testing process; training and education of staff, clients, and patients; and required treatment interventions. In many states, monthly reporting of the number of employees tested and the number of employees who convert to positive is required. A positive tuberculin (TB) test result must be reported to the department of health in all states.

Check Your Understanding 10.1

1. Healthcare organizations conduct regular campaigns and educational sessions for all employees on the proper methods and procedures for working with patients with blood-borne pathogens such as hepatitis or HIV. The procedures that healthcare staff must follow to protect patients and employees from possible exposure to infectious agents are called _____.
   a. Infectious deterrents
   b. Standard measures
   c. Standard precautions
   d. Infectious measures

2. David was admitted to the hospital following an automobile accident in which he suffered a fractured femur. Two days after surgery to repair the fracture, he developed pneumonia and was transferred to the ICU. The pneumonia was not present at the time of admission to the hospital so it is considered a:
   a. Healthcare-associated infection
   b. Hospital sickness
   c. Community-acquired infection
   d. Community sickness

QI Toolbox Technique: Flow Chart

Flow charts are analytical tools used to represent standard functions within processes and to illustrate the sequence of activities in a complex process. Their use allows a PI team to examine the process under investigation from all directions. The technique makes it possible for the team to gather the most important details so everyone on the team can understand the process and its contributing subprocesses in the same way. When a flow chart is well designed, few misconceptions can survive. Following is a discussion of commonly used **icons**, which are graphic symbols used to represent a critical event in a process flow chart:

- **Process icons**: Process icons represent periods in the process when actions are being performed by participants. It is important to break down the actions into their most detailed procedural bundles without adding as much detail as narrative description would include. In Real-Life Example #1 that follows this section, in Becky's first flow chart, the first process icon reads "Nurse triage of patient needs." The concept of triage is represented by the icon, but the description does not specify all the steps that the nurse would have to go through to triage a patient.

- **Decision icons**: Decision icons represent the points in the process at which participants must evaluate the status of the process. Depending on the outcome of the evaluation, the participant performs different subsequent courses of action. For example, in Becky's flow chart, the first decision point asks, "Need urine specimen?" When the triage evaluation returns a response of "No" to that question, the patient waits for their appointment with the physician. When the triage evaluation returns a response of "Yes," then the alternative courses of action to obtain a urine specimen are undertaken.

- **Predefined process icons**: Predefined process icons represent the formal procedures that participants are expected to carry out the same way every time. They are procedures that are formalized in manuals. For example, in Becky's flow chart, one of the first predefined procedures is "Procedure reviewed by lab tech." The use of this icon implies that the manner in which the lab tech explains the procedure to the patient is formalized. The lab tech must perform the explanation in the same way every time.

- **Connector icons**: Connector icons represent points in the flow chart description of the process where the analysis skips to another common point of the process. Connector icons are most often used at the edges of a page, where there is insufficient space for continuation of the description. For example, in Becky's flow chart (see figure 10.2), a connector icon follows the process icon labeled "Wait for physician." The icon is labeled "1." Review of figure 10.3 reveals another connector icon labeled "1." At that point, the physician's process continues. Farther down in figure 10.2, two icons are labeled "2." Both of these icons refer to the continuation of the path of the flow chart in figure 10.4.

- **Start/end icons**: Start/end icons mark the start or end of a process. For example, in Becky's flow chart (see figure 10.3), when no urine specimen is needed, the patient leaves the clinic after seeing the physician. The process ends there.

- **Manual input icons**: Manual input icons represent points in the flow chart description of the process where the participants must record data in paper-based or computer-based formats. For example, Becky's flow chart (see figure 10.5) includes a manual input icon labeled "Document UA results in patient record." The subprocess represented by the manual input icon follows the dipstick analysis performed in the clinic by either a nurse or a member of the house staff. When the clinician performing the dipstick analysis does not find blood, bacteria, or white blood cells (WBC) in the specimen, the analysis is complete, the findings are documented and then communicated to the physician.

- **Line connector icons**: Line connector icons direct the flow of processes from one step to another from decision points to subprocesses.

Real-Life Example #1

Becky is an RN working as the nurse manager of the outpatient clinics at Western States University Hospital. She was responsible for managing PI activities in the clinics, facilitating PI teams, and supporting PI activities with the various resources available to her. At that time, the medical center had recently embarked on a benchmarking program. Recall that Benchmarking is the systematic comparison of one organization's outcomes or processes with the outcomes or processes of similar organizations.

Becky and some of her colleagues began the benchmarking process by comparing the outcomes of the clinic's patients with published information on the outcomes of other organizations and with clinical trends apparent in the literature. In the course of examining pharmacy and therapeutics data, Becky and her clinical colleagues recognized that their organization appeared to be treating a significantly higher number of urinary tract infections (UTIs) than other, similar organizations. To identify the reason for the apparent discrepancy, the team first examined the published literature on the frequency of UTIs in ambulatory care practice. Next, they contacted clinicians at other ambulatory care centers in the country to gather information on their experiences. The team's investigations confirmed that, although the sex-specific distribution of the incidence of UTI was similar to other institutions (mostly occurring in females), the overall incidence was significantly higher at Western States University Hospital than at any of the other medical centers contacted. The situation appeared to provide an excellent PI opportunity—the kind of improvement that clinicians would see as important and valuable to patients as well as one that had important cost implications for the organization.

Becky convened a PI team, which included the director of the outpatient pharmacy, the director of the outpatient clinic laboratories, and leaders of the nursing teams from each of the ambulatory clinics in which patients with UTIs were commonly treated: internal medicine, family practice, obstetrics and gynecology, urology, general surgery, and pediatrics.

The team's initial discussion of the situation revealed the complexity of the processes in place to evaluate urinary tract function. Because the clinics are affiliated with a major university medical center, a number of caregivers might be involved in any one patient's care. First, there were providers from a variety of specialties and areas of expertise. Next, there were the nurses and medical assistants in each clinic. Because the medical center was a teaching facility, there also were house staff members rotating through the clinics on a monthly basis. Finally, there were the technicians who performed urinalysis procedures in the clinical laboratory. Where, when, and by whom a patient's urinalysis was performed could take any one of a number of paths in the organization.

Becky and her colleagues decided to develop flow charts for the various care paths. (See figures 10.2 through 10.6.) They collected data on the outcomes of each of the paths to see whether they could identify the organization's true experience with UTIs.

Figure 10.2. Example of a flow chart—page 1

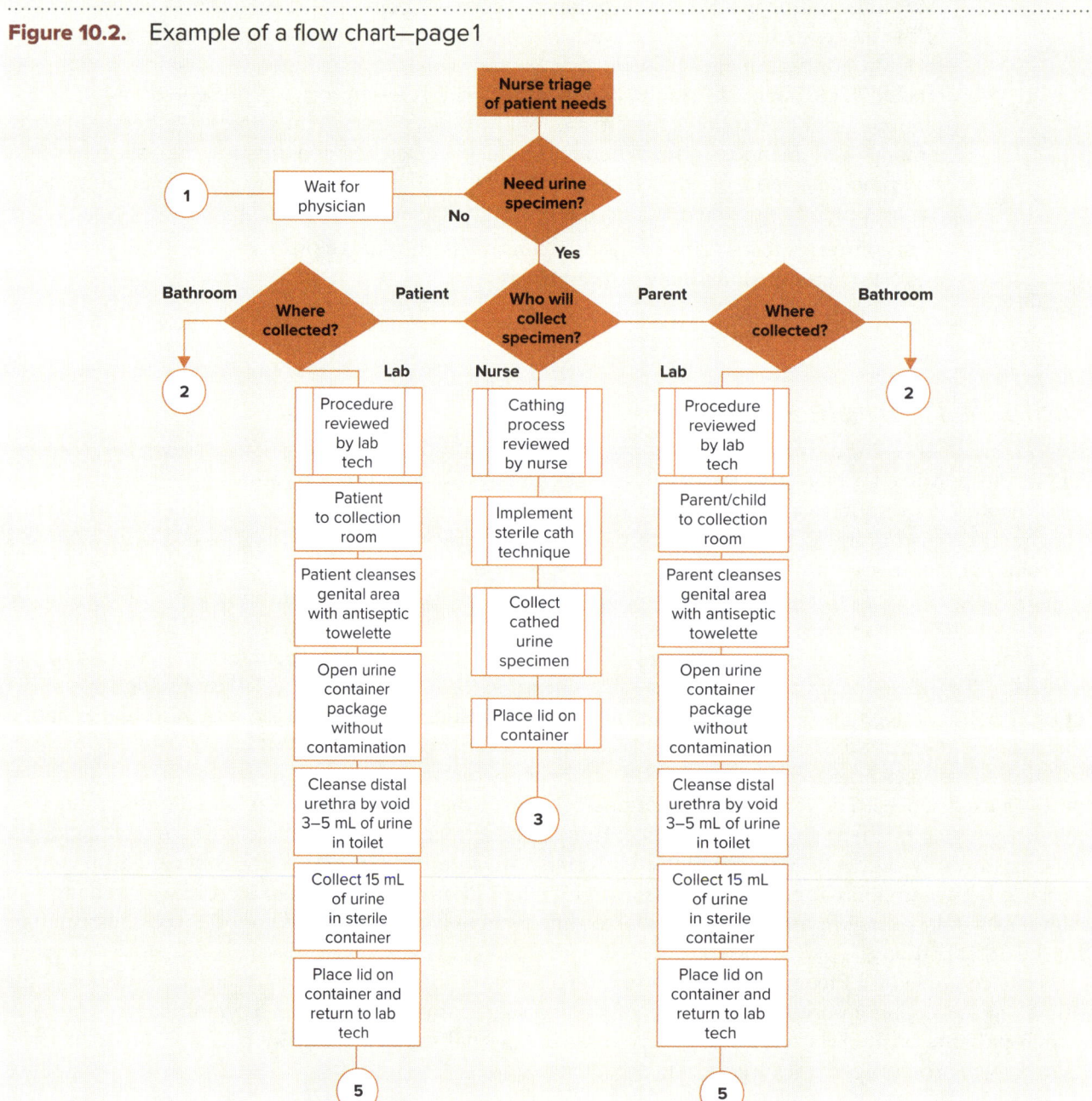

Figure 10.3. Example of a flow chart—page 2

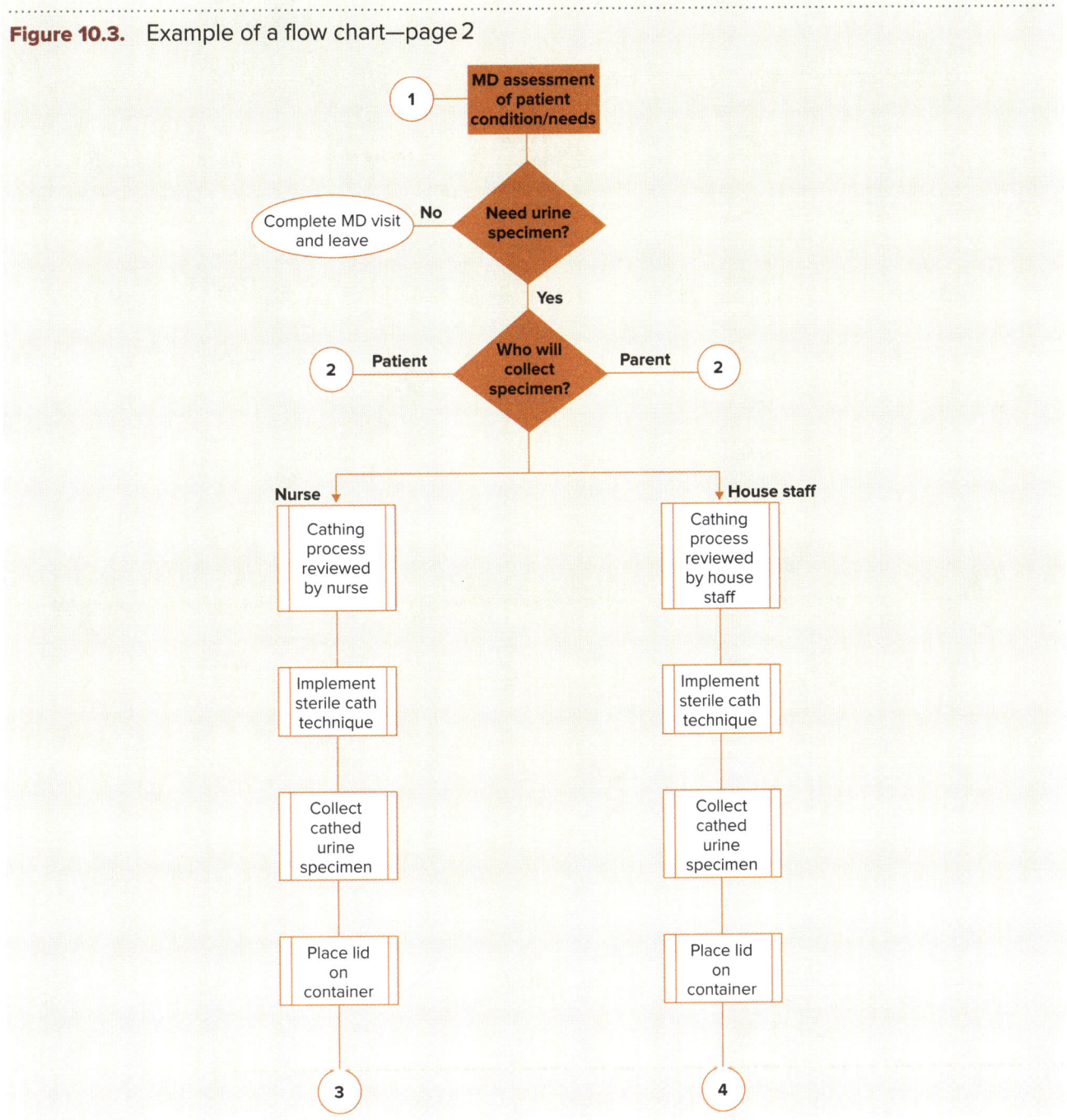

Figure 10.4. Example of a flow chart—page 3

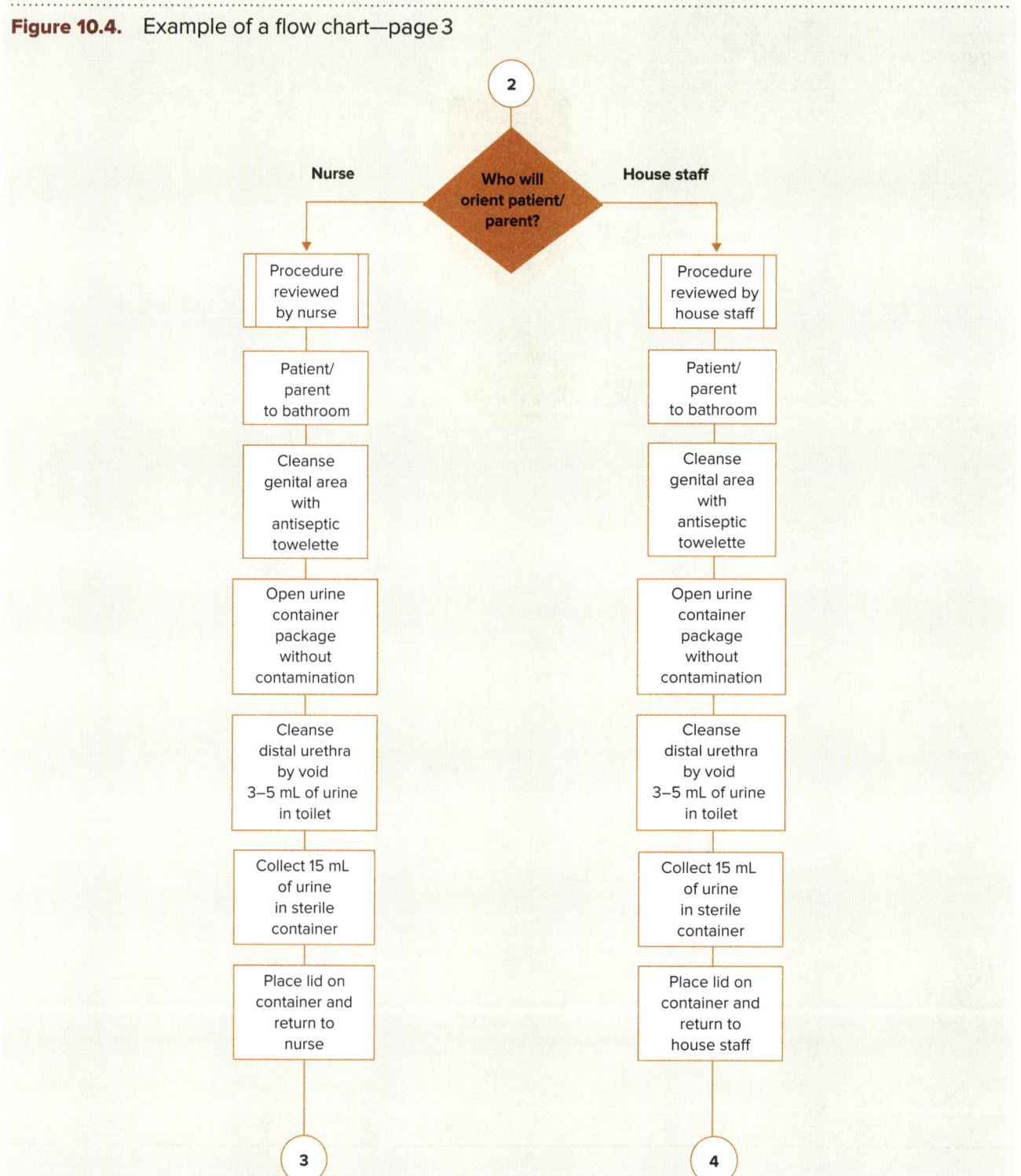

Managing Infectious Disease: Steps to Success 175

Figure 10.5. Example of a flow chart—page 4

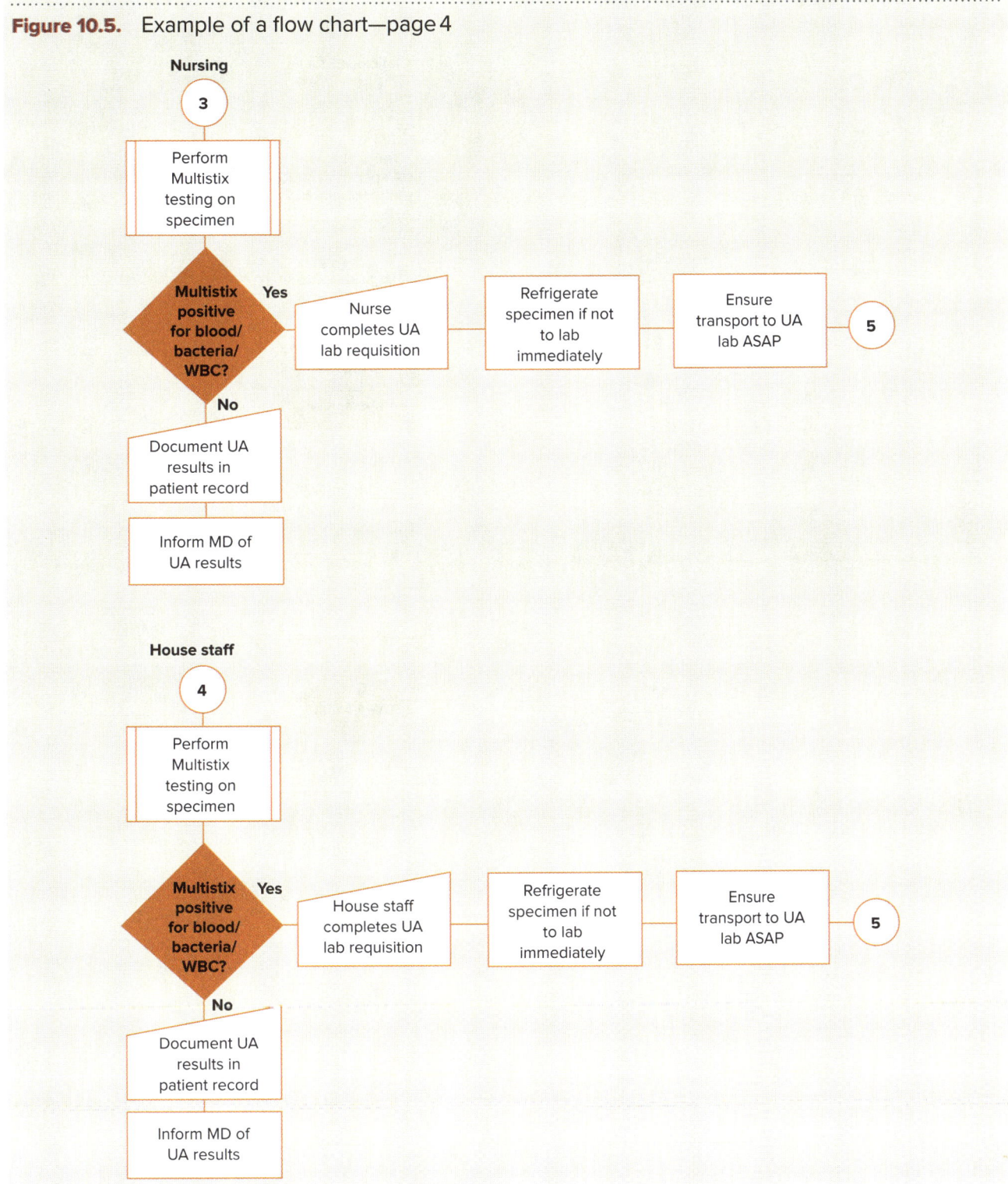

Figure 10.6. Example of a flow chart—page 5

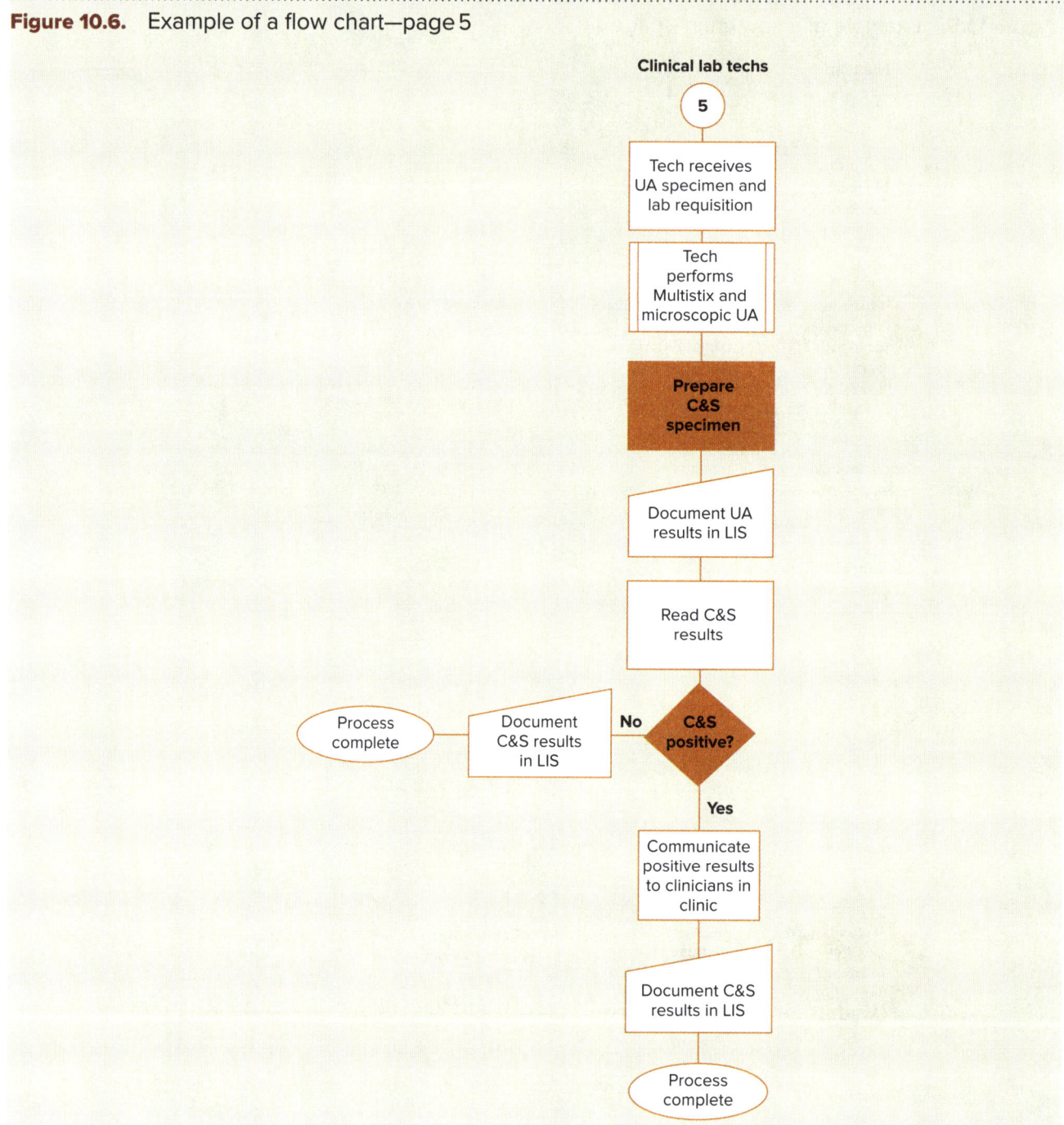

Real-Life Example #2

University Hospital is a Level 1 Trauma Center serving a large urban area and the surrounding urban counties and neighboring states. This large medical center had placed an increased emphasis on tracking and reducing the rates of hospital-acquired infections (HAIs). During the three years prior to the COVID-19 pandemic, the facility realized an average reduction of 2 percent in respiratory and 1 percent in bloodstream infections. In 2020, the hospital began to experience surges in admissions related to COVID-19. This increase in patient load challenged the hospital infrastructure not only because of volume but also because of the complexity of the patients being admitted. It became necessary to expand the intensive care units (ICU) into spaces that were not designed for that purpose. Based on the increased patient volume, the hospital had to reassign staff to the ICUs and also bring in contracted healthcare staff to the units. The hospital continued to track quality patient care indicators including infection rates. During the first three months of the pandemic surge, the hospital experienced a 12 percent increase in bloodstream HAIs along with a 25 percent increase in respiratory HAIs. The facility IPC team quickly conducted a root cause analysis and identified several issues that needed to be quickly addressed. First, the physical rooms being used for the ICU expansion did not allow for proper negative pressure ventilation. Second, because of the acuity of the patients, fatigue of the clinical staff, and adding clinical staff from outside the unit, the established bloodstream infection control protocols were not being followed appropriately. Finally, it was found that because of supply chain shortages, personal protective equipment such as masks and gowns were not being changed between patients. Using the root cause analysis findings, the IPC team addressed the issues in an effort to reduce the number of HAIs and bloodstream infections.

Case Study

The case study for this chapter is a continuation of Becky's investigation of the UTI issue in the ambulatory clinics of Western States University Hospital.

After flowcharting the process for collecting urine specimens (depicted in figures 10.2 through 10.6), Becky and her colleagues recognized how complex the issue was within their organization. They decided to collect data from all process paths evident in the flow chart. Because so many people were involved in the processes and because significant delays could be involved, they also began to wonder what role contaminated specimens played in the situation.

Although it was an expensive project, the team designed an investigative study to collect data. Urine specimens were routinely tested by nursing personnel or house staff in the clinic to determine each specimen's pH and specific gravity and to classify each specimen according to its color, clarity, and presence of gross hematuria. Each specimen was then tested with Multistix to determine whether microscopic bacteria, red blood cells (RBCs), or white blood cells (WBCs) were present. When a specimen failed any of the Multistix screens, it was referred to the laboratory for microscopic analysis, culture, and sensitivity analysis by a laboratory technician.

First, the team collected data regarding time elapsed between collection of the specimen, point-of-care testing with Multistix, and receipt of the specimen in laboratory. In addition, the team investigated the sequence of events that occurred in the interim. A summary of the data collected is provided in table 10.1.

Table 10.1. Average time to point-of-care screening with confidence intervals (in minutes)

Point-of-Care Training & Processing	Internal Medicine Clinic	Pediatrics Clinic	General Surgery Clinic	Orthopedic Surgery Clinic	Obstetrics Clinic	Gynecology Clinic	Specialty Clinic
Nurse	5.0 (4.0, 6.0)	4.25 (3.0, 5.5)	6.25 (5.0, 7.5)	6.0 (5.0, 7.0)	3.25 (2.75, 3.75)	3.0 (2.0, 4.0)	3.0 (2.0, 4.0)
House staff	10.0 (7.0, 13.0)	8.0 (6.0, 10.0)	12.13 (10.0, 14.25)	11.0 (9.0, 13.0)	6.5 (4.0, 9.0)	6.0 (4.0, 8.0)	7.5 (5.5, 9.5)

Second, on a temporary and random basis, the team obtained urine specimens from each clinic immediately following collection and had a complete analysis performed STAT in the clinic labs. This analysis identified pH, specific gravity, color, clarity, cell counts, and bacterial counts almost immediately after the specimen was delivered by the patient or collecting clinician. All specimens that showed microscopic bacteria either on Multistix or on microscopic analysis were cultured. A summary of the data collected is provided in table 10.2.

Table 10.2. Random STAT processing of clean-catch/cath urine specimens (percentage of positive specimens for culture)

Collector	Internal Medicine Clinic	Pediatrics Clinic	General Surgery Clinic	Orthopedic Surgery Clinic	Obstetrics Clinic	Gynecology Clinic	Specialty Clinic
Nurse or patient	5.6	13.2	4.2	3.4	7.0	3.9	5.7
House staff or patient	4.2	12.1	3.4	5.2	6.8	4.2	6.2
Parent	—	27.5	11.7	9.0	—	25.2	—

Third, the team compared the incidence of UTI identified in the randomly collected specimens with the incidence identified in specimens going through the usual process. A summary of the data collected is provided in table 10.3.

Table 10.3. Routine processing of clean-catch/cath specimens (percentage of positive specimens for culture)

Collector	Internal Medicine Clinic	Pediatrics Clinic	General Surgery Clinic	Orthopedic Surgery Clinic	Obstetrics Clinic	Gynecology Clinic	Specialty Clinic
Nurse or patient	5.7	12.4	5.1	4.1	7.2	4.1	5.2
House staff or patient	36.8	25.6	10.2	8.7	10.0	9.2	14.2
Parent	—	25.6	12.2	8.0	—	23.0	—

Case Study Questions

1. Upon examination of the data sets, Becky and her colleagues identified several areas where the analysis revealed situations that were probably contributing to the clinic's high UTI rate. Look at the UTI rate for children whose parents had collected the specimen versus the rate for children who had been catheterized by nursing personnel to collect the specimen. What might be the reason for the higher rate in children whose parents had collected the specimen?

2. Are there any other areas in the data that reveal important aspects that may be contributing to the high UTI rates? Suggest some possible reasons for these higher rates?

3. Upon discussion of the findings and examination of the flowcharted processes, the laboratory manager noted a subtle change in clinic processes that probably was contributing to the problem. House staff had begun at some point to Multistix the specimens in the original collection containers. Thus, what had been a clean-catch specimen could become a contaminated specimen when staff opened the container to perform the Multistix. What should have been done was to pour off a small amount or *aliquot* of the specimen into another container, reseal the original container for the laboratory, and perform the Multistix on the aliquot container. This process would minimize the possibility of contaminating the original specimen. How would this change in process be represented in the flow charts presented in the case study?

Review Questions

1. Defend why healthcare organizations require their staff to have certain vaccinations to be employed at the facility.

2. This decision icon symbol is used in flowcharting to indicate _____.

   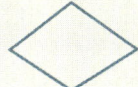

   a. a process in which actions are being performed by humans
   b. a point in the process at which participants must evaluate the status of the process
   c. formal procedures that participants are expected to carry out the same way every time
   d. a point in the process in which participants must record data in paper-based or computer-based formats

3. A patient was admitted with cough, fever, and shortness of breath through the emergency department. On day two, laboratory results confirmed the presence of bacteria in the sputum culture, and the physician documented a diagnosis of bacterial pneumonia. Based on this information, is the bacterial pneumonia a healthcare-associated infection or a community-acquired infection?

4. Which QI Toolbox Technique allows a PI team to examine the process under investigation from all directions?
   a. Cause-and-effect diagram
   b. Affinity diagram
   c. Flow chart
   d. Critical pathway

5. List the governmental organizations and federal law(s) that provide regulations in infection control. Describe how these regulations influence the healthcare facility's processes and activities regarding infection control (programs, policies, procedures).

References

CDC (Centers for Disease Control and Prevention). 2024. "HAIs: Reports and Data." https://www.cdc.gov/healthcare-associated-infections/php/data/index.html.

Forrester, J.D., P. M. Maggio, and L. Tennakoon. 2022. Cost of healthcare-associated infections in the United States." *Journal of Patient Safety* 18(2): e477–479, https://doi.org/10.1097/PTS.0000000000000845.

Joint Commission. 2024a. "National Patient Safety Goals." In *Hospital Accreditation Standards*. Oakbrook Terrace, IL: Joint Commission Resources.

Nelson, R. E, K. M. Hatfield, H. Wolford, M. H. Samore, R. D. Scott, S. C. Reddy, B. Olubajo, P. Paul, J. A. Jernigan, and J. Baggs. 2021. National estimates of healthcare costs associated with multidrug-resistant bacterial infections among hospitalized patients in the United States. *Clinical Infectious Diseases* 72 (Supplement_1): S17–26, https://doi.org/10.1093/cid/ciaa1581.

OSHA (Occupational Safety and Health Administration). 2024. "Standard 1910.1030: Bloodborne Pathogens." https://www.osha.gov/laws-regs/regulations/standardnumber/1910/1910.1030.

Utah Department of Health. 2023. "Utah Reportable Diseases." https://epi.utah.gov/wp-content/uploads/Rpt_Disease_List.pdf.

Resources

CDC (Centers for Disease Control and Prevention). 2024. "When and How to Wash Your Hands." https://www.cdc.gov/clean-hands/about/?CDC_AAref_Val=https://www.cdc.gov/handwashing/when-how-handwashing.html.

CDC (Centers for Disease Control and Prevention). 2024. "Infection Control: Transmission-Based Precautions." https://www.cdc.gov/infection-control/hcp/basics/transmission-based-precautions.html.

Joint Commission. 2024b. "Infection Prevention and Control." In *Hospital Accreditation Standards*. Oakbrook Terrace, IL: Joint Commission Resources.

Managing Risk Exposure

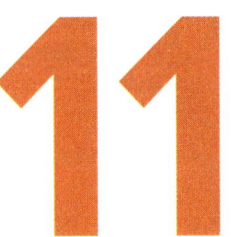

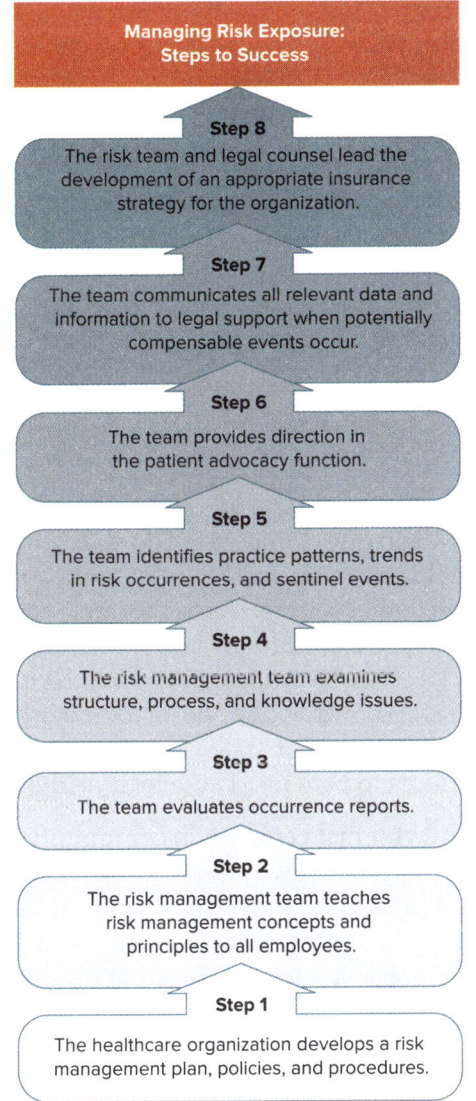

Managing Risk Exposure: Steps to Success

Step 8 — The risk team and legal counsel lead the development of an appropriate insurance strategy for the organization.

Step 7 — The team communicates all relevant data and information to legal support when potentially compensable events occur.

Step 6 — The team provides direction in the patient advocacy function.

Step 5 — The team identifies practice patterns, trends in risk occurrences, and sentinel events.

Step 4 — The risk management team examines structure, process, and knowledge issues.

Step 3 — The team evaluates occurrence reports.

Step 2 — The risk management team teaches risk management concepts and principles to all employees.

Step 1 — The healthcare organization develops a risk management plan, policies, and procedures.

Learning Objectives

- Assess the importance of managing risk exposure in today's healthcare organization
- Analyze the importance of using occurrence reporting to decrease risk exposure
- Describe how sentinel events can point to important opportunities to improve safety in healthcare organizations
- Explain how risk managers use their skills in patient advocacy to lessen the impact that potentially compensable events can have on healthcare organizations
- Evaluate the importance of the National Patient Safety Goals (NPSGs) for healthcare organizations and strategies for proactive risk-reduction activities

Key Terms

Cause-and-effect diagram
Medication error
National Patient Safety Goals (NPSGs)
Near misses
Occurrence report
Patient advocacy
Potentially compensable events (PCEs)
Risk
Risk manager
Root-cause analysis (RCA)

It is important to recognize that patients, residents, and clients have very special relationships with the healthcare organizations that provide their healthcare services. Those relationships are built on a set of mutual and very complex expectations, which, when not valued by either participant in the relationship, can lead to unanticipated negative occurrences that neither really desires. For patients, residents, and clients, the expectations are based on a set of rights that are willingly accorded by healthcare organizations with ethics-based practices and that have become codified by federal mandates for most US healthcare organizations.

Patient Rights

An example of the rights commonly accorded in acute-care settings can be found in figure 11.1. Patients also have responsibilities related to their care, which are addressed throughout the figure. Note that the list includes the majority of important issues that acute-care patients and their families need to be aware of when they accept care from providers in that setting. The rights are intended to educate patients and family members and to help them frame realistic expectations of the organization and its providers. In addition, they help providers remember to focus on their responsibilities that form the common basis of the provider–patient relationship in the US. Figure 11.2 shows an example of a resident's rights for a skilled nursing facility.

Other rights existing in the relationship are not stated in the federal mandate but are implicit when an organization provides healthcare services to patients. These include the following assertions:

- That care is provided concurrent with that common in community practice
- That all providers employed by or affiliated with the organization are credentialed, licensed, or certified as required by common practice or state licensing laws
- That the basic intent and vision of the organization is to effect outcomes deemed positive for patients, residents, or clients through the care processes employed in the organization

For the most part, these expectations are met. However, sometimes this is not the case. The risk of unanticipated negative occurrences is inherent in noncompliance with any of the issues discussed in this section or listed in figures 11.1 and 11.2.

Figure 11.1A. Example of patient rights and responsibilities from the Veterans Health Administration (VA)

1. Nondiscrimination and Respect
- You will be treated with dignity, compassion, and respect as an individual. Consistent with Federal law, VA policy, and accreditation standards of The Joint Commission, you will not be subject to discrimination for any reason, including for reasons of age, race, ethnicity, religion, culture, language, physical or mental disability, socioeconomic status, sex, sexual orientation, or gender identity or expression.
- You will receive care in a safe environment free from excess noise, and with sufficient light to ensure comfort and safety.
- You have a right to have access to the outdoors.
- We will seek to honor your cultural and personal values, beliefs, and preferences. We ask that you identify any cultural, religious, or spiritual beliefs or practices that influence your care.
- You or someone you choose has the right to keep and spend your money. You have the right to receive an accounting of any funds that VA is holding for you.
- We will respect your personal freedoms in the care and treatment we provide you. This includes trying to accommodate your normal sleep and wake cycles, food likes and dislikes, and other personal preferences.
- In the Community Living Center (CLC), you have the right to be free from chemical and physical restraints. In the inpatient acute care setting, and only in rare cases, the use of chemical and physical restraints may be used if all other efforts to keep you or others free from harm have not worked.
- In the Community Living Center (CLC), you may keep personal items and are expected to wear your own clothes. As an inpatient, you may wear your own clothes depending on your medical condition.
- You have the right to keep and use personal items as long as they are safe and legal.
- You have the right to social interaction and regular exercise. You will have the opportunity for religious worship and spiritual support. You may decide whether to participate in these activities. You may decide whether or not to perform tasks in or for the Medical Center or in the Community Living Center (CLC).
- You have the right to communicate freely and privately. You will have access to public telephones and VA will assist you in sending and receiving mail. You may participate in civic rights, such as voting and free speech.
- When a loved one is involved in support and care of a VA patient or CLC resident, VA considers a patient or CLC resident's family to include anyone related to the patient or CLC resident in any way (for example, biologically or legally) and anyone whom the patient or CLC resident considers to be family. If you are an inpatient, any persons you choose can be with you to support you during your stay. Medical staff may restrict visitors for inpatients if medical or safety concerns require it. You will be told promptly about any visitor restriction and the reason for it.
- In order to provide a safe treatment environment for all patients or CLC residents and staff, you and your visitors are expected to avoid unsafe acts that place others at risk for accidents or injuries. Please immediately report any condition you believe to be unsafe.

2. Health Information and Privacy
- Your privacy will be protected.
- You will be given information about the health benefits you can receive. The information will be provided in a way you can understand.
- You will receive information about the costs of your care (for example, co-payments), if any, before you are treated. You are responsible for paying your portion of any costs associated with your care.
- Your health record will be kept confidential. Information about you will not be released without your authorization unless permitted by law (an example of this is state public health reporting). You have the right to have access to or request a copy of your own health records.
- Please respect the privacy of other patients and CLC residents and do not reveal their health information that you may overhear or otherwise become aware of.

3. Partnering in Care
- You have a right to express your preferences concerning future medical care in an advance directive, including designating a health care agent to make health care decisions on your behalf when you can no longer do so.
- You, and any person(s) you choose, will be involved in all decisions about your care. You will be given information you can understand about the benefits and risks of treatment in your preferred language. You will be given other options. You can agree to or refuse any treatment. You will be told what is likely to happen to you if you refuse a treatment.
- Refusing a treatment will not affect your rights to future care but you take responsibility for the impact this decision may have on your health.
- Tell your provider about your current condition, medicines (including over-the-counter and herbals), and medical history. Also, share any other information that affects your health. You should ask questions when you do not understand something about your care. This will help us provide you the best care possible.

Figure 11.1B. Example of patient rights and responsibilities from the Veterans Health Administration (VA) (*Continued*)

- You will be given, in writing, the name and title of the provider in charge of your care. You have the right to be involved in choosing your provider. You also have the right to know the names and titles of those who provide you care. This includes students and other trainees. Providers will properly introduce themselves when they take part in your care.
- You will be educated about your role and responsibilities as a patient or CLC resident. This includes your participation in decision making and care at the end of life.
- If you believe you cannot follow the treatment plan, you have a responsibility to tell your provider or treatment team.
- You will be informed of all outcomes of your care, including any possible injuries associated with your care. You will be informed about how to request compensation and other remedies for any serious injuries.
- You have the right to have your pain assessed and to receive treatment to manage your pain. You and your treatment team will develop a pain management plan together. You are expected to help the treatment team by telling them if you have pain and if the treatment is working.
- As an inpatient or CLC resident, you will be provided any transportation necessary for your treatment plan.
- You have the right to choose whether or not you will participate in any research project. Any research will be clearly identified. Potential risks of the research will be identified and there will be no pressure on you to participate.
- You will be included in resolving any ethical issues about your care. If you have ethical issues or concerns, you may speak with the Medical Center's Ethics Consultation Service for help.

4. Concerns or Complaints

- You are encouraged and expected to seek help from your treatment team or a patient advocate if you have problems or complaints. Any privacy complaints will be addressed by the facility Privacy Officer. You will be given understandable information about the complaint process in your preferred language. You may complain verbally or in writing, without fear of retaliation.
- Your complaint, once received, will be provided to the identified department for review by a health care professional who may contact you to better understand your concern or ask clarifying questions. After the concern is understood, someone from the identified department will contact you to provide the final resolution.
- If you believe you or your family member has been neglected, abused, or exploited by VA staff, please report this promptly to the treatment team or patient advocate. You will receive help immediately.
- If you believe the organization has failed to address your concerns about health care quality and safety or suspected criminal activities, fraud, waste, abuse, or mismanagement, you may contact the VA Office of the Inspector General at 1-800-488-8244. For more information, visit va.gov/oig/hotline/.
- If you believe the organization has failed to address or satisfy your concerns about health care quality and safety, you may contact the Joint Commission's Office of Quality Monitoring at 1-800-994-6610. This does not apply to CLC Residents.

5. Additional Rights and Responsibilities of Community Living Center Residents

Because the CLC serves as your home for short or long-stay services, you have the following additional rights and responsibilities as a CLC resident:

- Staff will knock on your bedroom door prior to entry.
- You have the right to receive care from the same staff member every day to the extent that consistent assignment is possible.
- You may have visitors at any time of the day or night provided visitors are respectful of you, your need for privacy and the privacy of others. You may refuse visitors at any time.
- You have a right to consensual sexual activity and you have a right to privacy during those visits.
- Your care will be delivered in a setting that resembles home. Therefore, you will be invited to have your meals in a designated dining area and you will have access to those activities that contribute to meaningful use of time.
- In preparation for being discharged to your own home, you and/or your caregiver may be invited to participate in activities that prepare you to go home such as self-administration of medications and treatments.
- You and your caregivers have a right to attend treatment planning meetings and participate in household or resident council.

Source: Adapted from Veterans Health Administration 2023

Figure 11.2. Skilled nursing facility rights

As a resident of a skilled nursing facility (SNF), you have certain rights and protections under federal and state law. The SNF must provide you with a written description of your legal rights. By federal law, SNF residents have these rights:

- Freedom from discrimination—SNFs do not have to accept all applicants, but they must comply with Civil Rights laws that don't allow discrimination based on these: Race, Color, National origin, Disability, Age, Religion under certain conditions.
- Respect—You have the right to be treated with dignity and respect. You have the right to choose the activities you want to go to and make your own schedule. As long as it fits your care plan, you have the right to make your own schedule, including when you go to bed, rise in the morning, and eat your meals.
- Freedom from abuse and neglect—You have the right to be free from verbal, sexual, physical, and mental abuse, involuntary seclusion, and misappropriation of your property by anyone.
- Freedom from restraints— Physical restraints are any manual method or physical or mechanical device, material, or equipment attached to or near your body so that you can't remove the restraint easily. Physical restraints prevent freedom of movement or normal access to one's own body. A chemical restraint is a drug that's used for discipline or convenience and isn't needed to treat your medical symptoms. It's against the law for a SNF to use physical or chemical restraints, unless it's necessary to treat your medical symptoms. Restraints may not be used to punish or for the convenience of the SNF staff. You have the right to refuse restraint use except if you're at risk of harming yourself or others.
- Information on services and fees—You must be informed in writing about services and fees before you move into the SNF. The SNF cannot require a minimum entrance fee as a condition of residence.
- Money—You have the right to manage your own money or choose someone you trust to do this for you. If you designate the SNF to manage your money, it must meet specific terms when doing so.
- Privacy, property, and living arrangements—You have the right to privacy and to keep and use your personal belongings and property as long as they do not interfere with the rights, health, or safety of others.
- Medical care—You have the right to be informed about your medical condition, medications, and to see your own doctor.
- Visitors—You have the right to spend private time with visitors at any reasonable hour.
- Social services—The SNF must provide you with any needed medically related social services, including counseling, help solving problems with other residents, help in contacting legal and financial professionals, and discharge planning.
- Complaints—You have the right to make a complaint to the staff of the SNF, or any other person, without fear of punishment. The SNF must resolve the issue promptly.
- Protection against unfair transfer or discharge—You cannot be sent to another SNF or made to leave the SNF except in certain situations, including significant changes in your health status and failure to pay for services you are responsible for.
- Your family and friends—Your family members and legal guardians may meet with the families of other residents, participate in family councils, and help make sure you get good-quality care.

Source: Adapted from CMS n.d.a

Risk

The very nature of healthcare organizations makes them susceptible to risk. **Risk** is defined as an exposure to the chance of injury or financial loss and its associated liability. Claims associated with risk result from physical or psychological incidents that may adversely affect patients, visitors, or employees. Every day, employees in healthcare organizations work with equipment and substances that are dangerous even when used appropriately. Clinical laboratories perform analyses using chemicals that can cause burns. Radiological instruments deliver high doses of radiation. Hospital pharmacies package and deliver medications that may be harmful to patients when not administered precisely or in the correct dosages. Those involved in patient care are surrounded by numerous conditions and situations that could potentially cause injury.

Patients may also contribute to their own health risks through noncompliance with basic good-health practices. They may continue to smoke or overeat in spite of education about these risks to health. Some patients in the hospital setting may refuse to wait for assistance before getting out of bed to use the bathroom, or they may refuse to sleep with side rails on their beds and risk dangerous falls. Patients' personal belongings may disappear due to theft or negligence. Confused or sedated patients may pull out their own intravenous lines and expose nursing staff to blood-borne pathogens.

Patient care settings are places of complex and intense interactions that carry many potential opportunities for injury to patients, staff, and visitors. There also are the unintended consequences of treatment. Patients do not always respond to therapy as planned. The surgeon's knife sometimes nicks contiguous structures. The possibility of unintended injury is everywhere in healthcare organizations.

In 1999, the Institute of Medicine (IOM) published a landmark report on medical errors in healthcare titled *To Err Is Human: Building a Safer Health System*, which sent shock waves through the American healthcare industry. The IOM reported that "at least 44,000 [people], and perhaps as many as 98,000 [people], die in hospitals each year as a result of medical errors" that could have been prevented (Kohn et al. 1999, 26).

As a result of the IOM's report, both the government and the private sector increased their focus on safety issues in healthcare. The Clinton administration issued an executive order instructing government agencies that conduct or oversee healthcare programs to create a task force to find new strategies for reducing errors, and Congress appropriated $50 million to support efforts targeted at reducing medical errors. In response to these initiatives, the Patient Safety Improvement Act of 2003 was introduced to create a new system for voluntary reporting of medical errors. President George W. Bush signed into law the Patient Safety and Quality Improvement Act of 2005. The focus of the act was to provide federal protection across healthcare settings to promote cultures of safety by encouraging thorough reviews of errors and by developing effective solutions to prevent their recurrence. This act provided full federal privilege to patient safety information that is sent to a patient safety organization. There are many patient safety organizations, each with its own specific focus on creating better, safer healthcare. The act was designed to make healthcare information available to resources that can help develop and implement changes in processes that will reduce medical errors and save lives. In addition, state licensing agencies mandate that healthcare organizations report adverse medical events that result in death and serious harm.

In the private sector, businesses buying insurance coverage for their employees are encouraged to make safety a prime concern in their contracting decisions. Patients and their families are urged to take a proactive role in reducing medical errors by participating in safety initiatives established by healthcare providers.

In this atmosphere of complexity, danger, chance, and emotion, risk managers work to accomplish their professional objectives. The **risk manager** seeks to manage an organization's risk exposure and improve processes so the threat of injury and its associated liability is minimized. Occurrences involving liability for injury or property loss are called **potentially compensable events (PCEs)**.

Patients and clients come to healthcare facilities expecting improved physical and emotional health benefits for themselves and their family members. Employees come to work intending to provide the best quality healthcare they can deliver. Because most people come to the healthcare setting with the best intentions, negative occurrences can result in anger and guilt. Generally, faulty systems, ineffective processes, and conditions that lead healthcare employees to make mistakes or fail to prevent them cause errors. Such occurrences present healthcare organizations with opportunities for reducing errors and improving patient safety. The cornerstone of patient safety for healthcare organizations is to foster an environment that acknowledges the unintentional nature of human error and emphasizes how organizations can learn from their mistakes.

 Check Your Understanding 11.1

1. Katie is having abdominal pain and presents to the emergency department for treatment. While there, several procedures are performed, including imaging and laboratory testing. It is determined that Katie has appendicitis and she is transferred to the operating room for surgery. Due to her comorbidities, and the fact that her appendix ruptures prior to surgery, Katie spends two days in the hospital as an inpatient before being released. During this time, she receives treatment from numerous healthcare professionals. Describe the risks Katie may be exposed to during this hospitalization.

2. Describe the impact of the landmark study *To Err is Human* both in terms of awareness of medical errors and the increased focus on quality.

Managing Risk Exposure: Steps to Success

Most people think of risk management as the process of working through a malpractice suit. Although that is sometimes the case, risk managers are more often trying to identify organizational conditions that increase risk exposure *before* any injury occurs. Identification before injury allows the organization to be proactive in improving care processes prior to incurring the exposure.

Most healthcare organizations use an incident or occurrence reporting system to collect and report data. The system is set up to track all types of incidents and rate them anywhere from "near miss" and "no harm" to "severe harm or death." This performance improvement (PI) process is reported regularly to both the leadership team and the governing board. There is usually an assigned risk manager or team, depending on the size of the organization. This team is involved in investigating incidents and is usually directed by legal support from the healthcare facility or a contracted agency. Some risk management teams also participate in the patient advocacy program. They help track patient grievances and many times act as an intermediary between the patient and the organization to resolve conflicts that, if left unaddressed, could lead to legal issues. The goal of the risk management team is to spot patterns in incidents and, through an intense investigative process, identify problems or concerns. They work through the PI council to address the patterns and problems identified and develop interventions to resolve the problems.

Healthcare organizations' patient safety programs must include proactive error reduction activities to meet accreditation criteria. This means that healthcare organizations must identify and address underlying system problems that may result in adverse patient incidents. Healthcare organizations are integrating these proactive error reduction activities into their PI plans and goals. All healthcare settings are required to identify high-risk processes in which a failure of some type could jeopardize the safety of individuals to whom they provide services.

The Joint Commission defines a *sentinel event* as "a patient safety event (not primarily related to the natural course of the patient's illness or underlying condition) that reaches a patient and results in death, severe harm (regardless of duration of harm), or permanent harm (regardless of duration of harm). Sentinel events are a subcategory of adverse events" (Joint Commission 2024a, GL-38). A sentinel event includes any process variation for which a recurrence would carry a significant chance of a serious adverse outcome. Such events are called "sentinel" because they signal the need for immediate investigation and response. Examples of sentinel events include infant abduction from the nursery or a foreign body left in a patient after surgery.

An organization should include near misses in its definition of events that require intense investigation. **Near misses** include occurrences that do not necessarily affect an outcome, but if they were to recur they would carry significant chance of being a serious adverse event. Near misses are considered patient safety events and should be investigated by the healthcare organization. Near misses are a valuable tool for evaluation of processes and procedures, especially in high-risk or high-volume areas of facilities.

The Joint Commission established a Sentinel Event Alert notification and maintains a list of reported events in its Sentinel Event Database. This database includes detailed information on high-risk issues such as high-alert medication and bedrail-associated deaths and injuries, in addition to the occurrences noted previously. (A complete list is available on the Joint Commission website.) The website includes a detailed assessment of the problems, along with recommendations for changes to be implemented to prevent a sentinel event (Joint Commission 2024b).

Other initiatives related to patient safety and proactive error reduction include the Joint Commission's **National Patient Safety Goals (NPSGs)**. In 2003, the Joint Commission established six goals to help accredited organizations address specific areas of concern in relation to patient safety. The Sentinel Event Advisory Group determined these goals from the Sentinel Event Alerts. Each year, the goals are reevaluated and published for survey activities by midyear. Since 2009, the NPSGs have been accorded an entire chapter of the accreditation standards manuals. A small number of specific requirements for each of the goals will be identified for survey for each goal. Some of the patient safety goals may continue, while others may be adopted as standards of care or changed because of emerging new priorities and areas of focus in other chapters of the accreditation standards. All accredited organizations must implement the goals and associated recommendations that are relevant to the services their organization provides.

These goals and recommendations are the results of lessons learned from organizations that have experienced a sentinel event. Lessons learned are the findings from a **root-cause analysis (RCA)** that determined process issues and new solutions to prevent sentinel events from occurring. Additional information on sentinel events is addressed in step 5, and details related to conducting root-cause analysis are addressed in the QI Toolbox Techniques section of this chapter.

Step 1: The Healthcare Organization Develops a Risk Management Plan, Policies, and Procedures

The risk manager leads the development of risk management policies and procedures for the organization. The risk manager also helps the organization define and prioritize its own self-assessed risk factors for the population it serves. Policies and procedures in the risk management area include a policy describing the organization's malpractice and liability insurance strategy, procedures outlining its legal claims-tracking and negotiation system, and procedures outlining how its databases are maintained and risk management reports are developed. Risk managers also routinely review the operational policies and procedures of all departments to ensure that they have been designed in ways that reduce, rather than increase, the possibility of risk exposure. Risk management procedures also define requirements for occurrence reporting and reporting to insurers, licensing agencies, public health departments, governing bodies, the National Practitioners Data Bank, and other accrediting and regulatory agencies. In addition, risk managers review all approved policies and procedures across the organization to ensure that none of the activities will expose the organization to risk.

Step 2: The Risk Management Team Teaches Risk Management Concepts and Principles to All Employees

In conjunction with staff development coordinators, risk managers develop educational activities for employees, including the governing board. Examples of such activities include handwashing techniques, needle safety protocol, NPSGs including universal protocol, fall-risk prevention, surgical fire prevention, behavior treatment protocols, seclusion and restraint procedures, and incident documentation and reporting. Educational topics are based on data derived from risk management reports highlighting reoccurring events and issues. Program attendance for employees is tracked, and competency testing for comprehension and retention is performed.

Step 3: The Team Evaluates Occurrence Reports

The risk manager's principal tool for capturing the facts about PCEs is the **occurrence report**, a structured data collection tool that risk managers use to gather information (sometimes called the incident report). Effective occurrence reports carefully structure the collection of data, information, and facts in a relatively simple format. This process of reporting may be on paper (as shown in figure 11.3), but it is often completed electronically through a variety of risk management software programs. Note that the example in figure 11.3 captures information about the persons involved. It records information about the date and the time of day that the employees involved were working. Page 2 gathers information about the witnesses to the incident and gives the results of the patient's contact with and examination by a physician or nurse practitioner. Pages 3, 4, and 5 gather information regarding specific aspects of the most common incidents that occur in healthcare. For example, in section 7 on page 5, the report collects data on the type of burn. All data collected in these incident-specific sections are coded for easy checking and entry into a database management system for incident tracking.

Following completion by individuals in the department or facility area where the incident occurred, the occurrence report is routed to the risk manager. The risk manager reviews policy, procedure, and other aspects of the occurrence, and involves management and administrative staff as necessary. After the cause analysis and revision of policy, recommendations and/or corrective actions based on review of the incident are documented on page 6 of the report. This would include actions regarding policies and procedures, the outcome for the injured individual, contacts with manufacturers, and retraining of personnel.

The second important record for managing risk exposure is the patient's health record. Every response to an incident that relates to a patient must be documented in the patient's health record. If a case of injury should result in a malpractice suit or other legal action, this documentation becomes crucial. The clinicians involved in an incident must be certain that all appropriate clinical documentation regarding the occurrence is added to the health record and documented on the occurrence report.

Occurrence reports are generally not open to view by the plaintiff's attorney. Thus, to communicate the care given the patient in its entirety, and especially regarding an occurrence, the health record must be documented carefully because it will be used to portray the events to the public. The risk manager must

Figure 11.3. Sample occurrence report—page 1

Med Rec #: *00-05-45*
Name: *Jackson, Julia*
Date of Birth: *06-22-23*
Street: *6401 Fremont Ave*
City: *Western City, CA*

Risk Management use only: _____

Patient ID/Name of individual involved.
Use addressograph for patient.

INSTRUCTIONS: (1) Fill out the first page of the Incident Report Form. (2) Select the type of incident from the bottom of page 2. (3) Fill out all appropriate sections as directed. The report must be dated and filled out by the end of the shift in which the incident occurred or was discovered. **DO NOT COPY THIS FORM.** Please print; this report must be legible. **Please fill out all applicable parts of this form.** Upon completion of this form, route it to your Nurse Manager or Supervisor. Do not leave this form in the patient's chart.

Date of incident: *05 / 29 /* XX   Time (2400 Clock): *1645*   Hospital Unit: *Med/Surg*

What day of the week did it occur?
Sun [√]   Thurs [ ]
Mon [ ]   Fri [ ]
Tues [ ]   Sat [ ]
Wed [ ]

Did the incident occur during:
Day 0701–1500   [ ]
Evening 1501–2300 [√]
Night 2301–0700   [ ]

Employee involved worked a(n):
8 Hour shift   [√]
10 Hour shift [ ]
12 Hour shift [ ]
Double shift   [ ]
Other _____

Where did the incident occur? *patient room*

Description of incident. Include follow-up care given (i.e., vital signs, x-ray, laboratory tests, etc.).
Pt. developed a macular rash over trunk and extremities after 10 mg dose of Compazine given for postop nausea. Compazine stopped and Benadryl given IM.

IMMEDIATE EFFECT OF THE INCIDENT: *Severe macular rash over trunk*

Involved Person Data

Date of Admission: *05 / 29 /* XX
What sex is the person?
Male   [ ]
Female [√]

What is the person's age? _____

Current Diagnosis/Reason for visit: *Bowel Obstruction*

Inpatient [√]
Outpatient [ ]
Student   [ ]
Employee   [ ]
Visitor   [ ]
Volunteer [ ]
Other: _____

Is the involved person aware of the incident?   Yes [√]   No [ ]
Is the family aware of incident?   Yes [ ]   No [√]

Figure 11.3. Sample occurrence report—page 2

DO NOT COPY

**** **PLEASE PRINT** ****

Person preparing report (signature): *Gwen Nelson, R.N.*   Print: *Gwen Nelson, R.N.*
Name of individual witnessing incident (print): *Bob Patterson, R.N.*
Dept/Address: *Med/Surg Team Leader*
Name of employee involved in incident: *Gwen Nelson, R.N.* Dept/Address: *Med/Surg*
Name of employee discovering incident: *Gwen Nelson, R.N.* Dept/Address: *Med/Surg*

**** **STAFF TO NOTIFY ATTENDING PHYSICIAN AND/OR DESIGNATED RESIDENT/NURSE PRACTITIONER OF INCIDENT** ****

I notified Dr./NP: *Jeff Cook* at: *1650* (time).

M.D./NP responded ☐ in person ☑ by phone at: *1705* (time).

Was the attending physician notified?

Yes [√] Date: *05/29/XX* Time: *1650*

No [ ] Why not? _____

Examining Physician/Nurse Practitioner statement regarding condition/outcome of person involved:

Pt. was examined by me at 1700 hours. Trunk and extremities show a macular rash on them. One dose of Benadryl given IM to pt. and rash began to subside. Compazine stopped.

Examining MD/NP signature: *Tom Lander, M.D. House Staff*
Examining MD/NP name (print): *Tom Lander, M.D.*
Date: *05/29/XX* Time: *1700* Clinical Service: *Medicine*

CHOOSE THE TYPE OF INCIDENT YOU ARE REPORTING. Use the index below to locate the type of incident you are reporting, go to that section, and mark the appropriate box(es). THERE MAY BE MORE THAN ONE ITEM APPLICABLE IN A SECTION. CHECK BOX(ES) IN APPROPRIATE SECTIONS.

Medication/IV Incident	Page 3, Section 1	Patient Behavioral Incident	Page 5, Section 6
Blood/Blood Incident	Page 3, Section 2	Safety Incident	Page 5, Section 9
Burns	Page 5, Section 7	Security Incident	Page 5, Section 8
Equipment Incident	Page 5, Section 10	Surgery Incident	Page 5, Section 4
Falls	Page 4, Section 3	Treatment/Procedure Incident	Page 5, Section 5
Fire Incident	Page 5, Section 11		

CONFIDENTIAL: This material is prepared pursuant to Code Annotated, §26-25-1, et seq., and 58-12-43 (7, 8, and 9), for the purpose of evaluating healthcare rendered by hospitals or physicians and is NOT PART of the medical record.

Figure 11.3. Sample occurrence report—page 3

DO NOT COPY

SECTION 1 MEDICATION/IV INCIDENT

1A. TYPE OF MEDICATION
Fill in specific medication/solution on the adjacent line.
Analgesic _____
Anesthetic agent _____
Antibiotic _____
Anticoagulant _____
Anticonvulsant _____
Antidepressant _____
Antiemetic __*Compazine*_____
Antihistamine _____
Antineoplastic _____
Bronchodilator _____
Cardiovascular _____
Contrast media _____
Diuretic _____
Immunizations _____
Immunosuppressive _____
Insulin _____
Intralipids _____
Investigational drug _____
IV solution _____
Laxative _____
Narcotic _____
Oxytocics _____
Psychotherapeutic _____
Radionuclides _____
Sedative/tranquilizer _____
TPN _____
Vasodilator _____
Vasopressor _____
Vitamin _____
Other _____

1B. TYPE OF MEDICATION OR IV INCIDENT
Adverse reaction .... [√] 1B01
Allergic/contraindication. .... [ ] 1B02
Delayed stat order .... [ ] 1B03
Improper order (MD/NP) .... [ ] 1B04
Incompatible additive .... [ ] 1B05
Incorrect additive .... [ ] 1B06
Incorrect dosage .... [ ] 1B07
Incorrect drug .... [ ] 1B08
Incorrect narcotic count .... [ ] 1B09
Incorrect patient .... [ ] 1B10
Incorrect rate of flow .... [ ] 1B11
Incorrect route .... [ ] 1B12
Incorrect schedule .... [ ] 1B13
Incorrect solution/type .... [ ] 1B14
Incorrect time .... [ ] 1B15
Incorrect volume .... [ ] 1B16
Infiltration .... [ ] 1B17
Given before culture taken .... [ ] 1B18
Medication given before lab
　results returned .... [ ] 1B19
Medication missing from cart .... [ ] 1B20

Not documented .... [ ] 1B21
Not prescribed .... [ ] 1B22
Omitted .... [ ] 1B23
Outdated .... [ ] 1B24
Out-of-sequence .... [ ] 1B25
Patient took unprescribed medication ..... [ ] 1B26
Repeat administration .... [ ] 1B27
Transcription error .... [ ] 1B28
Other_____ 1B29

1C. ROUTE OF MEDICATION ORDERED:
IM .... [ ] 1C01
IV .... [ ] 1C02
PO .... [ ] 1C03
Other__*Suppository*_____ 1C04

1D. MEDICATION DISPENSING INCIDENT
Meds not sent/delayed from pharmacy ...... [ ] 1D01
Incorrectly labeled .... [ ] 1D02
Incorrect dose .... [ ] 1D03
Incorrect drug sent .... [ ] 1D04
Incorrect IV additive .... [ ] 1D05
Incorrect IV fluid .... [ ] 1D06
Incorrect route (IV, PO, IM, PR) .... [ ] 1D07
Mislabeled .... [ ] 1D08
Other_____ 1D09

SECTION 2
BLOOD/BLOOD COMPONENT INCIDENT

2A. BLOOD/BLOOD COMPONENT TYPE
Albumin .... [ ] 2A01
Cryoprecipitate .... [ ] 2A02
Factor VIII (AHF) .... [ ] 2A03
Factor IX (Konyne) .... [ ] 2A04
Fresh frozen plasma .... [ ] 2A05
Packed red blood cells (PRBC) .... [ ] 2A06
Plasmanate® .... [ ] 2A07
Platelets .... [ ] 2A08
RhoGAM® .... [ ] 2A09
Washed red blood cells (WRBC) .... [ ] 2A10
Whole blood .... [ ] 2A11
Other_____ 2A12

**2B. TYPE OF BLOOD/BLOOD COMPONENT
　　INCIDENT**
Crossmatch problem .... [ ] 2B01
Improper unit verification .... [ ] 2B02
Inappropriate IV fluids administered
　with blood components .... [ ] 2B03
Inappropriate documentation .... [ ] 2B04
Inappropriate storage .... [ ] 2B05
Incomplete patient ID .... [ ] 2B06
Incorrect patient .... [ ] 2B07
Incorrect rate .... [ ] 2B08
Incorrect type .... [ ] 2B09
Incorrect volume .... [ ] 2B10
Patient refused .... [ ] 2B11
Other_____ 2B12

CONFIDENTIAL: This material is prepared pursuant to Code Annotated, §26-25-1, et seq., and 58-12-43 (7, 8, and 9), for the purpose of evaluating healthcare rendered by hospitals or physicians and is NOT PART of the medical record.

Figure 11.3. Sample occurrence report—page 4

DO NOT COPY

SECTION 3
FALLS

3A. FALL CODE STATUS OF PATIENT
Attended .... [ ] 3A01
Unattended .... [ ] 3A02

3B. LOCATION OF FALL
Bathroom in patient's room .... [ ] 3B01
Bathroom (other location) .... [ ] 3B02
Elevator .... [ ] 3B03
Examining/treatment room .... [ ] 3B04
Hallway/corridor .... [ ] 3B05
Nursing station .... [ ] 3B06
Parking lot .... [ ] 3B07
Patient's room .... [ ] 3B08
Recreation area .... [ ] 3B09
Shower/tub room .... [ ] 3B10
Stairs .... [ ] 3B11
Waiting room .... [ ] 3B12
Walkway/sidewalk .... [ ] 3B13
Other_____   3B14

3C. FALL OCCURRED IN CONJUNCTION WITH:
Bedside commode .... [ ] 3C01
Chair .... [ ] 3C02
Due to toy .... [ ] 3C03
During transfer .... [ ] 3C04
Exam table .... [ ] 3C05
Fainting/dizzy .... [ ] 3C06
Fall/slip .... [ ] 3C07
From bed .... [ ] 3C08
Improperly locked device .... [ ] 3C09
Recreational activity .... [ ] 3C10
Scales .... [ ] 3C11
Stretcher .... [ ] 3C12
Table .... [ ] 3C13
Tripped .... [ ] 3C14
While ambulating unattended .... [ ] 3C15
While ambulating with assist .... [ ] 3C16
While entering or leaving bed .... [ ] 3C17
While using ambulatory device .... [ ] 3C18
Other_____   3C19

3D. PATIENT ACTIVITY PRIVILEGES
    (As per medical order)
Ambulate with assistance .... [ ] 3D01
Ambulate with walker .... [ ] 3D02
Ambulate without assistance .... [ ] 3D03
Bathroom privileges with assistance ...... [ ] 3D04
Bathroom privileges without assistance ... [ ] 3D05
Bedrest .... [ ] 3D06
Up Ad lib .... [ ] 3D07
Up in chair/wheelchair .... [ ] 3D08
Other_____   3D09

**3E. PATIENT MENTAL CONDITION AT THE
    TIME OF THE FALL**
Confused/poor judgment .... [ ] 3E01
Language barrier .... [ ] 3E02
Oriented .... [ ] 3E03
Unconscious .... [ ] 3E04
Uncooperative .... [ ] 3E05
Unresponsive/medicated .... [ ] 3E06
Other_____

3F. PATIENT'S CALL LIGHT WAS:
On .... [ ] 3F01
Off .... [ ] 3F02
Not within reach .... [ ] 3F03
Patient unable to use .... [ ] 3F04
Not applicable .... [ ] 3F05

3G. POSITION OF BED
High .... [ ] 3G01
Low .... [ ] 3G02
Intermediate .... [ ] 3G03
Not applicable .... [ ] 3G04

3H. BED ALARM
On .... [ ] 3H01
Off .... [ ] 3H02
Not applicable .... [ ] 3H03

3I. POSITION OF SIDE RAILS
(At the time of the fall)
    Half Rails [ ] 3I01   Full Rails [ ] 3I06
       1 Up   [ ] 3I02   1 Up   [ ] 3I07
       2 Up   [ ] 3I03   2 Up   [ ] 3I08
       3 Up   [ ] 3I04
       4 Up   [ ] 3I05
Not applicable [ ] 3I09

3J. PATIENT RESTRAINTS
Removed by patient .... [ ] 3J01
Restraints intact .... [ ] 3J02
Not applicable .... [ ] 3J03
Other_____   3J04

**3K. CONDITION OF AREA WHERE FALL
    OCCURRED**
Normal/dry .... [ ] 3K01
Wet floor .... [ ] 3K02
Ice condition .... [ ] 3K03
Other_____   3K04

**3L. FALLS IN CONJUNCTION
    WITH MEDICATION**
Narcotic or sedative received by patient
in the past 12 hours? .... [ ] 3L01
When was the last dose? _____   3L02
What was the drug? _____   3L03
What was the route of administration? ___ 3L04

CONFIDENTIAL: This material is prepared pursuant to Code Annotated, §26-25-1, et seq., and 58-12-43 (7, 8, and 9), for the purpose of evaluating healthcare rendered by hospitals or physicians and is NOT PART of the medical record.

Figure 11.3. Sample occurrence report—page 5

DO NOT COPY

SECTION 4
SURGERY INCIDENT
Anesthesia occurrence . . . . [ ] 0401
Contamination . . . . [ ] 0402
Incorrect needle count . . . . [ ] 0403
Incorrect sponge count . . . . [ ] 0404
Informed consent absent . . . . [ ] 0405
Informed consent incorrect . . . . [ ] 0406
Instrument lost/broken . . . . [ ] 0407
Retained foreign body . . . . [ ] 0408
Other_____ 0409

SECTION 5
TREATMENT/PROCEDURE INCIDENT
Adverse reaction . . . . [ ] 0501
Allergic response . . . . [ ] 0502
Application/removal of cast/splint . . . . [ ] 0503
Cancellation of procedures . . . . [ ] 0504
Catheter or tube related . . . . [ ] 0505
Delay . . . . [ ] 0506
Dietary problem . . . . [ ] 0507
Dressing/wound occurrence . . . . [ ] 0508
Informed consent absent . . . . [ ] 0509
Informed consent incorrect . . . . [ ] 0510
Injection site . . . . [ ] 0511
Invasive procedure/placement . . . . [ ] 0512
Mislabeled specimen . . . . [ ] 0513
Missing specimen . . . . [ ] 0514
Not documented . . . . [ ] 0515
Omitted . . . . [ ] 0516
Patient/site identification . . . . [ ] 0517
Positioning . . . . [ ] 0518
Prep problem . . . . [ ] 0519
Repeat procedure . . . . [ ] 0520
Reporting of test results . . . . [ ] 0521
Thermoregulation problem . . . . [ ] 0522
Transcription error . . . . [ ] 0523
Transfer/moving of patient . . . . [ ] 0524
Other_____ 0525

SECTION 6
PATIENT BEHAVIORAL INCIDENT
Attempted AWOL . . . . [ ] 0601
AWOL . . . . [ ] 0602
Inappropriate sexual behavior . . . . [ ] 0603
Injured by other patient . . . . [ ] 0604
Patient altercation . . . . [ ] 0605
Self-inflicted injury . . . . [ ] 0606
Suicide gesture . . . . [ ] 0607
Other_____ 0608

SECTION 7
BURNS
Chemical . . . . [ ] 0701
Electrical . . . . [ ] 0702
Inhalation . . . . [ ] 0703
Radioactive . . . . [ ] 0704
Thermal . . . . [ ] 0705

SECTION 8
SECURITY INCIDENT
Bomb threat . . . . [ ] 0801
Breaking and entering . . . . [ ] 0802
Drug theft . . . . [ ] 0803
Secure area key loss/missing . . . . [ ] 0804
Major theft (over $250) . . . . [ ] 0805
   Amount:_____
Minor theft . . . . [ ] 0806
   Amount:_____
Personal property damage/loss . . . . [ ] 0807
   Amount:_____
Hospital property damage . . . . [ ] 0808
   Amount:_____
Other_____

SECTION 9
SAFETY INCIDENT (patients and visitors only)
Body fluid exposure . . . . [ ] 0901
Chemical exposure . . . . [ ] 0902
Chemotherapy spill . . . . [ ] 0903
Drug exposure . . . . [ ] 0904
Hazardous material spill . . . . [ ] 0905
Needlestick . . . . [ ] 0906
Other_____ 0907

SECTION 10
EQUIPMENT INCIDENT
Disconnected . . . . [ ] 1001
Electrical problem . . . . [ ] 1002
Improper use . . . . [ ] 1003
Malfunction/defect . . . . [ ] 1004
Mechanical problem . . . . [ ] 1005
Not available . . . . [ ] 1006
Electrical shock . . . . [ ] 1007
Electrical spark . . . . [ ] 1008
Struck by . . . . [ ] 1009
Wrong equipment . . . . [ ] 1010
Tampered with
   By patient . . . . [ ] 1011
   Non-patient . . . . [ ] 1012
Other_____ 1013

SECTION 11
FIRE INCIDENT
Equipment caused . . . . [ ] 1101
Cigarette caused . . . . [ ] 1102
Laser caused . . . . [ ] 1103
Other_____ 1104

CONFIDENTIAL: This material is prepared pursuant to Code Annotated, §26-25-1, et seq., and 58-12-43 (7, 8, and 9), for the purpose of evaluating healthcare rendered by hospitals or physicians and is NOT PART of the medical record.

Figure 11.3. Sample occurrence report—page 6

DO NOT COPY

**EMPLOYEES DO NOT COMPLETE BELOW,
FOR NURSE MANAGER/SUPERVISOR USE ONLY.**

Recommendations and/or corrective actions based on review of report and discussion with employee:
NURSE MANAGER/SUPERVISOR Follow-Up [Check appropriate box(es)/Corrective action]

Policy/Procedure:

Evaluate	[ ] 1201	**Discussed with:**	
Recommend change	[ ] 1202	Physician	[ ] 1209
Changed	[ ] 1203	Staff	[ ] 1210
No action taken	[ ] 1204	Patient	[ ] 1211
Noncompliance	[ ] 1205	Other	[ ] 1212
Inadequate	[ ] 1206		
Needs enforcement	[ ] 1207	Date: _____	
Review with involved individual(s)	[ ] 1208	Time: _____	

Describe specific follow-up actions taken (if applicable include names of depts). _____
_____

SIGN AND DATE: (Indicates review of report)

1. Quality Management/Risk Management_____ ___/___/___
2. Nurse Manager/Supervisor (as applicable) _____ ___/___/___
3. Department Head/DON (as applicable) _____ ___/___/___
4. QM Coordinator (as applicable)_____ ___/___/___
5. Other: Title_____ Name _____ ___/___/___

BIOENGINEERING USE ONLY

Manufacturer contacted .... [ ] 1301
Manufacturer instructions followed .... [ ] 1302
Needs enforcement of policy/procedure .... [ ] 1303
Include instructions in staff education and training .... [ ] 1304
Preventative maintenance or biomedical evaluation of equipment ordered ... [ ] 1305
Recommend repair or replacement .... [ ] 1306
Removed from service .... [ ] 1307
Other _____ [ ] 1308

RISK MANAGEMENT USE ONLY
IMMEDIATE EFFECT OF THE INCIDENT

Alteration in skin integrity	[ ] 1401	Patient discomfort/inconvenience	[ ] 1411
Birth related injury	[ ] 1402	Psycho/social trauma	[ ] 1412
Breach of confidentiality	[ ] 1403	Reproductive injury or loss	[ ] 1413
Death	[ ] 1404	Sensory impairment	[ ] 1414
Disability	[ ] 1405	Severe internal injuries	[ ] 1415
Disfigurement	[ ] 1406	Substantial disability	[ ] 1416
Drug/blood reaction	[ ] 1407	Unanticipated neuro deficit	[ ] 1417
Fluid imbalance	[ ] 1408	Unanticipated systemic deficit	[ ] 1418
Neuro deficit	[ ] 1409	Indeterminate	[ ] 1419
Orthopedic injury	[ ] 1410	None	[ ] 1420
		Other_____	[ ] 1421

Description_____

CONFIDENTIAL: This material is prepared pursuant to Code Annotated, §26-25-1, et seq., and 58-12-43 (7, 8, and 9), for the purpose of evaluating healthcare rendered by hospitals or physicians and is NOT PART of the medical record.

develop a careful balance while overseeing the documentation of a PCE. Complete details on all persons involved, actions taken, and condition and responses of the patient should be documented in the occurrence record. However, in the patient's health record, the details should be limited to those documenting care given to the patient in an objective manner. No details about how or what contributed to the occurrence should be included. No mention should be made in the patient's health record of an incident or occurrence report having been completed (see figure 11.4).

The documentation of a **medication error**, a mistake that involves an accidental drug overdose, administration of an incorrect substance, accidental consumption of a drug, or misuse of a drug or biological during a medical or surgical procedure, in the sample occurrence report (shown in figure 11.3) is a good example. The Joint Commission has a patient rights standard related to disclosing outcomes. The standard requires that all patients be informed of any outcomes, unanticipated or otherwise, from an error such as a decrease in medication dosage due to a reaction from an ordered medication or a medical intervention initiated because of the original error (Joint Commission 2024c, RI 8-9). For instance, suppose a patient received an inaccurate dose of Lasix, causing excess fluid depletion from the body and concomitant lightheadedness requiring oxygen. The initial error may be a medication error caused by the prescriber or a dosing error caused by the personnel giving the medication. It also may simply be the patient's adverse reaction to the particular medication. Generally, the patient is not informed that an incident report has been completed. The patient will be informed that due to a reaction from the medication, they will need oxygen for a period of time.

Step 4: The Risk Management Team Examines Structure, Process, and Knowledge Issues

As department members and PI teams begin to identify customers and review performance, issues in organizational structures, processes, outcomes, and knowledge may become apparent. Commonly, these issues are documented in department or team communications to a PI or leadership council. Risk managers are members of the council and routinely review communications from the departments and teams for this purpose. Issues, in turn, should be documented in risk management databases so that corrective action may be initiated if and when they meet a performance threshold (the level above which the occurrence is not occurring by chance and cannot be tolerated). If it becomes apparent that members of the organization do not have an appropriate understanding of procedure or policy, the risk manager may have to initiate training sessions to educate staff regarding the issue. These training sessions must also be documented.

Step 5: The Team Identifies Practice Patterns, Trends in Risk Occurrences, and Sentinel Events

Using aggregate data summarized from the occurrence report discussed in step 3, the risk manager attempts to identify trends in risk occurrences within the organization. For example, if there were an increase in occurrence reports documenting patient falls on a particular nursing unit, the risk manager might ask the nurse manager on that unit to be sure that staff understand how to identify a patient at risk for falls, that assessments for fall risks are completed, and that appropriate preventive measures are instituted with identified patients.

Another important PI activity that contributes to the risk manager's databases is the credentialing of physicians and the validation of nurses' and other clinicians' licenses to practice. Committees of the medical staff and other disciplines standardize monitoring of clinicians' practice patterns and outcomes. Documentation of these reviews is analyzed by these committees and the risk manager to identify clinicians who may be practicing outside their scope of licensure, or who may benefit from additional education regarding policy, procedure, or the current standard of practice in the region where the healthcare organization does business. A critical area of liability for a healthcare organization is the process of verifying staff clinical competency

Figure 11.4. Sample progress note in a patient's record

	PROGRESS NOTES	Med Rec# 00-05-45 Jackson, Julia
	DATE & TIME	NOTES MUST BE DATED AND TIMED
	5/29/XX 1650	Patient developed a macular rash over entire trunk and extremities after 10 mg of Compazine given for nausea. Dr. Cook and house staff notified. Gwen Nelson, R.N.
	5/29/XX 1700	Called to pt. for rash on trunk & extremities. Pt. examined, adverse reaction to Compazine most likely. Patient to receive 20 mg of Benadryl IM now. If nausea continues, Dramamine 50 mg IV prn. T. Lander, M.D.
	5/29/XX 1700	Dr. Lander examined patient and ordered Benadryl 20 mg IM. Patient injected IM 20 mg of Benadryl. Gwen Nelson, R.N.
	5/29/XX 1810	Rash is subsiding and nausea less. Gwen Nelson, R.N.

PROGRESS NOTES

and practitioners working outside their scope of licensure or approved privileges. Malpractice claims against a provider would be in favor of the plaintiff if unfavorable information related to competency or privileging is revealed during the discovery process of a lawsuit.

Step 6: The Team Provides Direction in the Patient Advocacy Function

The first major objective of a proactive risk management program is to minimize the organization's exposure to risk or legal action. The second major objective is to minimize the economic impact of indemnity and expense payments related to malpractice and liability claims. The economic impact of a quality risk program should be measured by the development of goodwill and the satisfaction of its customers. Historically, this second objective has been a function of risk management and is known as patient advocacy. **Patient advocacy** is the function performed by patient representatives (sometimes called ombudsmen) who respond personally to complaints from patients and/or their families. Some healthcare organizations have removed this responsibility from the risk manager and established a separate patient advocate service that works with the risk manager on complaints specific to PCEs.

The objective of patient advocacy is to support the patient through difficult interactions with the healthcare organization. A patient advocate is "a hospital employee whose job is to speak on a patient's behalf and help get any information or services needed" (CMS n.d.b). Most businesses can be somewhat bureaucratic, and healthcare organizations are no exception. Add the confusion, complexity, danger, and chance of PCEs, and the patient may feel shunned and isolated by the organization at a time of great personal strife. The patient needs to express their anger to lessen it and needs someone in the organization to validate their right to feel it. All licensed healthcare organizations are required to inform patients of their rights to initiate a complaint or grievance and to have their complaints reviewed and, if possible, resolved.

The risk manager as patient advocate must be sure that the patient knows the facts associated with an occurrence. The patient advocate must accept responsibility for the occurrence in the customer's eyes when the organization's employees were responsible for the situation during which the incident occurred. If the organization's employees were not responsible for the situation but the customer believes that they were, the patient advocate should continue to serve a neutral role in resolving the situation. The challenge for the patient advocate is to investigate the complaint and address the issues specific to the event in such a way as to avoid legal action against the organization. Sometimes just listening to the patient's concerns, offering an apology, or negotiating monetary compensation can resolve the complaint without any legal action against the organization.

Step 7: The Team Communicates All Relevant Data and Information to Legal Support When PCEs Occur

Inevitably, some claims of liability involve formal legal action. The facility's attorneys, representatives of the facility's insurance company, and the plaintiff's attorneys then become involved.

The risk manager continues to function as the organization's representative in such legal environments. They coordinate all requests for information by *subpoena duces tecum* from attorneys or from the courts. The risk manager explains the organization's perspective to attorneys regarding the completion of interrogatories and coordinates the appearance of employees at depositions or at trial. They remain open to negotiation of an appropriate settlement to conclude the action before it goes to trial.

The risk manager is responsible for communicating all relevant data and information to the organization's insurer as soon as possible after a PCE is recognized. The risk management department routinely provides the organization's insurance company with copies of occurrence reports for all PCEs. The timeliness and efficiency of such communications are extremely important if PCEs are to be resolved rapidly and without litigation. Subsequently, the risk manager must keep the insurer informed of important communications with the patient or the patient's attorneys. Insurance company representatives must have complete information to make appropriate resolution decisions.

Step 8: The Risk Team and Legal Counsel Lead the Development of an Appropriate Insurance Strategy for the Organization

In addition to transmitting information regarding PCEs, the risk manager also takes the lead in designing a malpractice and liability insurance strategy that meets the needs of the healthcare organization. To be effective in this area, the risk manager must have an in-depth knowledge of the organization's services, facilities, equipment, procedures, and staff capabilities.

The insurance strategy is developed with reference to the healthcare service lines of the organization. For example, the perinatal service is one of the service lines that has the greatest inherent risk of liability. Numerous complications can occur during a woman's pregnancy, labor, and delivery, and many of these complications cannot be foreseen. The fact that the organization provides perinatal services would be taken into consideration by the organization's management and insurer.

Check Your Understanding 11.2

1. Explain why the occurrence report is a risk manager's principal tool for capturing the facts about potentially compensable events (PCEs) and explain why these reports are not shared publicly or filed in the patient's health record.

2. Yolanda is a nursing supervisor in the newborn intensive care unit. During her shift, several parents of newborns in the unit are visiting, and the neonatologist has also recently been in and provided orders for several of the newborns. Because of the current workload, Jackie, another nurse in the unit, has asked Yolanda to help her complete the orders. Yolanda is asked to administer a medication to one of the newborns that Jackie has already retrieved for the patient. Jackie tells Yolanda that she has double checked the medication both through bar coding and with the order. Before Yolanda goes to administer the medication, she scans both the medication and the newborn's patient ID band and learns that she has the incorrect medication for this patient. Yolanda does not administer that medication but goes back to the order and through the proper steps administers the correct medication. Based on this scenario, which of the following occurred?
   a. Time-out
   b. Serious event
   c. Sentinel event
   d. Near miss

QI Toolbox Techniques

At Community Hospital of the West, Dr. Low, an obstetrician, delivered Mrs. Yu's infant with relatively little difficulty. However, when the placenta was delivered, a rush of blood appeared at the patient's cervical os. Dr. Low attempted to explore the patient's uterus to see whether there were still pieces of the placenta inside that were causing the bleeding, but there was so much blood that she could not adequately explore the uterus. After several minutes of trying to deal with the situation, she realized that the bleeding did not appear to be abating even though the uterus was contracting appropriately. Dr. Low decided to take Mrs. Yu to surgery to perform an exploratory laparotomy and possible emergency hysterectomy. The physician knew that if she could not stop the bleeding, the patient's life would be in danger. She packed the uterus as tightly as possible, instructed nursing staff to find blood for a transfusion, covered the patient with a sheet, placed the patient on oxygen, and began wheeling the patient's gurney to the elevator.

Community Hospital of the West is a major tertiary care facility in a large US city. It has always provided obstetrical delivery and neonatal services in the north wing of the second floor of the facility. Delivery rooms were developed in this wing. Surgical services and the ORs were developed in the north wing on the third floor. When patients required cesarean section deliveries or other surgical treatment, they had to be transferred from the delivery rooms on the second floor to the ORs on the third floor.

Dr. Low and the obstetrical nurses assisting her waited for approximately one minute before an elevator arrived. Most of the hospital staff found the elevators very slow and had commented on this many times over the years. Dr. Low, the nurse, and Mrs. Yu arrived in about another minute and a half on the third floor, and they rushed into an OR. Crash induction of anesthesia was begun. As the OR staff tried to get a line in to start the blood transfusion and Dr. Low began to remove the packing from the uterus, a massive amount of blood gushed from the organ. The patient's heart went into ventricular fibrillation, and despite emergency resuscitative efforts, Mrs. Yu died.

Because the death occurred during a surgical procedure, it was reportable to the county coroner's office. The coroner accepted the case and performed an autopsy. Mrs. Yu was found to have an anomalous uterine artery that had been opened upon delivery of the placenta, and she bled to death.

Common toolbox techniques that PI teams use to evaluate and assess the causes of unexpected or adverse events include cause-and-effect diagrams and root-cause analysis. These tools help focus PI teams on the underlying source and factors that led to the unexpected or adverse event.

Cause-and-Effect Diagram

The death of a patient as described in the case of Mrs. Yu is always classified as a sentinel event. In such cases, the organization should perform a root-cause analysis of the event to discover what processes in the organization led to the occurrence. There is always the possibility that unusual and unexpected events will occur. No one really could have known that Mrs. Yu's uterus was anomalous in its blood supply. Does that mean that Mrs. Yu's death was truly inadvertent? Could the death of this patient have been averted despite the anomaly in her anatomy?

The toolbox technique used most often in RCA is the cause-and-effect diagram. A **cause-and-effect diagram**, also called a fishbone diagram, is an investigational technique that facilitates the identification of the factors or causes that contribute to a problem. This technique structures the root-cause inquiry and ensures that investigators examine the situation from all perspectives. As figure 11.5 shows, the effect is at the head of the fish, and the fish bones delineate the causes of the situation. The causes are classified into four categories. In the structure shown, the categories all begin with the letter *M*. This design was intended to make it easier to remember the categories as "the four Ms": *Manpower*, *Material*, *Methods*, and *Machinery*. Other approaches use other names for the categories; for example, *People*, *Policies*, *Procedures*, and *Equipment*.

- *Manpower* examines influences of the human worker on the situation. In the case of Mrs. Yu's death, a human worker influence was the obstetrical nurses' lack of training in surgical procedures. This lack of training meant that emergency surgical procedures could not be performed in the delivery room.
- *Material* examines the influences of supplies and equipment on the situation. In the real-life example, surgical supplies and equipment were not available to Dr. Low in the delivery room, so she could not perform the necessary exploratory procedure there.
- *Methods* examines influences of policies and procedures on the situation. In Mrs. Yu's case, it was the policy of the institution to take all obstetrical cases requiring surgical delivery or other surgical procedures to the OR on the third floor of the hospital. This policy caused a fairly long period of time to elapse during transport and in this situation led to the patient's death from blood loss.
- *Machinery* examines influences of machines or other major pieces of equipment on the situation. In this case, the slowness of the hospital elevator contributed to the delay in effective treatment.

Figure 11.5. Sample cause-and-effect diagram

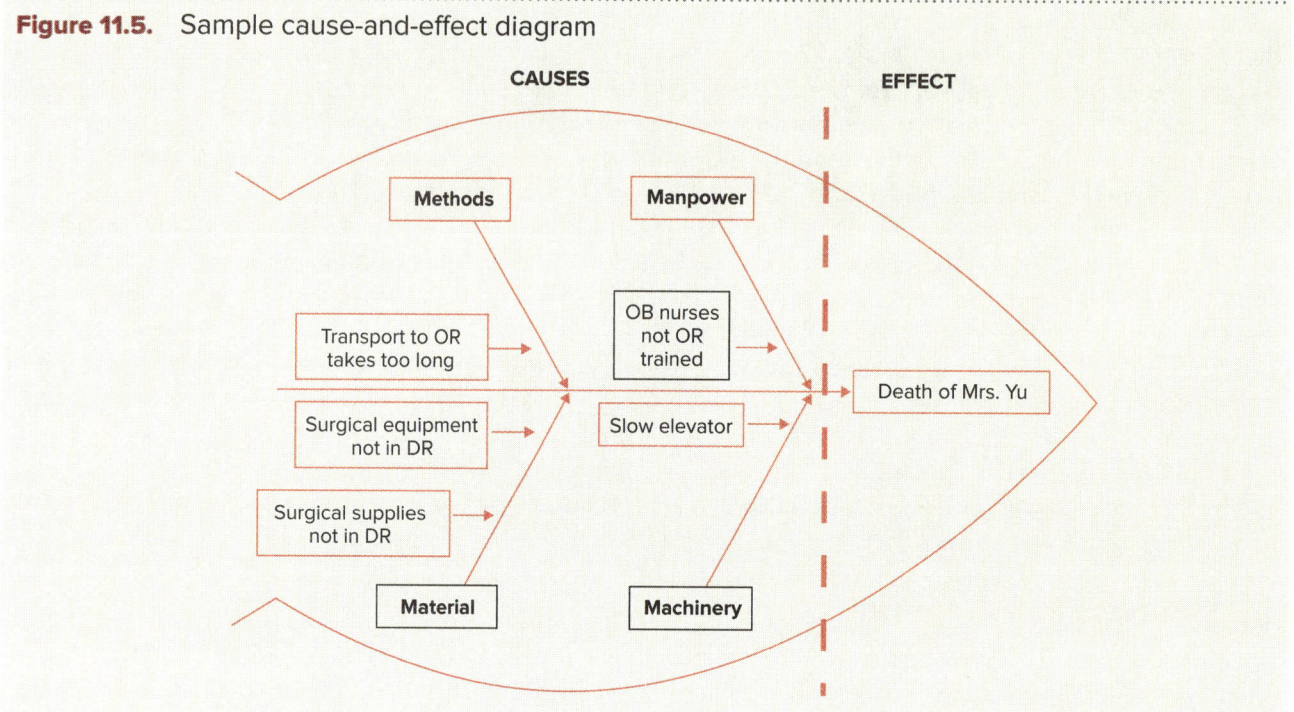

Root-Cause Analysis

Root-cause analysis (RCA) is a process in which a sentinel event is evaluated from all aspects (human, procedural, machinery, and material) to identify how each contributed to the occurrence of the event and to develop new systems that will prevent recurrence. In RCA, it is important to continue to ask the question *Why?* until the absolute root cause has been discovered. *Proximate causes* are those that can be pointed to directly and are usually identified first in the RCA process. In the case of Mrs. Yu, a proximate cause was the inability of the obstetrical nurses to assist in emergency surgical procedures. However, that proximate cause has, in turn, many underlying causes, some of which may be the root cause of the sentinel event. Those underlying causes must be identified, because their existence is what really allowed the sentinel event to happen.

Investigators of Mrs. Yu's death had to ask *Why?* many times to get to the root causes of all the problems contributing to that occurrence. With respect to the lack of expertise in surgical procedures of obstetrical nursing staff, asking *Why?* uncovered significant negative attitudes on the part of all involved. Obstetrical nurses were reluctant to take on new responsibilities. Nursing administration was unwilling to commit the funds to train nurses in new expertise. Obstetrical physicians were skeptical that the obstetrical nurses could develop acceptable levels of competence. The institution's administration recognized that significant remodeling of the delivery suites would be required to provide surgical services there. If an RCA had not been performed, all of these contributing factors would have remained under the surface and would not have been dealt with. As is often the case, many different situations came together at the same time to contribute to a patient's unnecessary death.

In any situation, several levels of proximate causes must be identified and worked through to finally uncover the root causes. Repeatedly asking *Why?* helps investigators arrive at root causes. (See figure 11.6.)

Figure 11.6. Sample root-cause analysis

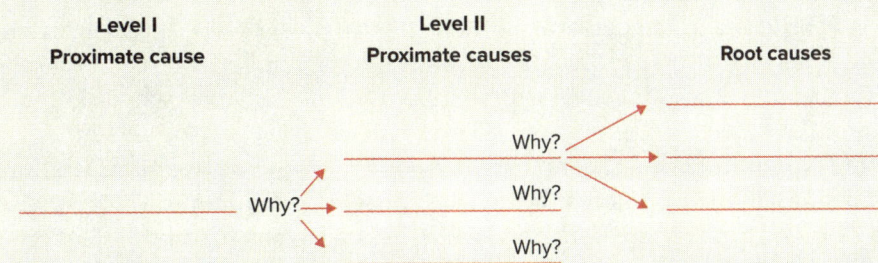

After the investigation and RCA of the factors that contributed to Mrs. Yu's death, administrators at Community Hospital of the West recognized that the current configuration of the delivery suite in the facility had directly contributed to a patient's death. In a situation in which her anomalous uterine anatomy presented the care team with dangerous and unexpected consequences, she need not have died. If the exploratory laparotomy and possible emergency hysterectomy procedures could have been performed in the delivery room, Mrs. Yu's life probably could have been saved.

The administrators recognized that every transport of a patient from the delivery room to the OR exposed the patient to unnecessary risk. The time wasted in transport in this case had proved fatal. The administrators undertook reconfiguration of the environment and processes to prevent a recurrence of this situation. The delivery rooms were rapidly remodeled and equipped with all the equipment and supplies necessary to support the performance of surgical procedures. Obstetrical nurses were retrained to assist on surgical procedures so that these procedures could be performed in the delivery room just as they would be performed in the OR. Following that episode, all cesarean sections and other obstetrical emergency procedures were performed without requiring the patient to be transported to an OR.

Check Your Understanding 11.3

1. After a recent adverse event at a skilled nursing facility, the facility's administrator and director of nursing used a tool to determine the contributing factors of the event. Which of the following tools did they use to analyze the situation?
   a. Affinity diagram
   b. Cause-and-effect diagram
   c. Flow chart
   d. Pareto chart

2. What is the role of root-cause analysis in healthcare?
   a. Improving employee satisfaction
   b. Enhancing hospital infrastructure
   c. Reducing patient safety incidents and improving quality of care
   d. Streamlining administrative processes

Case Study

Dr. Reid, has been an anesthesiologist at General Hospital for 15 years. He is 45 years old. The physician is board certified to perform all kinds of anesthesia procedures, including those for every type of surgical and obstetrical procedure. His colleagues have noticed for some time that he has become more and more haggard looking, but they ascribe this to the hectic work schedule that anesthesiologists often must maintain.

One day, Dr. Reid was admitted to the intensive care unit at General Hospital. The news quickly spread through the organization. It was found that he had a compromised immune system and was close to dying from septicemia that had developed from abscesses in his arm as a result of injections. Some of the OR nurses discussed the situation on their break and speculated that Dr. Reid was a drug addict.

Dr. Hansen, another anesthesiologist, noticed a pattern of irregularities in the seals of vials of the powerful anesthetic drug Fentanyl being used in the OR. To Dr. Hansen, it appeared that the manufacturer's seals had been tampered with. Dr. Hansen and some of the OR nurses had also noticed over the past year that Dr. Reid's appearance and behavior had changed.

Dr. Hansen had mentioned to the chief of the anesthesia service that Dr. Reid was "not acting like himself" and that it seemed that some vials of Fentanyl in the OR may have been tampered with. Not wanting to challenge or accuse a fellow physician, the chief of anesthesia disregarded the comment and terminated the conversation. Dr. Hansen did not discuss the problem with anyone else—not the director of surgical services, the chief of surgery, the director of nursing, or an administrator.

The possibility of personal addiction among healthcare workers is a job-related issue. Individuals who have access to controlled medications can become caught in an addictive cycle themselves, especially when system processes fail to hold professionals accountable for controlled substance use or abuse. Most organizations offer employees access to confidential counseling. Unfortunately, many times those who have problems with alcohol or drugs are unable to see their problem and justify their use in a variety of ways. The facility should have a mechanism in place for confidential reporting of suspected abuse. The ability to offer Dr. Reid, or any provider, a professional intervention could save them physically and mentally from severe trauma.

Case Study Questions

1. What observations were made or what evidence was there to indicate that Dr. Reid had a drug problem?
2. Does General Hospital bear any responsibility for Dr. Reid's predicament? Why or why not?
3. What are the root causes of this situation? Build a cause-and-effect diagram on the basis of the findings in this case study.
4. What are the costs to the organization in terms of reputation, patient and employee safety, and organizational culture? What would you recommend General Hospital do to mitigate the impact of these costs?

Review Questions

1. George was walking into the hospital on his way to visit his wife who had just delivered their first child. His arms were loaded with flowers, balloons, and a teddy bear for the baby. As George was crossing the lobby, he slipped, dropped what he was carrying, and cried out in pain as he fell to the floor. Prior to George entering the hospital, housekeeping had just mopped the lobby floor and failed to put out a "wet floor" sign. George ended up in the emergency department with a fractured wrist. What is the role of the risk manager in this scenario, and how should the risk manager respond?

2. A person who represents the rights and interests of another individual as though they were the person's own is referred to as a patient _____.
   a. Advocate
   b. Friend
   c. Advisor
   d. Manager

3. Explain how risk managers use their skills in patient advocacy to lessen the negative impact that potentially compensable events can have on healthcare organizations.

4. A patient was taken into surgery at a local hospital for treatment of colon cancer. A large section of the colon was removed during surgery, and the patient was taken to the medical floor after surgery. Within the first 24 hours post-op, the patient developed fever, chills, and abdominal pain. An abdominal CT scan revealed the presence of a foreign body. This situation describes a _____.
   a. Near miss
   b. Sentinel event
   c. Security incident
   d. Time-out

5. Explain the importance of patients' rights as they receive services at a healthcare facility.

References

CMS (Centers for Medicare and Medicaid Services). n.d.a. "Skilled Nursing Facility Rights." Accessed January 11, 2024. https://www.medicare.gov/what-medicare-covers/what-part-a-covers/skilled-nursing-facility-rights.

CMS (Centers for Medicare and Medicaid Services). n.d.b. "Glossary." Accessed January 15, 2024. https://www.cms.gov/glossary?term=patient+advocate&items_per_page=10&viewmode=grid.

Joint Commission. 2024a. "Glossary." In *Hospital Accreditation Standards*. Oakbrook Terrace, IL: Joint Commission Resources.

Joint Commission. 2024b. "Sentinel Event Policy and Procedures." https://www.jointcommission.org/resources/sentinel-event/sentinel-event-policy-and-procedures/.

Joint Commission. 2024c. "Rights and Responsibilities of the Individual." In *Hospital Accreditation Standards*. Oakbrook Terrace, IL: Joint Commission Resources.

Kohn, L. T., J. M. Corrigan, and M. S. Donaldson, eds. 1999. "Committee on Quality of Health in America, Institute of Medicine." In *To Err Is Human: Building a Safer Health System*. Washington, DC: National Academies Press.

Veterans Health Administration. 2023. "Rights and Responsibilities of VA Patients and Residents of Community Living Centers." https://www.va.gov/health/rights/patientrights.asp.

Resources

ASHRM (American Society for Healthcare Risk Management). 2010. *Risk Management Handbook for Health Care Organizations*, 6th ed. Edited by R. Carroll. San Francisco: Jossey-Bass.

Patient Safety and Quality Improvement Act of 2005. Public Law 109-41.

Spath, P. L., ed. 2011. *Error Reduction in Health Care: A Systems Approach to Patient Safety*, 2nd ed. San Francisco: Jossey-Bass.

Wessels, R. and L.M. McCorkle. 2021. Analysis of patient safety risk management call data during the COVID-19 pandemic. *Journal of Healthcare Risk Management* 40(4), 30–37.

Wu, D. D. and D. L. Olson. 2020. *Pandemic Risk Management in Operations and Finance*. Vol. 10. New York: Springer International Publishing.

Building a Safe Medication Management System 12

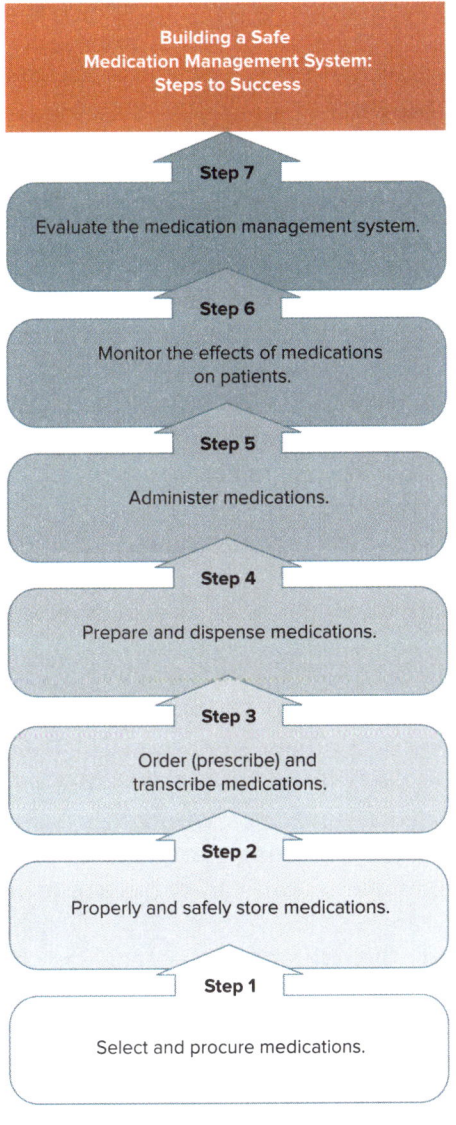

Chapter 12 Building a Safe Medication Management System

Learning Objectives

- Distinguish how health policy, national initiatives, the private sector, and professional advocacy all contribute to the design of safe medication management systems
- Identify the important functions in a safe and effective medication management system
- Use the failure mode and effects analysis (FMEA) tool as a proactive risk-reduction strategy in anticipating medication system failures
- Apply the process of monitoring and reporting medication errors and adverse drug events
- Describe patient safety issues and the legal consequences associated with medication errors and adverse drug events

Key Terms

Adverse drug event (ADE)
Adverse drug reaction (ADR)
Brand name
Diversion
Drug pedigree
Failure mode and effects analysis (FMEA)
Formulary
Generic
Medication administration record (MAR)
Medication reconciliation
Pharmacy and therapeutics (P&T) committee

Federal laws provide a foundation for the state laws that govern pharmacy practice. In addition to the specific drug laws enforced by the Food and Drug Administration (FDA) and the Drug Enforcement Administration (DEA), there are federal laws regulating the approval, storage, and dispensing of medications and controlled substances that apply to various aspects of pharmacy practice. In each state, the Department of Professional Licensing (DOPL) or its equivalent is responsible for regulating the practices of those who prescribe and dispense medication. There are instances in regulating pharmacy practice in which state law may be more stringent than federal law or vice versa. These regulations have been developed to protect the patient and to provide for minimum standards of practice. The rules and regulations that govern pharmacy practice are continually evaluated and updated as new technologies, new medications, and new protocols are developed and adopted.

In the US, drug regulation is performed by the FDA. FDA activity is a major factor in the nation's public health and safety. Before a drug can be marketed, testing must show that it is safe and effective for its intended use. Once marketed, the drugs are monitored by the FDA to make sure that they work as intended and there are no serious negative (adverse) effects from their use. If drugs on the market are found to have significant adverse effects, the FDA can recall them (take them off the market). Bringing a new drug to market is a long and difficult process in which the vast majority of research does not produce a successful drug. Thousands of chemical combinations must be tried to find one that might work as hoped. Once a potentially useful drug is created, it must undergo an extensive testing and approval process before it can be made available to the public. In the US, the length of time from the start of development through testing and ultimate FDA approval can often be more than 10 years.

The sheer number of available drugs; their different names and costs; multiple prescriptions from different providers; and the potential for system errors in the ordering, preparing, dispensing, and administration of medications are among the many factors that make using prescription drugs a complex process filled with many risks. A landmark study (Leape et al. 1995) identified system failures as fundamental to errors that cause an **adverse drug event (ADE)**. An ADE is defined as patient injury that results from a medical intervention related to a medication, including harm from an adverse reaction or medication error. This study found that 39 percent of errors occurred in prescriber ordering and 38 percent in nurse administration. The most common type of errors were dosing errors, which occurred more than three times as frequently as any other error, and which most commonly included wrong-dose errors and errors in drug choice. More importantly, Leape and colleagues identified lack of knowledge about the drug as the most common proximal cause of drug errors, accounting for 22 percent of ADEs. Of particular concern to health professionals involved in the medication-use process was a later study that showed that adverse medical events originate more frequently from errors and accidents in the processes of prescribing, ordering, dispensing, administering, and monitoring medication than from any other sources (Bates et al. 1995).

Since the much-publicized 1999 report by the Institute of Medicine (IOM), *To Err Is Human: Building a Safer Health System*, numerous initiatives have emerged to address the problems associated with medical errors. The IOM orchestrated the drive to improve safety and quality in US healthcare by publishing a series of reports on various problems associated with the healthcare delivery system (Kohn et al. 1999).

The Leapfrog Group, founded in 2000 by the Business Roundtable (a national association of Fortune 500 chief executive officers), mobilized the purchasing power of 150 large employers. The group's intent was to leverage its influence to initiate and advance safety improvements in healthcare, thereby giving consumers information to make more informed healthcare choices. The Leapfrog Group advocated for a variety of quality improvement standards, including computerized provider order entry and evidence-based medicine.

Since 2000, the Joint Commission has engaged in significant efforts to redesign standards and survey processes to better reflect national initiatives aimed at quality improvement and patient safety. The Joint Commission made medication management a top priority by increasing the stringency of its standards and aligning them with a survey process that uses a tracer methodology to track the care, treatment, and services that patients receive. Using this tracer activity allows surveyors to assess how staff from various departments and disciplines work together and communicate across services to provide safe, high-quality care.

Medication reconciliation is a National Patient Safety Goal (NPSG) (Joint Commission 2024a) aimed at addressing a major cause of medication-related sentinel events and medication errors due to a lack of information. This goal encourages healthcare professionals, including physicians, nurses, and pharmacists, as well as the patient and family, to work together to safely prescribe medications and assess for a potential allergic or **adverse drug reaction (ADR)**. Medication reconciliation is the process of identifying the most accurate list of all medications a patient is currently taking (including prescription and nonprescription drugs, vitamins, herbal agents, and nutritional supplements) and then comparing (reconciling) the list to the physician's admission, transfer, and discharge orders at each transition point along the patient's continuum of care. For example, when a patient is transferred from one facility to another, the complete and reconciled list of medications is communicated to the next provider of service, and the communication is documented. Alternatively, when the patient leaves a facility's care and goes directly to their home, the complete and reconciled list of medications is provided to the patient's primary care provider, the original referring provider, or a known next provider of service. It may also be provided to the patient.

The list of organizations involved in patient safety efforts continues to grow. Research on the nature, frequency, and preventability of adverse medical events has begun to bear fruit as health insurance payers become more insistent that providers demonstrate they are implementing strategies to ensure patients' safety.

Building a Safe and Effective Medication Management System: Steps to Success

The medication management system is complex and involves many processes. (See figure 12.1.) Medications are prescribed by providers, dispensed by pharmacists, and administered by nurses. All efforts in the design and implementation of a medication management system must be collaborative and multidisciplinary to be fully effective. The Joint Commission standards define a well-planned and well-implemented medication management system as one that supports patient safety and improves the quality of care by doing the following:

- Reducing variation, errors, and misuse
- Using evidence-based practices to develop medication management processes
- Managing critical processes to promote safe medication management throughout the [healthcare organization]
- Monitoring medication management processes with regard to efficiency, quality, and safety
- Standardizing equipment and handling processes, including those for sample medications across the [healthcare organization] to improve the medication management system
- Monitoring the medication management process for efficiency, quality, and safety (Joint Commission 2024b, MM 2)

Figure 12.1. Steps in medication management

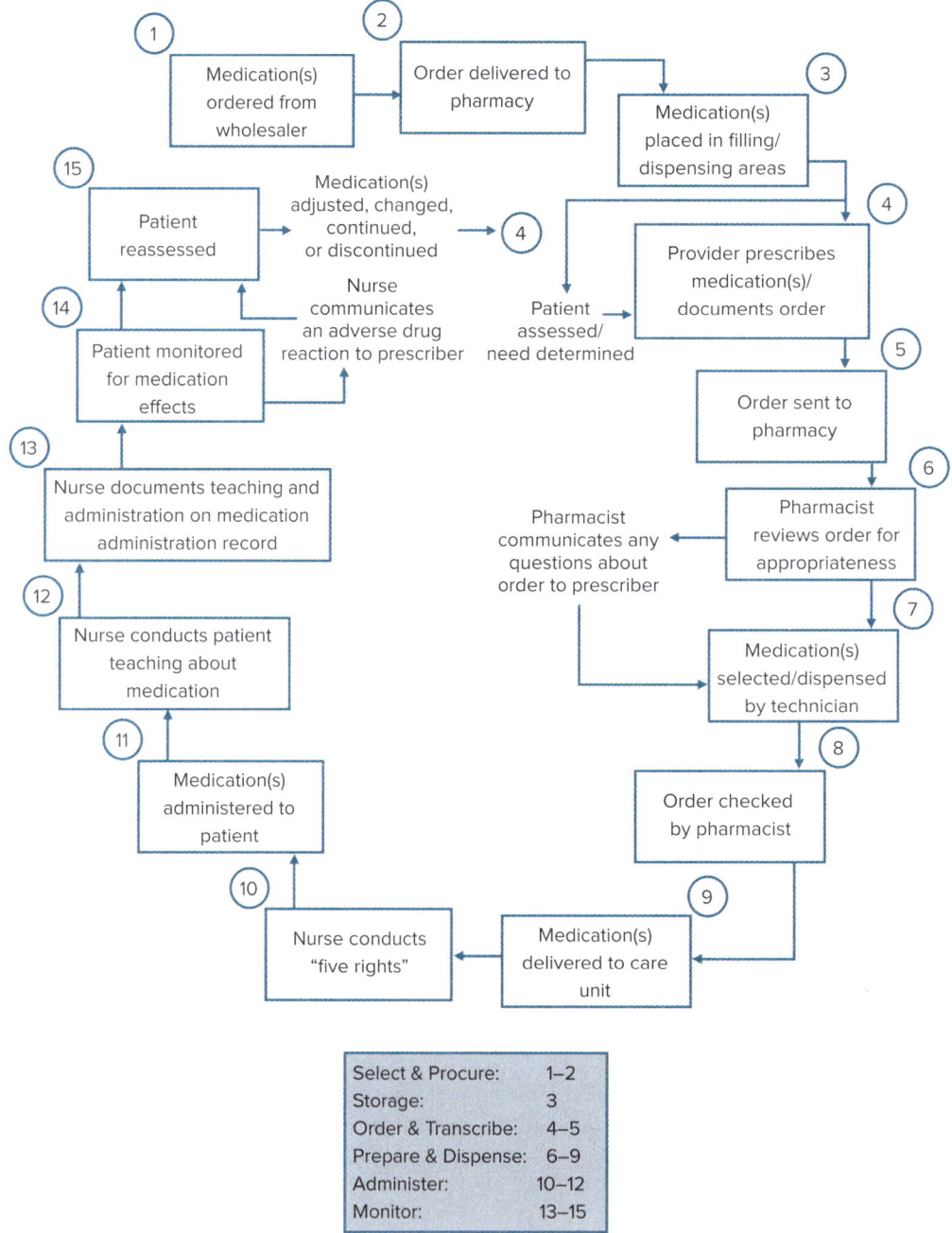

Step 1: Select and Procure Medications

Pharmacies in most healthcare organizations have processes in place to select, purchase, store, and evaluate medications. The list of medications maintained in the healthcare organization is generally referred to as a **formulary** and includes medications selected by members of the healthcare team—those involved in ordering, dispensing, or administering medications or monitoring their use. The formulary is composed of medications used for commonly occurring conditions and diagnoses treated in the healthcare organization. Organizations are required to maintain a formulary and document that they review it at least annually for each medication's continued safety and efficacy.

Criteria used to determine an organization's formulary may include indications for when a medication is to be used, the medication's effectiveness, risks associated with the medication, and its cost. Due in large part to the costs associated with medication use, the management of drug purchases (or inventory control) is an essential process that most healthcare organizations have to address to stay solvent.

The pharmacy purchases medications from a licensed drug wholesaler or directly from a drug manufacturer. The pharmacy will stock thousands of medications from many manufacturers. Obtaining medications directly from individual manufacturers is a difficult and costly process. Wholesalers stock inventories of the most-used medications, obtain less-used medications as they are needed, and make frequent deliveries, often on a daily basis. They also provide value-added services such as emergency delivery, automated inventory systems, automated purchasing systems, generic substitution options, private label products, and many other options. Obtaining most medications from a single wholesaler simplifies the purchasing process.

The FDA established requirements related to the distribution of prescription drugs to counteract the introduction of counterfeit drugs into the US drug distribution chain. Manufacturers, wholesalers, repackagers, and pharmacies must maintain a **drug pedigree**, which is a record of the chain of custody of the drug as it moves through the supply chain from manufacturer to pharmacy (FDA 2024).

Step 2: Properly and Safely Store Medications

Medications stored in the pharmacy and in patient care areas are tightly controlled, and policies clearly delineate who has access to these storage areas. Federal and state laws require that all medications be stored in a manner that prevents access by unauthorized individuals. These same laws require that controlled medications (those classified as narcotics) be maintained in double-locked storage. Tracking and recordkeeping in the purchasing, prescribing, and dispensing of controlled medications are more regulated than that for noncontrolled medications because of their potential for abuse and diversion. Automated storage and dispensing devices are common technologies used to control unauthorized access to medications.

Medications approved for use in an organization are routinely stored under conditions suitable for product stability as recommended by the drug manufacturer. This includes storing medications at certain temperatures—for example, room temperature (68°–77°F), refrigeration (36°–46°F), or freezing (4°–14°F)—in refrigerators designated "medication only." Refrigerator temperatures must be monitored and recorded daily to ensure safe storage. A schedule to inventory all medications stored in the facility to check for expired medications also should be considered when addressing policies related to product stability. Additional storage considerations related to product stability and safety include storing medications for external use separately from medications for internal use and storing extremely flammable products in a specially designed area.

Each healthcare organization must determine whether a patient's own medications may be used and how they will be stored, controlled, and administered. These medications, if allowed, can be administered only in response to orders that permit their administration, and only after they have been evaluated and identified as correct. Some organizations may prohibit patients from using their own medications if the medication is on the facility's formulary and available for use. A facility may allow a patient to use their own medication when it is a nonformulary medication or when an alternative is not available. The organization must define its responsibilities for the safe use and proper storage of these medications. An organization must ensure that medications and the chemicals used to prepare medications are accurately labeled with contents, expiration dates, and warnings; limit or standardize the number of drug concentrations available in the organization; remove concentrated electrolytes from care units or areas; and maintain medications in patient care areas in the most ready-to-administer forms available from the manufacturer (unit doses prepackaged by the pharmacy).

Ensuring proper and safe storage of medications requires periodically inspecting all medication storage areas (including areas where emergency medications and supplies are kept and where sample medications are used) to confirm controls are in place and working. Inspections should focus on storage conditions (for example, refrigeration and protection from light), security (especially for controlled substances), removal of expired and other unusable medications, identification of hazardous conditions, and labeling errors. Findings from inspections should be documented, communicated to appropriate stakeholders in the organization, and corrected as appropriate.

Step 3: Order (Prescribe) and Transcribe Medications

Many medication errors occur while communicating or transcribing medication orders. Clear understanding and communication among staff involved in the medication process are essential. The healthcare organization is responsible for taking steps to reduce the potential for error or misinterpretation when orders are written or verbally communicated. To reinforce the skills and judgment needed for safe medication ordering, organizations often provide training and orientation to providers involved in this step of medication use management.

The required elements of how orders are written or communicated must be specified in policies and procedures. State and federal laws require medication orders to include the patient's name, medication, strength, route, rate, and frequency. Medication orders should clearly state administration times or time intervals between doses. The organization must be very clear about which abbreviations are *not acceptable to use* when writing or communicating medication orders. The Joint Commission published a list of abbreviations classified as "Do Not Use" that healthcare organizations cannot use in writing or communicating medication orders (Joint Commission 2024c). (See figure 12.2.) Organization policy should also define whether or when the diagnosis, condition, or indication for use is included on a medication order. Some organizations require an indication for use or special precautions when ordering medications to be taken "as needed," or for medications specified as confusing or high risk (for example, those with look-alike, sound-alike names).

Figure 12.2. The Joint Commission "Do Not Use" abbreviation list for medication orders

Official "Do Not Use" List[1]

Do Not Use	Potential Problem	Use Instead
U, u (unit)	Mistaken for "0" (zero), the number "4" (four) or "cc"	Write "unit"
IU (International Unit)	Mistaken for IV (intravenous) or the number 10 (ten)	Write "International Unit"
Q.D., QD, q.d., qd (daily) Q.O.D., QOD, q.o.d., qod (every other day)	Mistaken for each other Period after the Q mistaken for "I" and the "O" mistaken for "I"	Write "daily" Write "every other day"
Trailing zero (X.0 mg)* Lack of leading zero (.X mg)	Decimal point is missed	Write X mg Write 0.X mg
MS MSO$_4$ and MgSO$_4$	Can mean morphine sulfate or magnesium sulfate Confused for one another	Write "morphine sulfate" Write "magnesium sulfate"

[1]Applies to all orders and all medication-related documentation that is handwritten (including free-text computer entry) or on pre-printed forms.

*Exception: A "trailing zero" may be used only where required to demonstrate the level of precision of the value being reported, such as for laboratory results, imaging studies that report size of lesions, or catheter/tube sizes. It may not be used in medication orders or other medication-related documentation.

Source: Joint Commission 2024c.

During accreditation surveys an organization's staff may be asked to discuss efforts made to minimize the use of verbal medication orders. Policies should define when verbal (spoken) orders are acceptable and how "read-back" requirements are met. Some organizations prohibit verbal orders for nonurgent, high-risk medications or for high-risk patients. The healthcare organization must also have policies in place for the management of written medication orders. The Joint Commission has defined several types of orders to consider and address in organization policy as "acceptable to use." For example, "as needed" or prn orders, taper orders, or orders for medications at discharge or transfer (Joint Commission 2024b).

Additional policy considerations specific to ordering medications may include determining when generic or brand name medications are acceptable or required as part of a medication order. **Generic** drugs are those with a name representing the chemical composition; they have the same active ingredient as a brand-name drug. The **brand name** is a distinct drug name given by the manufacturer for marketing/sales purposes. Other policies may specify when weight-based dosing for pediatric populations is required and what actions to take when medication orders are incomplete, illegible, or unclear.

Step 4: Prepare and Dispense Medications

Joint Commission standards specify procedures for pharmacist prescription review prior to administration of any medication (see figure 12.3). No medication or patient care area is exempt from this requirement, unless a provider controls the ordering, preparation, and administration of the medication or when a delay would harm the patient in an urgent situation (Joint Commission 2024b, MM 15). For example, this applies to standing orders for labor and delivery, orders for respiratory therapy medications, orders for emergency department patients awaiting transfer to an inpatient room, and orders for preoperative patients in an ambulatory surgery unit.

Increased pharmacist involvement in the review of patient allergies, laboratory test results, and medication orders for appropriateness have been shown to significantly reduce ADEs. Types of errors prevented by pharmacist review include prescribing errors (inappropriate dose, nonformulary agent, and medication errors related to transfer), administration errors (inappropriate timing of dose, transcription errors, missed doses, extra doses given, and doses administered after discontinuation), pharmacy errors (inappropriate dose recommendations, incomplete dispensing instructions), and discharge errors. Pharmacists providing patient education can help reduce errors that may occur after discharge because the patient does not understand how to take a medication. At a minimum, any concerns, issues, or questions a pharmacist may have in reviewing a medication order are clarified with the individual prescriber *before* dispensing the medication.

Figure 12.3. The Joint Commission's minimum criteria for pharmacist reviews

Pharmacist-required review elements for each prescription or medication order:

- Patient allergies or potential sensitivities
- Existing or potential interactions between the medication ordered and food and medications the patient is currently taking
- Appropriateness of the drug, dose, frequency, and route of administration
- Current or potential impact as indicated by laboratory values
- Therapeutic duplication
- Other contraindications

Source: Joint Commission 2024b. Reprinted with permission.

Activities associated with medication preparation and dispensing pose one of the greatest opportunities for error within the pharmacy. Preparation includes the selection, compounding (sterile or nonsterile), packaging, and labeling of the medication. For each of these steps it is critical that technical and professional staff understand the importance of following appropriate procedures and double-checking their work. Selecting the incorrect medication is the most common type of error that other healthcare professionals and the general public associate with the pharmacy. Safeguards must be instituted to ensure that the appropriate medication is selected 100 percent of the time. Practices such as separating look-alike and sound-alike medications and using bar-coded storage technology have improved medication selection safety.

Compounding for sterile and nonsterile medications often requires calculations to determine the amounts of medications and other ingredients to be used. All sterile compounding is performed in a clean environment, so pharmacy personnel need to be trained in aseptic technique and product handling. In particular, antineoplastic (anticancer) agents require even greater safeguards because of their caustic nature and potential for harm.

The order delivery process also has potential for error. As with selecting and compounding, standard safeguards can be employed to decrease the likelihood of errors in order delivery. Standardizing medication labeling and ensuring that medications are delivered to the correct patient care unit and stored in a secure, patient-specific area labeled with the patient's name helps to minimize errors.

Step 5: Administer Medications

In many healthcare organizations, medication administration is the step in the process that has the fewest safeguards because it typically relies on a single healthcare professional to perform it correctly. Healthcare organizations use at least two patient identifiers (such as the patient's name and date of birth) prior to administering medications as a safety precaution to ensure that patients receive the correct medication. Hospitals also require a second check for certain medications, such as insulin, chemotherapy drugs, and other high-alert or high-risk drugs, prior to administering. Identifying ways that the patient, along with family members, can be involved in their own care is an important patient safety strategy. The patient can be an important source of information about many aspects of care and treatment.

One of the most effective ways to prevent administration errors is to provide all medications used within the organization in ready-to-administer form (e.g., the unit dose system). All medications should remain intact in labeled packaging until the point of administration. Maintaining an accurate **medication administration record (MAR)**, which is the record used to document each dose of medication administered to a patient, is critical. Procedures must be in place to periodically review the accuracy of the MAR, particularly with respect to controlled substances such as narcotics.

The "five rights" of medication administration—right patient, right drug, right dose, right route, and right time—should be observed at all times (Hanson and Haddad 2023). (See figure 12.4.) This practice should be monitored periodically for validation. The pharmacy should provide appropriate administration instructions (such as "take with food") for each medication. A pharmacist should be readily available to answer questions related to a particular drug or its administration. Pharmacists also should participate in the design of a medication administration course for nursing staff and other healthcare professionals responsible for drug administration.

Figure 12.4. Five rights of medication administration

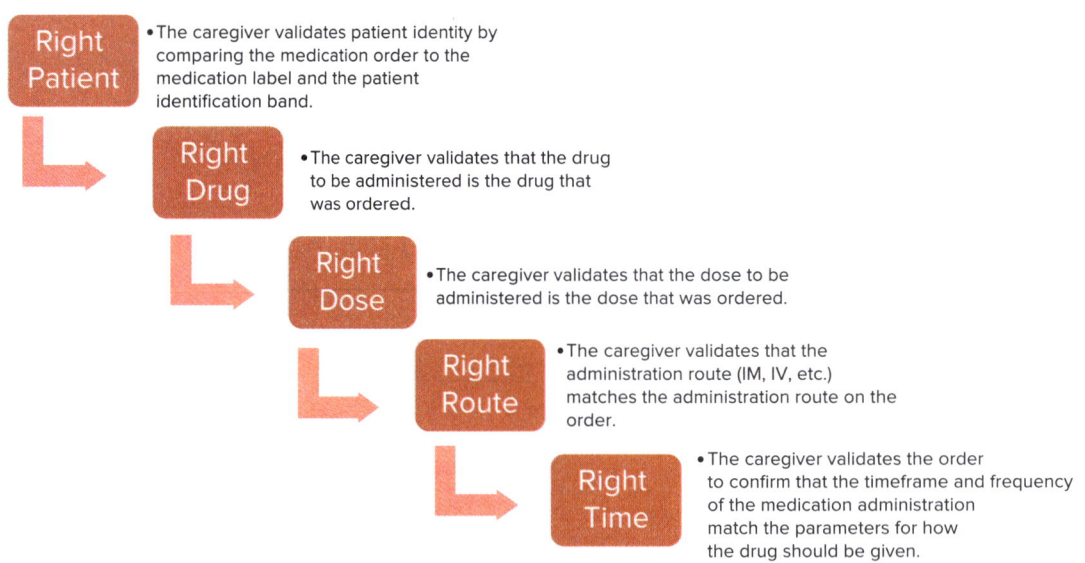

Source: Adapted from Hanson and Haddad 2023

Automated bedside point-of-care (BPOC) scanning uses bar code technology to guarantee that the five rights are followed. Using a scanning device, the nurse scans their badge and the medication to be administered and then scans the patient's bar-coded identification bracelet. Because the system is integrated with the MAR, it will alert the nurse if an error is detected (such as wrong patient, wrong administration time, or wrong medication). These systems are considered "best practice" because of their ability to reduce medication errors associated with drug administration.

Even though a caregiver follows the five rights of medication administration and uses bar-coding technology, errors during medication administration still commonly occur. One of the factors in medication errors is that the caregiver can be easily distracted through interruption or due to the complex nature of the healthcare environment. This interruption may be due to noise, other people, or electronic devices and often leads to a delay in treatment or a loss of concentration. Healthcare organizations often have distraction-free zone policies for all caregivers while completing high-risk tasks such as medication administration. These policies are an attempt to not only limit distraction but also to educate caregivers in understanding that distractions do occur and that they must learn to manage these distractions. One method being taught is mindfulness. A distraction-free zone policy typically includes direction to employees to avoid distraction while preparing or administering medication.

Step 6: Monitor the Effects of Medications on Patients

Monitoring the effects of medications helps ensure that medication therapy is appropriate for the patient and minimizes the occurrence of an ADE. Each patient's response to medication is monitored according to their clinical needs. Monitoring a medication's effect on a patient includes gathering the patient's own perceptions about side effects and, when appropriate, perceived efficacy, and referring to information from the patient's health record, relevant lab results, clinical response, and medication profile. A healthcare organization should have a well-defined process for monitoring a patient's response to the first dose(s) of a medication.

The most widely recognized and studied adverse event involving drug therapy is an **adverse drug reaction (ADR)**. The World Health Organization (WHO) defines an ADR as "any response that is noxious, unintended, and undesired and that occurs at doses normally used in man for prophylaxis, diagnosis, or therapy" (WHO 1970). Healthcare organizations using medication therapy as a treatment intervention need to have processes in place to respond to actual or potential ADRs. Reporting requirements may include external reporting to the United States Pharmacopeia (USP), the FDA, and/or the Institute for Safe Medication Practices (ISMP). Internal reporting requirements should be incorporated into the organization's performance improvement (PI) program and integrated into activities of the **pharmacy and therapeutics (P&T) committee**.

High-risk or high-alert drugs are those involved in a high percentage of medication errors and sentinel events and medications that carry a higher risk for abuse, errors, or other adverse outcomes. Lists of high-risk and high-alert drugs are developed by the organization based on external resources, the organization's unique drug utilization patterns, and internal data about medication errors and sentinel events. Examples of high-risk drugs include investigational drugs, controlled medications, medications not on the approved FDA list, medications with a narrow therapeutic range, psychotherapeutic medications, and look-alike or sound-alike medications that are new to the market or new to the facility.

The National Coordinating Council for Medication Error Reporting and Prevention (NCC MERP) developed a widely used taxonomy for medication error reporting (NCC MERP 1998). The taxonomy provides a logical framework for the development of internal error reporting programs as well as a means to classify and analyze medication errors.

Step 7: Evaluate the Medication Management System

The key to an effective medication management system is having mechanisms for reporting potential and actual medication-related errors and a process to improve patient safety based on this information. Most care settings have an organization-wide PI process to identify and analyze medical errors, medication errors, and near misses. A near miss can be described in the following way: if the error had not been identified, could it have caused patient harm? Many organizations treat near misses in the same way they treat sentinel events, using error reduction tools such as root-cause analysis (RCA) or failure mode and effects analysis (FMEA) in an effort to prevent future occurrences. Reporting such adverse events should be nonpunitive, and each report should be reviewed and investigated.

The P&T committee has a key role in multidisciplinary safety improvement activities; its importance cannot be understated. The committee consists of pharmacists, providers, nurses, hospital administrators, and other healthcare professionals. The committee should have a leadership role in the organization's medication safety efforts. Improvement initiatives should be a major part of every P&T agenda.

Many hospitals have established a medication safety committee that may be a P&T subcommittee. The medication safety committee reviews and evaluates current literature, national error reports, internal reports, and hospital processes to assist with recommendations for improvement. Membership on this committee should be multidisciplinary and should include representatives from the hospital's risk management and quality departments. In some hospitals, this committee is charged with forming risk-reduction teams and developing auditing systems to investigate patterns of medication errors. From these findings, they identify and recommend system-based changes.

One very important aspect of medication management in healthcare facilities is the monitoring of the use and administration of controlled substances because of the use of these medications in treatment of patients of all kinds. Inpatient acute-care settings utilize various types of pain control medications, outpatient clinics may distribute narcotics for pain control, and substance-abuse treatment facilities may distribute psychotropics and synthetic opiates to their clients. Any of these uses and settings can be at risk of diversion. **Diversion** is the removal of a medication from its usual stream of preparation, dispensing, and administration by personnel involved in those steps for the purpose of using or selling the drug in nonhealthcare settings. An individual might take the medication for personal use or to sell or distribute to others. Documentation of the preparation, dispensing, and administration may still be entered in information systems or health records as though the medication were given as ordered.

The work of all staff involved in the medication processes must be regularly monitored to ensure that all policies and procedures are being followed to the letter and that every dose of medication can be accounted for through all steps of the process. When carelessness or infractions in following policy and procedure are identified, the individual involved must be counseled and must undergo disciplinary action. The organization must also determine whether to report the individual to law enforcement and licensing or credentialing agencies. State licensure is usually revoked for infractions of these policies, and professional discipline is instituted per the certifying agency. If the individual involved is diverting for personal use, the organization may have to be further involved as an employer to assist the individual in treatment for substance abuse issues.

Check Your Understanding 12.1

1. Dylan experienced a motorcycle accident and is being treated at a local hospital for multiple fractures and injuries. To help to alleviate his pain, he is given pain medication by his nurse Holly. Holly correctly followed all the steps of medication administration and the drug was administered correctly. Holly began monitoring Dylan, as this was the first administration of the medication. Within a few minutes of administration, Dylan begins experiencing respiratory distress. Even though the five rights of medication administration were followed, Dylan is experiencing a(n):
   a. Adverse drug event
   b. Drug error
   c. Adverse pharmacological
   d. Medication error

2. Give three examples from the list of "Do Not Use" abbreviations published by the Joint Commission. List the abbreviation, note what each could be mistaken for, and detail why these abbreviations are a patient safety issue.

QI Toolbox Technique: Failure Mode and Effects Analysis

There are two proven approaches to error analysis and reduction that are used by the healthcare industry. The first approach, root-cause analysis (RCA), is a retrospective (reactive) tool used to analyze the true cause of error. The second approach, **failure mode and effects analysis (FMEA)**, is a prospective (proactive) tool useful in analyzing potential problems when introducing new systems or equipment or when looking anew at an existing process. Organizations are increasingly using RCA as one step of a proactive risk-reduction effort combined with FMEA. One step of FMEA involves identifying the root causes of failures (failure mode).

FMEA includes defining high-risk processes using flow charts; identifying potential failure points in current processes; and scoring each potential failure by considering factors such as the frequency of failure, potential harm, and the likelihood that the failure will be detected before it reaches the patient. Both tools are used frequently in analyzing potential or real medication errors.

Healthcare organizations investigate medication-related problems using methods such as FMEA, a technique that promotes systems thinking (ASQ 2024). Potential failures with the highest criticality score become the focus of process redesign. Figure 12.5 illustrates the potential risks to medication safety and prioritizes areas for improvement when administering medication to hospital patients. In this example, four potential failure modes are identified: wrong medication administered, incorrect dosage given, allergic reaction not detected, and inadequate patient education on medication.

The potential effects of each failure mode are determined and a severity (S) rating assigned. The potential causes of each failure mode are identified and an occurrence (O) rating is assigned, followed by assignment of the detection (D) ratings of each failure mode. Finally, the risk priority number (RPN) is calculated by multiplying the severity rating by the occurrence rating and then by the detection rating (RPN = S ×O ×D). For the potential failure mode of incorrect dosage given, the severity rating is high (3), as the patient may receive too much or too little of the medication leading to adverse effects or inadequate treatment. The occurrence rating of this failure mode (incorrect dosage given) is moderate (2), and may be attributed to misinterpretation of prescription orders. The detection rating for this failure mode (incorrect dosage given) is moderate (2), as it may be caught during regular patient checks. The RPN score for this potential failure mode is calculated as severity (3) times occurrence (2) times detection (2) equals 12 (3×2×2= 12). The higher the risk priority number (RPN), the higher the priority for addressing that particular failure mode. In figure 12.5, two of the four potential failure modes for administering medication to hospital patients have a risk priority number of twelve (12), indicating that both potential failure modes, incorrect dosage given and inadequate patient education on medication, should be addressed to ensure ongoing improvement and patient safety.

Figure 12.5. Sample FMEA for administering medication to patients in a hospital

Sample Failure Mode and Effects Analysis for Potential Problems for Medication Safety								
Process	Severity of Failure Mode (S)		Cause of Failure Mode Occurrence (O)		Detection of Failure Mode (D)		RPN Score (S×O×D)	
Wrong medication administered	Patient may experience adverse effects or no therapeutic benefit.	High (3)	Similar medication packaging or labeling	Low (1)	Low (may not be immediately apparent)	Low (1)	3×1×1 = **3**	
Incorrect dosage given	Patient may receive too much or too little of the medication, leading to adverse effects or inadequate treatment.	High (3)	Misinterpretation of prescription orders	Moderate (2)	Moderate (may be caught during regular checks)	Moderate (2)	3×2×2 = **12**	
Allergic reaction not detected	Patient may experience an allergic reaction, which can be severe.	High (3)	Lack of patient allergy history verification	Low (1)	Moderate (can be detected through proper verification)	Moderate (2)	3×1×2 = **6**	
Inadequate patient education	Patient may not understand how to take the medication, leading to noncompliance or misuse.	Moderate (2)	Insufficient patient education resources	Moderate (2)	High (can be addressed through education checks)	High (3)	2×2×3 = **12**	

Real-Life Example

In 1962, a new sleeping pill containing the drug thalidomide was found to cause severe birth defects when used by pregnant women. This included lost limbs and other major deformities that affected thousands of children in Europe, where the drug had been widely used. In the US, the drug had not been approved for marketing and was only being used in tests. However, the nature of the defects and the number of children affected created a public demand in the US for tighter drug regulations that resulted in the Kefauver-Harris Amendment, which changed the course of the drug approval process. From then on, manufacturers were required to provide proof of both safety and effectiveness of a drug before they could market it. Later studies found thalidomide to be safe and effective in treating multiple myeloma, and it is now approved for that use in individuals who are not pregnant or likely to become pregnant.

Case Study

Mike is a nurse working in the newborn intensive care unit (NICU) in a large tertiary care medical center. He has gone to the medication room to pick up a medication ordered for one of his newborn patients. While in the medication room, he scans the bar code on the medication to ensure that this is the correct drug for his patient. He also confirms that this medication matches the ordered drug. He returns to the NICU and scans the bar code on the medication again, as well as the bar code on the patient's identification band, confirming a match. The drug Mike needs to administer to this patient is considered a high-risk medication. Per hospital policy, Mike must have another nurse confirm the medication before administering it to his patient. As Mike is preparing to ask another nurse to confirm this high-risk medication, the respiratory therapist stops Mike to ask him a question about his patient. Mike and the respiratory therapist complete their conversation, and after this distraction, Mike administers the medication to his newborn patient without confirming the medication with another nurse.

Case Study Questions

1. What negative outcome could this patient experience because of this situation?
2. Which step in the medication administration process was missed?
3. How could Mike have used the skill of mindfulness to increase his awareness of distraction?
4. How could a distraction-free zone policy and subsequent culture have altered the circumstances presented in the case?

Review Questions

1. Provide two examples of possible patient safety issues related to medication errors and adverse drug events, and demonstrate how a healthcare organization could avoid these safety issues with effective policies and procedures.

2. In consideration of the "Do Not Use" abbreviation list for medication orders, which of the following medication orders would be considered acceptable?
   a. Take 1 tablet q.d.
   b. Take 1 tablet every 6 hours
   c. Administer 1 U of packed red blood cells
   d. Administer 200.0 m.g. of Tylenol if the patient's temperature was > 99.5 degrees F.

3. Detail how laws and regulations have improved the likelihood that a patient will receive medication that has been administered correctly.

4. A patent for a new drug gives its manufacturer an exclusive right to market the drug for a specific period of time under which type of name?
   a. Brand
   b. Generic
   c. Specific
   d. Patent

5. Inappropriate dose, nonformulary agent, and medication errors related to transfer are all examples of which type of medication error?
   a. Administration
   b. Pharmacy
   c. Discharge
   d. Prescribing

References

ASQ (American Society of Quality). 2024. "Failure Mode Effects Analysis (FMEA)." https://asq.org/quality-resources/fmea.

Bates, D. W., D. J. Cullen, N. Laird, L. A. Petersen, S. D. Small, D. Servi, G. Laffel, B. J. Sweitzer, B. F. Shea, and R. Hallisey. 1995. Incidence of adverse drug events and potential adverse drug events: Implications for prevention. *JAMA* 279:1200–1205.

FDA (Food and Drug Administration). 2024. "Drug Supply Chain Security Act Product Tracing Requirements | Frequently Asked Questions." https://www.fda.gov/drugs/drug-supply-chain-security-act-dscsa/drug-supply-chain-security-act-product-tracing-requirements-frequently-asked-questions.

Hanson A. and L. M. Haddad. 2023. "Nursing Rights of Medication Administration." In *StatPearls*. Treasure Island (FL): StatPearls Publishing. https://www.ncbi.nlm.nih.gov/books/NBK560654/.

Joint Commission. 2024a. "National Patient Safety Goals." In *Hospital Accreditation Standards*. Oakbrook Terrace, IL: Joint Commission.

Joint Commission. 2024b. "Medication Management." In *Hospital Accreditation Standards*. Oakbrook Terrace, IL: Joint Commission Resources.

Joint Commission. 2024c. "The official 'Do Not Use' list." https://www.jointcommission.org/resources/news-and-multimedia/fact-sheets/facts-about-do-not-use-list/.

Kohn, L. T., J. M. Corrigan, and M. S. Donaldson, eds. 1999. "Committee on Quality of Health in America, Institute of Medicine." In *To Err Is Human: Building a Safer Health System*. Washington, DC: National Academies Press.

Leape, L. L., D. W. Bates, D. J. Cullen, J. Cooper, H. J. Demonaco, T. Gallivan, R. Hallisey, J. Ives, N. Laird, and G. Laffel. 1995. Systems analysis of adverse drug events. *JAMA* 274:35–43.

NCC MERP (National Coordinating Council for Medication Error Reporting and Prevention). 1998. "NCC MERP Taxonomy of Medication Errors." https://www.nccmerp.org/sites/default/files/taxonomy2001-07-31.pdf.

WHO (World Health Organization). 1970. International drug monitoring: The role of the hospital—a WHO report. *Drug Intelligence & Clinical Pharmacy* 4:101–110.

Resources

Huckels-Baumgart, S., A. Baumgart, U. Buschmann, G. Schüpfer, and T. Manser. 2021. Separate medication preparation rooms reduce interruptions and medication errors in the hospital setting: A prospective observational study. *Journal of Patient Safety* 17(3):e161–e168, https://doi.org/10.1097/PTS.0000000000000335.

Kavanagh, A. and J. Donnelly. 2020. A lean approach to improve medication administration safety by reducing distractions and interruptions. *Journal of Nursing Care Quality* 35(4):e58–e62, https://doi.org/10.1097/NCQ.0000000000000473.

Kellogg, K. M., J. S. Puthumana, A. Fong, K. T. Adams, and R. M. Ratwani. 2021. Understanding the types and effects of clinical interruptions and distractions recorded in a multihospital patient safety reporting system. *Journal of Patient Safety* 17(8):e1394–e1400, https://doi.org/10.1097/PTS.0000000000000513.

Prescription Drug Amendment of 2007. Public Law 110-85.

WHO (World Health Organization). 2024. "Medication Without Harm." https://www.who.int/initiatives/medication-without-harm.

Managing the Environment of Care

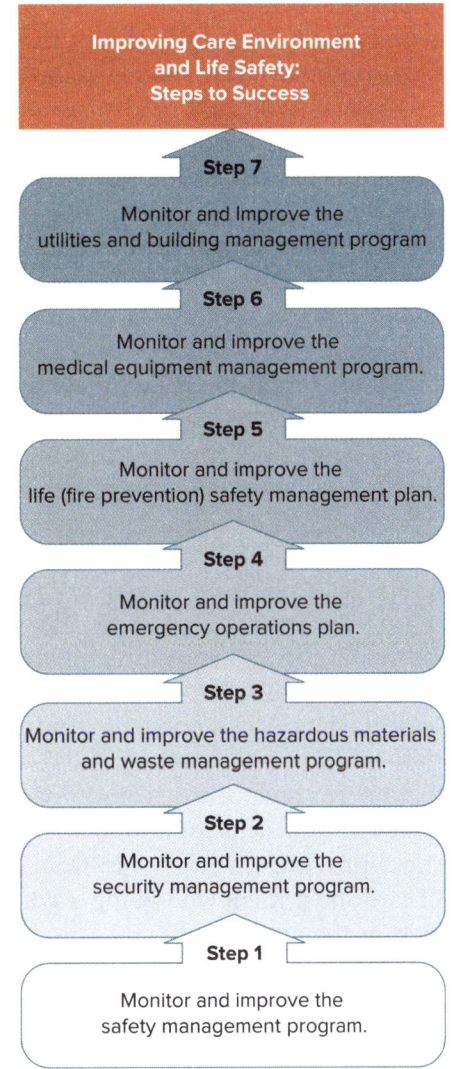

Chapter 13 Managing the Environment of Care

Learning Objectives

- Examine the seven programs and plans that are key elements in a healthcare organization's environment of care
- Explain how the relationship between accreditation standards and the National Incident Management System (NIMS) influences the development of an emergency operations plan
- Model risk assessment and hazard vulnerability analysis processes
- Apply the safety monitoring process

Key Terms

All-hazards approach
Emergency
Emergency operations plan (EOP)
Hazard vulnerability analysis (HVA)
National Incident Management System (NIMS)
Safety data sheets (SDSs)

The goal of managing the care environment in any healthcare organization is to provide a safe, functional, supportive, and effective environment for patients, staff, and visitors. By their nature, healthcare organizations have the potential to be dangerous environments. They house complex equipment, hazardous materials, toxic and flammable chemicals, infectious materials, and medical devices that can injure patients, visitors, and staff when inappropriately managed. Also of major importance, healthcare organizations need to be prepared for catastrophic emergencies such as natural, human-caused, or technology-caused events and the handling of an influx of injured individuals.

Healthcare workers provide care to individuals who may have family relationships or other visitor issues that may spill over into the healthcare environment. Issues in the lives of healthcare workers may also affect the work environment. Violence in the workplace is a threat that must be assessed and managed. Because of these and other safety issues, healthcare organizations must continuously monitor and evaluate their patient environments and the safety and security of the individuals receiving and providing care services. Developing plans to manage the healthcare environment, educating staff regarding their role in supporting a safe environment, monitoring and assessing performance, and making improvements based on these findings are all critical functions that contribute to effectively managing the environment of care (EC).

Improving the Environment of Care: Steps to Success

The Joint Commission requires a varying number of safety functions and plans, depending on the type of license or services provided by an organization. This chapter will review all seven safety programs required by the Joint Commission for an acute-care hospital. The standards require the assessment of safety features for staff and visitors, with patients being the largest visitor population. The EC includes the safety, security, and comfort of staff, patients, and other visitors. For the purposes of safety, a *visitor* is defined as any person who is not an employee of the healthcare organization. This group includes patients, patients' families and other guests, volunteers, independent contract providers, students in training, agency personnel, and vendors. A quality program emphasizes clinical care and patient well-being, as do the Joint Commission patient safety standards. (The patient safety standards, as they relate to the EC, are discussed later in this chapter.)

The seven written safety standards (plans) for the EC cover the following areas:

- Safety management
- Security management
- Hazardous materials and waste management

- Life safety management
- Medical equipment management
- Utilities management
- Smoking policy management (Joint Commission 2024a)

This chapter discusses the scope, goals, and objectives of each program or plan. Common to each plan is an orientation and education program for personnel, with their specific roles and responsibilities defined, as well as an annual evaluation of each plan's objectives, scope, performance, and effectiveness.

Step 1: Monitor and Improve the Safety Management Program

The safety management program is the overall plan for the EC. It demonstrates the master plan and outlines the design of the safety functions for the organization. The safety committee oversees all safety programs, including the following:

- Designating an individual or individuals to develop, implement, and monitor safety management activities
- Designating an individual or individuals to intervene whenever conditions immediately threaten life or health or threaten damage to equipment or buildings
- Overseeing the worker safety program
- Conducting comprehensive, proactive risk assessments that evaluate potential adverse impact on buildings, grounds, equipment, occupants, and internal physical systems
- Establishing safety policies and procedures that are practiced and reviewed as frequently as necessary
- Responding to product medical/equipment/pharmaceutical safety recalls
- Ensuring that all grounds and equipment are maintained appropriately (Joint Commission 2024a)

The overall safety plan describes the risk assessment of the physical environment, the design of services that support the therapeutic and work environment, and the education and preparation of the staff to safely and securely serve the patient population. The plan describes how to train staff on use of equipment and how to maintain an environment that is responsive to patient care needs, including responding to emergencies.

In addition, the plan includes organizational goals for monitoring and maintaining the physical components of the EC and for managing human activities. Reporting organizational incidents that are relevant to safety programs (such as reports of unusual occurrences, incident reports, and security reports) is integral to each safety function. Each safety program is evaluated annually, and plans are updated or revised to address current regulatory compliance, policy, and procedural changes based on the organizational experiences and staff training needs.

Step 2: Monitor and Improve the Security Management Program

The security management program is designed to manage the physical and personal security of patients, staff, and other individuals coming to the facility as well as the security of the building, equipment, supplies, and information.

The security management program is reflective of the security risk assessment conducted annually. Figure 13.1 shows an example of a security risk assessment and program evaluation. Included in the risk assessment is the trending of the prior-year statistics of security incidents in the facility and on the grounds, including any workplace violence against employees. If possible, the assessment should include a police grid of crime in the areas or neighborhoods surrounding the facility. Neighborhood crime statistics may be available on websites, through local hospital or merchants security associations, or by calling local police precincts. Security risks determined by the assessment are evaluated, and processes, procedures, and education are designed and implemented to avoid those risks. Efficacy of the security plan is monitored, trended, and reported to the safety committee, administration, medical staff, and the board of trustees. Staff are educated and trained to report or respond to security events.

Figure 13.1A. Security risk assessment and program evaluation

FACILITY DESCRIPTION

Name of facility: _____

Type of facility (e.g., acute-care hospital): _____

City and State: _____

Location: _____ inner city _____ suburban _____ rural _____ university

Licensed beds: _____

Avg. beds occupied: _____

Number of buildings: _____

Total square footage occupied: _____

Number of parking garages: _____

Total number of surface parking lots: _____

Total number of parking spaces: _____

Emergency room services? _____ yes _____ no

If yes, what level? _____

Birthing services? _____ yes _____ no

If yes, what is the annual number of births per year? _____

Psychiatry unit? _____ yes _____ no

Local crime rate (as determined by police statistics): _____ high _____ medium _____ low

SECURITY DEPARTMENT DESCRIPTION

Special authority? _____ yes _____ no

If yes, please describe: _____

Weapons carried? _____ yes _____ no

If yes, please describe: _____

To what department and position does security report? _____

Position	Number	FTEs
Director	_____	_____
Manager(s)	_____	_____
Coordinator(s)	_____	_____
Supervisor(s)	_____	_____
Officer(s)	_____	_____
Parking Officers	_____	_____
Administrative Assistant	_____	_____
Dispatch Coord.	_____	_____
Dispatch	_____	_____
Other	_____	_____

Figure 13.1B. Security risk assessment and program evaluation (*Continued*)

SECURITY PROGRAM EVALUATION

Date of last internal program evaluation: _____

Date of last external program evaluation: _____

High Risk Areas/Departments	Vulnerability/Risk

List major vulnerabilities/risks identified, actions taken, and status (use additional sheets, if necessary):

Vulnerability/Risk	Actions Taken	Status

SECURITY-RELATED STATISTICS			
Type of Incident	**Number**	**Increase from 2024**	**Value-Cost—N/A**
Homicide(s)			
Abduction(s)			
Abduction attempt(s)			
Arson(s)			
Rape(s)			
Other sexual assault(s)			
Robbery(ies)—armed			
• Facility departments			
• Public areas (internal)			
• Public areas (grounds)			
• Parking lot(s)			
• Parking garage(s)			
Robbery(ies)—unarmed			
• Facility departments			
• Public areas (internal)			
• Public areas (grounds)			
• Parking lot(s)			
• Parking garage(s)			
Auto theft(s)			

Figure 13.1C. Security risk assessment and program evaluation (*Continued*)

Type of Incident	Number	Increase from 2024	Value-Cost—N/A
Auto break-ins			
Assault(s)			
• Emergency room			
• Psychiatry			
• Patient care areas			
• Public areas (internal)			
• Public areas (grounds)			
• Parking lot(s)			
• Parking garage(s)			
Threats			
• Emergency room			
• Psychiatry			
• Patient care areas			
• Public areas (internal)			
• Public areas (grounds)			
• Parking lot(s)			
• Parking garage(s)			
Bombing(s)			
Bomb threat(s)			
Theft			
• Facility property			
• Patient property			
• Staff property			
• Visitor property			
• Contractor property			
Vandalism			
• Graffiti			
Fraud(s)			
Suicide(s)			
Unsecured doors			
Workplace violence			
Auto accidents			
Tickets issued			
Total number	_____	_____	
Total value			_____

SPECIAL EVENTS	DATE	# PARTICIPANTS
	—	
BACKGROUND CHECKS	_____ yes	_____ no
DRUG SCREENING	_____ yes	_____ no

Figure 13.1D. Security risk assessment and program evaluation (*Continued*)

SECURITY RISK ASSESSMENT			
Item	Yes	No	Comments
Is there a security plan for the entire organization?			
Is it reviewed and revised at least annually?			
Does it contain a mission statement that parallels the hospital mission?			
Is there a letter of authority from the CEO for the security director?			
Is the local geographic area deteriorating?			
Is crime in the area increasing?			
Is there a relationship between security and the state and local police?			
Do patients, staff, and visitors feel secure?			
Has the organization's patient mix changed since last year?			
Has security staffing increased, decreased, or stayed the same?			
Is the current staffing level adequate? If not, why?			
Can security resources be better utilized?			
Have security resources changed in relation to hospital resources?			
Have additional electronic security devices been installed, altering staffing needs?			
Are security staff competent to do their jobs? How do you know?			
Have security personnel performed to the expected level?			
Does security staff receive training and education as needed?			
Are education and training effective? How do you know?			
How are employees made aware of their security roles?			
Do you know how to respond to a security incident (how to contact security and complete an incident report)?			
Is security addressed in the hospital's onboarding process?			
Are security policies and procedures up to date?			
Do they accurately guide security staff on how to do their jobs?			
Is security addressed regularly by the safety committee?			
Does the safety committee make recommendations for security?			
Are security incidents tracked and analyzed as trends? Who does this?			
Are there performance standards in place that measure key aspects of the security program?			
Is security participating in any performance improvement projects?			
Has security improved, gotten worse, or stayed the same in the last year?			
Are security communication devices appropriate?			
Are there emergency communication devices in place?			
Is there a security hotline?			
Is security cameras/video monitoring, in place, functional, etc.?			
Are there alarms in place, with policies that explain them?			
Are patrol vehicles appropriate?			
Do officers carry protective weapons? Are they trained to do so?			
Do security personnel know and observe all applicable laws, standards, and guidelines?			
Do security staff participate in policy development?			
Are lighting levels appropriate throughout the facility?			
Are access control policies in place and adequate?			
Are doors checked and secured appropriately?			
Does the facility design allow for hiding areas?			
What are the sensitive, high-risk areas?			
How were they determined to be high risk?			
What measures were taken to reduce this risk? Have they worked?			
Are there security policies for infant abduction, workplace violence, bomb threats, hostage situations, emergency preparedness, fires, VIPs, hazardous spills, weapons, theft, trespassing, identification, and visitation?			
Are these policies enforced?			

The security management program and security policies describe procedures to manage door access, visiting hours, and after-hours access to the facility; security risks in parking areas, such as suspicious vehicles; high-risk patients, such as victims of crime or patients in police custody; high-profile patients or visitors; weapons in the facilities; suspicious individuals and disruptive visitors; and the issuing of trespass notices, to name a few. Healthcare organizations often use a color-code system (such as Code Green) to alert employees of a situation within the facility when a security threat has been identified. Employees are trained to recognize the color-code system, which can vary by healthcare organization, so that when an alert is given, they can respond appropriately based on their role and location.

Security emergency response may address phone threats, use of panic alarms, abduction of babies or children, civil unrest, bomb threats, active shooters, and hostage crises. In addressing terrorist activities, plans may include handling of suspicious packages and mail or securing ventilation systems. If animal research is conducted at the facility, the research lab may be vulnerable to activist groups from the community, and security should address securing the labs and protecting personnel.

Security management is a technology-rich field, and an organization needs to describe the technology it uses in its plan or policies. The security office is usually responsible for issuing employee identification badges and keys and authorizing electronic access to doors. In addition, it is usually responsible for video surveillance and monitoring.

The security management program identifies security-sensitive areas in the hospital; for example, cash-handling areas (such as the cafeteria, pharmacy, and gift shop), registration or clinic areas where copays are collected, and the cashier's office. Other security-sensitive areas include clinical areas where newborns and their mothers are located; in the obstetrics department, patient wristbands serve as a tracking system that alerts hospital personnel when a newborn is taken out of the designated area. Other sensitive areas are the inpatient and outpatient pharmacies, where drugs and controlled substances are stored for dispensing. The emergency department can be a high-risk area for violence, as police may bring crime victims or perpetrators there for medical treatment. Gang violence may spill into the treatment area as rivals try to finish criminal activity that began on the streets.

Care providers in the nursery, pediatric units, and labor and delivery may be forced to handle domestic disputes or violence as family members carry their arguments into the healthcare organization. An abused child or domestic partner may need protection from the abuser, or a child may be at risk from a parent faced with losing custody to a state family protection agency.

Security addresses the multiple forms of workplace violence that occur within the healthcare organization. A plan may coordinate activities with the human resources department, social work, employee assistance programs, and/or the senior leadership of an organization.

Most people think of violence as a physical assault or battery. However, workplace violence is a much broader problem, comprising any act in which a person is abused, threatened, intimidated, or assaulted in their employment. Workplace violence includes the following:

- **Threatening behavior**: Making menacing gestures such as shaking fists, destroying property, or throwing objects
- **Verbal or written threats**: Making a threat to harm another individual or destroy property
- **Harassment**: Any behavior that demeans, embarrasses, humiliates, annoys, alarms, or verbally abuses a person that is known or would be expected to be unwelcome; includes words, gestures, intimidation, bullying, or other inappropriate activities
- **Verbal abuse**: Swearing, insulting, or using condescending language
- **Physical attacks**: Hitting, shoving, pushing, or kicking
- **Employee-to-employee harassment**: Rumors, swearing, verbal abuse, pranks, arguments, or property damage

- **Domestic violence**: Domestic violence does not stay home when its victims go to work. It can follow them, resulting in violence in the workplace.
- **Stranger violence**: Violence perpetrated by clients, visitors, or complete strangers who come to the workplace

Security education should include defining workplace violence and training employees how to defuse potentially violent situations, how to protect against them, and what methods to use to alert security or other personnel. Employees experiencing domestic violence should be encouraged to notify security, their supervisor, or the human resources department. Support and backup can be provided to the employee, such as an escort to and from the car and surveillance of the facility and grounds for a stalker.

Security events should be trended and reported to the safety committee at least quarterly. (See table 13.1.) The prior year's security events are reviewed annually with the risk assessment. The evaluation and analysis of event trends and concerns determine the need for new security equipment, technology, and procedures, along with education for the staff. The annual appraisal is submitted to the safety committee, medical staff, and board of trustees for recommendations and approval.

Step 3: Monitor and Improve the Hazardous Materials and Waste Management Program

Healthcare facilities manage toxic and hazardous materials and wastes by identifying chemicals and materials that need special handling and disposal. Organizations are required by regulations of the US Department of Labor, Occupational Safety and Health Administration (OSHA), to have a written hazards communication program and to educate and train staff about the unique hazards in the workplace.

OSHA Hazard Communication Standard 1910.1200(g) is based on the premise that employees who may be exposed to hazardous chemicals in the workplace have a right to know about the hazards and how to protect themselves. For this reason, the Hazard Communication Standard is sometimes referred to as the Worker Right-to-Know Legislation, or more often as the Right-to-Know Law.

The Hazard Communication Standard sets forth guidelines and requirements in the following areas:

- **Chemical labeling provision**: Requires that all chemicals in the workplace be labeled. The label includes a signal word, pictogram, hazard statement, and precautionary statement for each hazard class and category. All chemicals should maintain their proper label(s) and warning signs associated with the chemical(s).

- **Safety data sheets (SDSs)**: Documents that give detailed information about a material, including any associated hazards. SDSs should be provided by the chemical manufacturer, distributor, or importer to any downstream user to provide details about any hazards of their products. SDSs are based on a 16-section format, are presented in a user-friendly manner, and must be available to employees at locations where hazardous materials are used. They must include the following information:
  - **Identification**: Name of the chemical (same name as that on the container's label) and any other common names or synonyms used for the substance; contact information (including emergency telephone number) of the manufacturer or importer; recommended use or restrictions on use of the chemical
  - **Hazard(s) identification**: Chemical classification, signal word, pictogram, hazard statement, listing of hazards not otherwise classified, and precautionary statements
  - **Composition/information on ingredients**: Identifies product ingredients listed on the SDS, as well as impurities and stabilizing additives. If a trade secret is claimed, information on substances, mixtures, and all chemicals is also included.
  - **First-aid measures**: Recommendations for initial care by first responders that should be given to individuals exposed to the chemical

Table 13.1A. Security risk assessment and program evaluation

	Information Collection & Evaluation System Safety Committee					
SECURITY MANAGEMENT	1st quarter	2nd quarter	3rd quarter	4th quarter	YTD	GOAL
WORKER SAFETY						
Total industrial accidents						
OSHA reportables						
Type of injury						
• Back injury						
• Needlestick total						
* Employees						
* Student/contract staff						
* # Avoidable						
* # Not avoidable						
• Blood fluid exposure						
• Chemical exposure						
• Repetitive motion injury						
• Patient related						
Productive hours						
Hours lost						
Rate						
Modified duty hours						
PPDs, hep B, and flu shots						100%
Safety inspections						1/yr non-patient 2/yr clinical areas
Security investigations						
Theft						
Unsecured doors						
Narcotic discrepancy/drug diversion						

Table 13.1B. Security risk assessment and program evaluation (*Continued*)

SECURITY MANAGEMENT	1st quarter	2nd quarter	3rd quarter	4th quarter	YTD	GOAL
Vehicle accidents						
Vandalism						
Suspicious individual/trespass						
Code Pink/missing child						
Elopement						
Psych assists						
Visitor injury						
Missing patient belongings						
Calls to police						
Total helipad landings						
Night helipad landings						

HAZARDOUS MATERIALS MGT	1st quarter	2nd quarter	3rd quarter	4th quarter	YTD	GOALS
Inventory updated						Minimum annually
Number of hazmat spills						
Biohazard waste found in landfill						
Air quality sampling						

LIFE SAFETY MGT	1st quarter	2nd quarter	3rd quarter	4th quarter	YTD	GOALS
# Fire drills						1/shift/quarter
# Participants						
Staff demonstrate knowledge of fire safety						
Staff describe evacuation procedures						
Annual fire extinguisher inspection						
Monthly fire extinguisher inspection						
Fire alarm system inspections						
# Items listed in SOC						

Table 13.1C. Security risk assessment and program evaluation (Continued)

EQUIPMENT MANAGEMENT	1st quarter	2nd quarter	3rd quarter	4th quarter	YTD	GOAL
Equipment PMs						
Equipment scheduled for PM						
% of PMs completed						
PMs not completed						
Malfunctioning equipment						
% of malfunctioning equipment						
Abuse errors						
Unduplicated errors						
% of unduplicated errors						
Patient injured						
Alarm testing						
% of alarm testing						
UTILITIES MANAGEMENT	**1st quarter**	**2nd quarter**	**3rd quarter**	**4th quarter**	**YTD**	**GOAL**
Utility failures						
Emergency generator testing						
Medical gas testing (annual)						
RECALLS REQUIRING ACTION	**1st quarter**	**2nd quarter**	**3rd quarter**	**4th quarter**	**YTD**	**GOAL**
Equipment						
Medical devices						
Pharmaceuticals						
EDUCATION	**1st quarter**	**2nd quarter**	**3rd quarter**	**4th quarter**	**YTD**	**GOAL**

- **Firefighting measure**: Specifications and special instructions, such as conditions when the material might catch fire or explode and what should be done to deal with the hazard, including recommendations on extinguishing equipment, protective equipment, and precautions for fire-fighters
- **Accidental release measures**: Identifies appropriate actions to be taken in the event of a spill, leak, or release of a chemical to contain and minimize exposure
- **Handling and storage**: Detailed instructions for safe handling of the substance, including how to store, move, and use the materials; provides advice on general hygiene practices
- **Exposure controls/personal protection**: Details the personal protective equipment to use when working with the material, lists safe work procedures, and indicates exposure limits and engineering controls
- **Physical and chemical** properties: Additional information such as the material's appearance, odor, boiling point, vapor pressure, vapor density, solubility in water, melting point, and evaporation rate
- **Stability and reactivity**: Includes the hazards and stability of the chemical and identifies certain conditions under which a reactive material becomes dangerous. Reactive materials can burn or explode when exposed to air or water or when mixed with other substances. This section provides information to help prevent exposure of such materials to these conditions.
- **Toxicological information**: Identifies the routes of exposure, short- and long-term effects of exposure, symptoms of exposure, and an indication of whether the chemical is listed in the National Toxicology Program (NTP) report on carcinogens or has been found to be a potential carcinogen
- **Ecological information (nonmandatory)**: Includes information on how the chemical would affect the environment if it were released
- **Disposal considerations (nonmandatory)**: Provides guidance on proper disposal, reclamation of the chemical or its container, and safe handling practices
- **Transport information (nonmandatory)**: Includes guidance on shipping and transporting of hazardous chemical(s) for all transportation methods
- **Regulatory information (nonmandatory)**: Identifies safety, health, and environmental regulations for the specific product that are not listed elsewhere on the SDS
- **Other information**: Includes information on when the SDS was prepared or when revisions were last made to it

- **Hazard determination provision**: Requires an employer to identify and maintain an inventory of all hazardous chemicals used in the workplace
- **Written implementation program**: Requires an employer to have a written hazard communication program plan
- **Employee training**: Requires that employers train employees how to handle hazardous materials, how to use and interpret SDSs, and how to understand hazardous materials labeling and information about the Hazard Communication Standard (OSHA 2012)

The Joint Commission surveys organizations to ensure compliance with the OSHA standard and requires a written safety management plan for hazardous materials and waste. A healthcare organization designs its plan to do the following:

- Develop an inventory (see table 13.2 for an example) of all hazardous materials and wastes used, stored, or generated. This includes vapors and gases used in surgery and medical gases used throughout the facility.

- Specify how it will maintain safety information for employees in the form of SDSs. This SDS information may be maintained as hard copy or via electronic means. Various contract service companies provide electronic or fax copies of SDSs to organizations as needed.

Table 13.2. Sample hazardous materials inventory

Department:	Chemotherapy Drugs		Hazardous	Materials Inventory	
Product Name	Manufacturer	Class	Type Haz	Spill Response	Quantity
				If fire, SCBA required. Call fire department.	
Cytarabine (ARA-c) 2 gm	Bedford 55390-0134-01				10
Dactinomycin (Cosmegen®) 0.5 mg/mL vial	Ovation Pharmaceuticals				8
Daunorubicin 20 mg/4 mL vial	Bedford 55390-0108-10				10
Docetaxel Taxotere® 80 mg/2 mL	Sanofi-Adventis 00075-8001-80				
Docetaxel (Taxotere) 20 mg/0.5 mL	Sanofi-Adventis 00075-8001-80				
Doxorubicin (Adriamycin®) 200 mg/100 mL	Bedford 55390-0238-01			Small spills—Wipe liquids with spill pad. Wipe solids with wet spill pad/ sheet. Clean using detergent/water. Large spills—Cover liquid with spill pads/pillows, etc. Cover powder with damp cloth/spill sheet. Clean using detergents/water. Treat cloth, clothes, contaminated materials as hazardous materials. Incinerate.	
Fludarabine Phosphate (Fludara®) 50 mg vial	Berlex Labs 0015-511-06				4
Fluorouracil® 500 mg/10 mL (50 mg/mL)	Valeant Pharmaceuticals 63323-0117-10				10
Gemcitabine HCL (Gemzar®) 1 gm	Eli Lilly & Co 0002-7502-01				Order as needed
Hydroxyurea 500 mg capsule	Bristol Labs 00003-0830-50				100
Imiglucerase (Cerezyme) 400 units 200 units	Genzyme 58468-4663-01				
Idarubicin Hydrochloride 5 mg/5 mL	Pharmacia Upjohn				3

- Develop and implement written procedures to follow in the event of hazardous materials and waste spills or exposure.
- Develop policies and procedures for selecting, handling, storing, transporting, using, and disposing of the hazardous materials and waste.
- Manage the following materials and minimize risks, as described in the hazardous materials and waste plan or policy, as applicable:
    - Hazardous energy sources
    - Hazardous medications
    - Radioactive materials
    - Infectious and regulated medical waste, including sharps
    - Vapors and medical gases
- Review results of staff dosimetry monitoring at least quarterly to assess whether staff radiation exposure levels are as low as reasonably achievable. (Joint Commission 2024a, EC 9–10)

The hazardous materials plan should specify supervisors' responsibility to provide adequate and appropriate space, containers, and personal protective equipment for the safe handling and storage of hazardous materials and wastes. Supervisors are to ensure that employees receive appropriate training on the hazardous materials and wastes in their work area, know how to obtain an SDS, and know how to report hazardous material or waste spills or exposure. In addition, healthcare organization employees must be educated on regulations regarding the proper disposal of all hazardous and nonhazardous waste and controlled substances that pose a potential threat to the environment.

Step 4: Monitor and Improve the Emergency Operations Plan

An **emergency** is a situation created by a natural disaster, pandemic, or human-caused event. When an emergency occurs, it can impede a healthcare organization's ability to care for patients. The demand for care can significantly increase during an emergency, and the healthcare organization's resources may be stretched, limiting its ability to respond. Additionally, healthcare facilities may experience damage from an emergency and may also be challenged by an electrical outage or lost means of communication (Joint Commission 2024b, EM 1).

Terrorist activity or mass shootings, natural disasters such as hurricanes, and public health crises such as the COVID-19 pandemic have focused the nation's attention on emergency preparedness and the ability of the community, including hospitals, to respond. Response may consist of handling a large influx of patients or the need to evacuate patients from hospitals and extended-care facilities to safer sites.

In response to these catastrophic emergencies, the **National Incident Management System (NIMS)**, a system that provides guidelines for common functions and terminology to support clear communication and effective collaboration in an emergency situation, has evolved to include standardization of an **all-hazards approach** for disaster and emergency management and business continuity programs in the private and public sectors. The "all-hazards approach supports a general response capability that is sufficiently nimble to address a range of emergencies of different duration, scale, and cause. For this reason, the plan's response procedures address the prioritized emergencies but are also adaptable to other emergencies that the organization may experience" (Joint Commission 2024b, EM 4). This standardization has required healthcare organizations to reevaluate their **emergency operations plan (EOP)**, and the Joint Commission to redefine standards that address six critical areas of emergency management, with a focus that includes a linkage to community resources. The EOP is an organization's written document that describes the process it would implement for managing the consequences of emergencies, including natural and human-made disasters, which could disrupt the organization's ability to provide care, treatment, and services (Joint Commission 2024c, GL 13). Following are the six critical areas an organization must address in its EOP:

- **Communication**—In the event that community infrastructure is damaged and/or a healthcare organization's power or facilities experience debilitation, communication pathways are likely to fail. The healthcare organization must develop a plan to maintain communication pathways both within the organization and to critical community resources.

- **Resources and assets**—A solid understanding of the scope and availability of a healthcare organization's resources and assets during an emergency is important. Materials and supplies, vendor and community services, as well as state and federal programs, are some of the essential resources that hospitals must know how to access in times of crisis in order to ensure patient safety and sustain care, treatment, and services.

- **Safety and security**—The safety and security of patients is the prime responsibility of the healthcare organization during an emergency. As emergency situations develop and parameters of operability shift, organizations must provide a safe and secure environment for their patients and staff.

- **Staff responsibilities**—During an emergency, the probability that staff responsibilities will change is high. As new risks develop along with changing conditions, staff will need to adapt to their roles to meet new demands on their ability to care for patients. If staff cannot anticipate how they may be called to perform during an emergency, the likelihood that the organization will not sustain itself during an emergency increases.

- **Utilities management**—A healthcare organization is dependent on the uninterrupted function of its utilities during an emergency. The supply of key utilities, such as power or potable water, ventilation, and fuel, must not be disrupted or adverse events may occur as a result.

- **Patient clinical and support activities**—The clinical needs of patients during an emergency are of prime importance. The organization must have clear, reasonable plans in place to address the needs of patients during extreme conditions when the infrastructure and resources are taxed. (Joint Commission 2024b, EM 12-26)

With sufficient planning for these six critical areas of emergency management, a healthcare organization will have developed an all-hazards approach. Achieving this all-hazards approach to preparedness means that the organization has planned and prepared for a wide spectrum of possible emergencies (Joint Commission 2024b, EM 12).

The Joint Commission further requires organizations to conduct an annual **hazard vulnerability analysis (HVA)** to identify potential hazards, threats, and adverse events and assess their impact on the care, treatment, and services that must be sustained during an emergency. See table 13.3 for a sample HVA form. Once the top hazard vulnerabilities are identified, situational plans need to be developed for events such as utility failures, earthquakes, hurricanes, floods, tornadoes, and airline disasters.

Table 13.3A. Sample hospital hazard vulnerability assessment tool

Event	PROBABILITY	ALERTS	ACTIVATIONS	SEVERITY = (MAGNITUDE - MITIGATION)						RISK
				HUMAN IMPACT	PROPERTY IMPACT	BUSINESS IMPACT	PREPARED-NESS	INTERNAL RESPONSE	EXTERNAL RESPONSE	
	Likelihood this will occur	Number of Alerts	Number of Activations	Possibility of death or injury	Physical losses and damages	Interruption of services	Preplanning	Time, effectiveness, resources	Community/ mutual Aid staff and supplies	*Relative threat
SCORE	0 = N/A 1 = Low 2 = Moderate 3 = High			0 = N/A 1 = Low 2 = Moderate 3 = High	0 = N/A 1 = Low 2 = Moderate 3 = High	0 = N/A 1 = Low 2 = Moderate 3 = High	0 = N/A 1 = High 2 = Moderate 3 = Low	0 = N/A 1 = High 2 = Moderate 3 = Low	0 = N/A 1 = High 2 = Moderate 3 = Low	0–100%
Active Shooter										
Acts of Terrorism										
Air Quality Issues										
Bomb Threat										
Building Move										
Chemical Exposure, External										
Chemical Exposure, Internal										
Chemical Spill										
Child Abduction										
Civil Unrest/ Protesting										
Communication / Telephony Failure										
Dam Failure										
Drought										
Earthquake										
Epidemic										
Evacuation										
Explosion										
Fire, External										

Table 13.3B. Sample hospital hazard vulnerability assessment tool (*Continued*)

Event	PROBABILITY	ALERTS	ACTIVATIONS	SEVERITY = (MAGNITUDE - MITIGATION)						RISK
				HUMAN IMPACT	PROPERTY IMPACT	BUSINESS IMPACT	PREPARED-NESS	INTERNAL RESPONSE	EXTERNAL RESPONSE	
Fire, Internal										
Flood, External										
Flood, Internal										
Forensic Admission										
Gas/Emissions Leak										
Generator Failure										
Hostage Situation										
Hurricane										
HVAC Failure										
Inclement Weather										
Infectious Disease Outbreak										
IT System Outage										
Landslide										
Mass Casualty Incident - Hazmat										
Mass Casualty Incident - Medical										
Mass Casualty Incident - Trauma										
Natural Gas Disruption										
Natural Gas Failure										
Pandemic										
Patient Elopement										
Patient Surge										
Picketing										
Planned Power Outages										
Power Outage										

Table 13.3C. Sample hospital hazard vulnerability assessment tool (*Continued*)

Event	PROBABILITY	ALERTS	ACTIVATIONS	SEVERITY = (MAGNITUDE - MITIGATION)						RISK
				HUMAN IMPACT	PROPERTY IMPACT	BUSINESS IMPACT	PREPARED-NESS	INTERNAL RESPONSE	EXTERNAL RESPONSE	
Radiation Exposure										
Seasonal Influenza										
Sewer Failure										
Shelter in Place										
Strikes/Labor Action/Work Stoppage										
Suicide										
Supply Chain Shortage/Failure										
Suspicious Package/Substance										
Temperature Extremes										
Tornado										
Transportation Failure										
Trauma										
Tsunami										
Utility Failure										
VIP Situation										
Water Contamination										
Water Disruption										
Weapon										
Workplace Violence/Threat										

Source: Adapted from Kaiser Permanente 2021. Reprinted with permission.

Emergency preparedness planning should be systematic and comprehensive. Planning should include activities that mitigate, prepare for, respond to, and provide recovery information from an emergency event. Table 13.4 lists some of these planning activities.

Emergency planning begins with an HVA to determine the types of disasters that the organization may face. Disasters may be technological, man-made, or natural. A good starting point for gathering information is the state health department website, which usually includes an analysis of the state's potential risk sites, such as earthen dams, industrial sites with hazardous or toxic chemicals, and the type and frequency of past natural disasters. An HVA may be found by county in some larger states, and the county websites will provide emergency preparedness for their locale.

The group conducting the HVA also should assess the organizational experience of the prior year (and longer, if available) taken from the safety monitoring and trending data. Events emanating from within the organization, such as security events, utility failures, information systems failures, hazardous material spills or exposures, or findings from disaster drill critiques, will provide direction as to which situational plans should be written or revised.

The organization's disaster coordinator should be involved with the county or state emergency management committees to provide another mechanism to obtain information regarding local concerns and to coordinate disaster response with local healthcare facilities and emergency response agencies. When developing the EOP, the healthcare organization communicates its needs and vulnerabilities to community emergency response agencies and identifies the capabilities of the community in meeting the organization's needs.

An important element of emergency planning is the implementation of an incident command structure that can link and coordinate with community authorities and their incident command structures. National initiatives require standardization of incident command structure and nomenclature at all levels of response: emergency medical services, fire and police, hospitals, and city and state emergency management agencies.

Improving the Environment of Care: Steps to Success 239

Table 13.4. Hazard vulnerability planning activities

Hazard	Mitigation (long-term)	Preparedness (to respond)	Response (to emergency)	Recovery (short- and long-term)
	Definition: Any activities that actually eliminate or reduce the occurrence of a disaster, including long-term activities that reduce the effects of unavoidable disasters.	Definition: Preparedness activities are necessary to the extent that mitigation measures cannot prevent disasters. Preparedness measures also seek to enhance disaster response operations.	Definition: Generally, responses are designed to provide emergency assistance for casualties. Responses also seek to reduce the probability of secondary damage and to speed recovery operations.	Definition: Recovery continues until all systems return to normal or better. Short-term recovery returns vital life support systems to minimum operating standards. Long-term recovery may continue for a number of years after a disaster. Recovery's purpose is to return life to normal.
Earthquake	Secure moveable objects that may cause injury Fasten shelves Take pictures off walls Place heavy objects on low shelves Store sufficient fuel, medical supplies, pharmaceutical supplies, food, and water to sustain patients and staff for a short period of time Prepare 72-hour kits for offices Adhere to building codes Store hazardous chemicals in appropriate cabinets Contract/make arrangements with a building inspector Educate staff	Have utility schematics available Encourage staff preparedness at home through provision of home disaster information	Protect self Protect patients Activate plan Conserve resources Unplug nonessential equipment Review need for rotating staff	Have building inspection Return utilities to normal Assess and repair structural damage Replace equipment Restock supplies Evaluate economic impact Activate Incident Stress Debriefing Team
Hazardous Materials Facility	Store hazardous chemicals appropriately Educate staff on handling hazardous chemicals Review possible alternative to hazardous chemicals Routine removal for disposal Lock hazmat disposal storage Use nonsparking tools	Have spill kits on hand Use SDS hotline number to obtain SDS, as needed Know chemical inventory in department Train appropriate staff on use of ETO sniffer	Secure area of spill Evacuate if necessary Notify security Notify fire department, if appropriate	Dispose of waste properly Evaluate cause of spill Replenish spill kit/supplies
Information Systems	Back up systems nightly Maintain off-site backups of business records Maintain updated virus protection and firewalls			

The incident command structure is used in each type of emergency event and is as elaborate or simple as the size of the organization or event requires. In other words, it is an all-hazards command structure. Figure 13.2 shows an example of an incident command structure for a small organization, and figure 13.3 shows one for a larger, more complex organization.

Figure 13.2. Incident command structure for a small healthcare organization

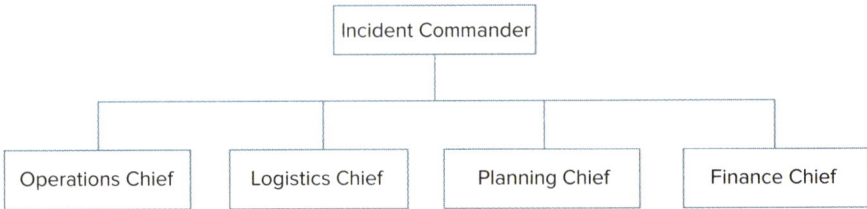

The basic EOP describes the management of space, supplies, staff, and security (see figure 13.4) and describes the following processes in detail:

- Assignment of authority for notifying staff, notifying and communicating with external authorities, communicating with patients and their families, and communicating with the community when emergency response measures are initiated
- Setup of command center and identification of individuals to serve in the incident command structure
- Assignment of staff to cover all essential functions
- Management of activities related to the following:
    - Care and treatment of patients
    - Modifying or discontinuing services
    - Staff support (housing, incident stress, and debriefing)
    - Staff family support, childcare
    - Obtaining supplies (pharmaceuticals, linens, food, and water)
    - Security
    - Communications with news media
    - Evacuation (including transportation of patients, staff, equipment, and health records)
    - Establishing alternative care sites
    - Tracking patients (disaster log)
- Credentialing of volunteers (physicians, nurses, and others not associated with the facility)
- Interhospital cooperation or transfer agreements
- Situational plans, including the following:
    - Radioactive, biological, and chemical isolation and decontamination
    - Communication emergencies
    - Utility failures, alternative means of meeting essential building utility needs
    - Natural disasters as identified in the HVA
    - Human-caused disasters as identified in the HVA
    - Fire response

The EOP is practiced twice a year in response to either an actual disaster or a planned drill. Exercises should stress the limits of the organization's emergency management system to assess preparedness capabilities and performance. Exercises should be plausible scenarios that are realistic and based on the organization's HVA. In organizations providing emergency services, one drill must simulate the influx of patients, and the organization must participate in one community-wide practice drill a year.

Figure 13.3. Incident command structure for a large healthcare organization

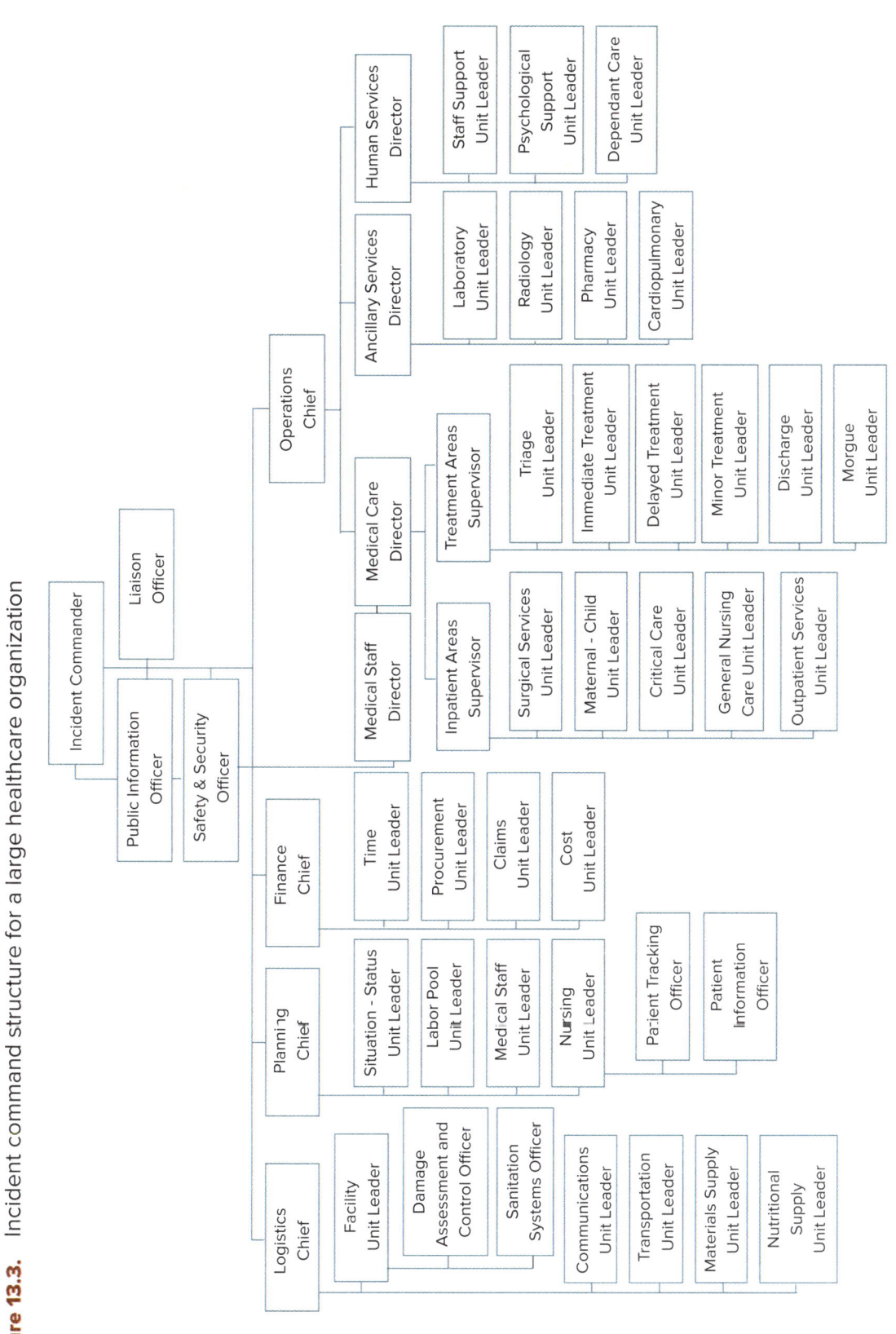

Figure 13.4A. Emergency management plan

Community Hospital of the West
EMERGENCY OPERATIONS PLAN

MISSION STATEMENT:
Community Hospital of the West supports the Emergency Operations Plan to ensure effective response to mitigate, prepare, respond, and recover from disasters or emergencies affecting the facility internally or from external events.

OBJECTIVES:
Community Hospital of the West has established, supports, and maintains an emergency preparedness program (Disaster Manual) that implements specific procedures in response to a variety of internal disasters. In the event of any type of disaster that places an unusual demand on space, supplies, security, or the facility staff, the emergency preparedness plan will be implemented.

The program integrates the center's role with the disaster plans of local, county, state, and federal emergency management authorities and facilities in proximity to Community Hospital of the West. The facility will assist external disaster victims within the capability and mission of the hospital.

SCOPE:
The emergency preparedness plan provides a mechanism to augment normal operation of the facility during an incident. The plan represents a principle-based (all hazards) response to any event, which may compromise facility operations. It may be implemented in whole or in part, or it may represent merely the first step in a more comprehensive mobilization of resources. It is intended that disaster situations be managed with as little variation from normal facility policies and procedures as possible. However, since no amount of planning can foresee every circumstance, flexibility within the guidelines of the plan is crucial.

Emergency preparedness includes the following:

1. Potential emergencies are identified from a hazard vulnerability analysis.
2. Procedures are identified for disaster readiness and management of a variety of disasters.
3. Procedures are identified for informing staff of "disaster alert" or need for disaster response.
4. Procedures are identified for individual department response to disaster.
5. Procedures are identified for evacuation.
6. Definition of the "all hazards" command structure is provided for responding to and recovery from emergencies. The command structure is referred to as the Incident Command system. The Incident Command personnel in the command center integrate the hospital's role with community-wide emergency response agencies and promote interoperability between the hospital and the community.
7. Descriptions of procedures are provided for mitigation, preparedness, response, and recovery.
8. The plan addresses four phases of emergency management: mitigation, preparedness, response, and recovery. At a minimum, the Emergency Operations Plan has been developed with the involvement of facility leaders, including the Medical Director.

AUTHORITY:
The Safety Officer has the authority to intervene whenever conditions exist that pose an immediate threat to life or health or pose a threat of damage to equipment or the building.

Figure 13.4B. Emergency management plan (*Continued*)

Community Hospital of the West
EMERGENCY OPERATIONS PLAN

RESPONSIBILITY:

Board of trustees:

- Supports the Emergency Operations Program through providing staff and resources for preparedness planning
- Receives recommendations for mitigation, preparedness, evaluation of response to disaster/drill (critiques), and recovery

Safety committee administration medical director:

- As a member of the Administration, chairs the Safety Committee
- Convenes committee twice a year (at a minimum) to implement the plan(s), train, and critique staff on their response
- With Administration and Safety Officer, assumes roles in the Incident Command Center during disasters and drills providing direction to the hospital and communicating with the community's incident command structure
- Recommends educational needs of staff, additional equipment, supplies, etc., pertaining to emergency management response
- Plans, designs, measures, assesses, and improves processes through ongoing receipt of monitoring data, written formal review of disasters/disaster drills and annual performance evaluation
- Submits reports at least quarterly to the Board, to include critiques of disasters/drills, recommendations for preparedness response, and education needs
- Updates Emergency Operations Plan (Disaster Manual) as needed

Safety officer:

- Oversees emergency management planning and reports updates and revisions to the Safety Committee
- Directs planning, implementation, and evaluation of disaster drill response
- Accepts assignment as a section chief in the incident command structure
- Attends community emergency management committees as appropriate
- Provides training to department staff in department response to disasters/drills

Department managers:

- Support participation of their staff in the implementation of the plan/drills
- Monitor staff compliance with the plan and participation in drills, event/incident reporting, and implementation of appropriate corrective actions

Figure 13.4c. Emergency management plan (*Continued*)

Community Hospital of the West
EMERGENCY OPERATIONS PLAN

Employees:

- Annually review disaster procedures through participation in mandatory training/education
- Take drills seriously and respond appropriately
- Take prompt action in identifying and reporting internal disasters
- Support the Emergency Operations Plan by following policies and procedures, participating in drills and appropriately responding to actual events, reporting deficiencies and problems promptly, and participating in training and demonstrating competence

TRAINING/EDUCATION:
New employee orientation includes information relative to the hospital response to disasters:

- Access to the hospital
    - Employee identification
    - Situational events
    - Evacuation

- The Safety Officer will provide disaster critique feedback annually and after each disaster/drill and education for employees on disaster response and disaster-specific procedures and evacuation.

ANNUAL EVALUATION:
An evaluation of objectives, scope, performance, and effectiveness of the emergency preparedness plan and staff response is conducted annually and after each disaster/drill. This evaluation is accomplished by reviewing data sources and reports as follows:

1. Analysis of Disaster Drills; debriefing with disaster participants, involved facility staff and departments, county/state Emergency Operations staff, volunteers, etc.
2. Actual incidents within or outside the facility
3. Disaster literature/research findings
4. Information from the community, state, and/or federal agencies
5. Disaster Drill critiques
6. Department Evaluation Reports
7. Activity Log

The Safety Committee will analyze the data sources and implement appropriate actions to be taken and update the Disaster Manual.

PERFORMANCE IMPROVEMENT GOALS:
Performance goals will be established for each drill implemented, and objectives of each drill will be reviewed by the Safety Committee and submitted to the Board.

Performance Standards/Quality Improvement projects have been established for a minimum of 2 of the Safety Management programs in the Environment of Care Management.

Finally, each disaster response, whether an actual emergency or a practice drill, must be critiqued. Problems identified and lessons learned during an actual event or drill should be assessed and, as appropriate, addressed in the written EOP. Administrators, medical staff, and the board of trustees should approve emergency preparedness planning. In addition to drills, the organization's personnel should receive education and training as needed (at least annually).

Step 5: Monitor and Improve the Life (Fire Prevention) Safety Management Plan

Building and fire codes require facilities to be designed, constructed, maintained, and operated to minimize a fire emergency and protect patients, visitors, staff, and property from fire, smoke, and other products of combustion. The major component of the life safety management plan is a fire prevention plan that is based on appropriate design and construction of the building, fire detection, alarm and extinguishment systems, and training to provide for appropriate safety for all occupants.

The following activities should be components of a fire prevention program (for detailed information refer to National Fire Protection Association standards):

- Inspect, test, and maintain fire detection, alarm, and protection equipment such as audible alarm systems, fire and smoke detectors, extinguishers, water flow devices, evacuation route exit signs, fire doors, and air handling and smoke management systems. This inspection, testing, and maintenance must be conducted within the time frames required by the Life Safety Code of the National Fire Protection Association (NFPA) and other codes required by state and local agencies.
- Identify, investigate, and report deficiencies and failures in the fire prevention program.
- Evaluate proposed acquisition of bedding, window coverings, furnishings, room decorations, wastebaskets, and equipment in the context of fire safety.
- Develop and implement a fire response plan through drills, education, and training of staff. Staff is trained regarding:
    - Their roles and responsibilities at the fire's point of origin and away from the point of origin
    - When and how to sound fire alarms
    - Use of fire extinguishers
    - Smoke and fire containment
    - Preparing for evacuation
- Use an easy method to train staff, such as *RACE* and *PASS*.
    - RACE stands for
        - **R** = Rescue anyone in immediate danger of the fire
        - **A** = Activate alarms
        - **C** = Confine fires (close doors and windows)
        - **E** = Extinguish fires using PASS and prepare to evacuate patients
    - PASS, which is training for the use of fire extinguishers, stands for
        - **P** = Pull pin
        - **A** = Aim nozzle
        - **S** = Squeeze handle
        - **S** = Sweep from side-to-side
- Conduct fire drills for each shift. A realistic fire scenario should be prepared for each drill, and staff knowledge is evaluated. All fire drills are critiqued to identify problems and opportunities for improvement. Figure 13.5 is an example of a tracking form used to document fire drills. A separate evaluation of staff response to each drill is documented and used in the annual evaluation of the fire safety plan.
- Oversee safety of construction and remodeling activities, including inspection for appropriate installation of fire protection systems and equipment and enforcement of safety requirements of contractors, such as hot work permits and above-ceiling permits. The facility must comply with all federal, state, and local rules, regulations, and laws.

- Conduct a life safety assessment in addition to the infection control risk assessment prior to beginning construction to determine whether the construction will interfere with life safety codes. If deficiencies or hazards are identified, appropriate activities from the Interim Life Safety Measures (ILSMs) policy will be instituted. Some examples of the 11 ILSMs are:
    - Smoke-tight barriers between construction areas and the rest of the facility
    - Increased surveillance
    - Additional firefighting equipment
    - Increased number of fire drills conducted
    - Organization-wide fire safety education
- Use the Joint Commission's Statement of Conditions (SOC) form to note when building code deficiencies affecting life safety are identified (Joint Commission 2024d, LS 5–9).

Figure 13.5A. Fire drill tracking summary

Fire Drill Summary: (Building's name) _____ With (number of) _____ smoke compartments

Complete the table below: (A) Date of fire drill; (B) Day of week; (C) Time of day drill was held; (D) Smoke compartment from which fire drill initiated; (E) Total number of compartments observed during drill; (F) Total number of observers; (G) Was another smoke compartment monitored on the same floor and immediately adjacent to the drill site (if applicable)? (H) Was another smoke compartment monitored on the floor immediately above/below the drill site (if applicable)?

For the fire drills, did you elect to observe all areas?   YES   NO   N/A   (Please circle)

Or did you elect to randomly observe different locations using the four criteria?   YES   NO   N/A   (Please circle)

Fire Drill Summary		Morning Drills		Afternoon Drills		Night Drills
Date of fire drill	A		A		A	
Day of week	B		B		B	
Time of day	C		C		C	
Where initiated?	D		D		D	
Number of compartments observed	E		E		E	
Number of observers	F		F		F	
Adjacent compartment observed?	G	Yes No N/A	G	Yes No N/A	G	Yes No N/A
Was adjacent compartment above/ below compartment observed?	H	Yes No N/A	H	Yes No N/A	H	Yes No N/A

Figure 13.5B. Fire drill tracking summary (*Continued*)

Fire Drill Summary		Morning Drills		Afternoon Drills		Night Drills	
Date of fire drill	A		A		A		
Day of week	B		B		B		
Time of day	C		C		C		
Where initiated?	D		D		D		
Number of compartments observed	E		E		E		
Number of observers	F		F		F		
Adjacent compartment observed?	G	Yes No N/A	G	Yes No N/A	G	Yes No N/A	
Was adjacent compartment above/below compartment observed?	H	Yes No N/A	H	Yes No N/A	H	Yes No N/A	
Date of fire drill	A		A		A		
Day of week	B		B		B		
Time of day	C		C		C		
Where initiated?	D		D		D		
Number of compartments observed?	E		E		E		
Number of observers	F		F		F		
Adjacent compartment observed?	G	Yes No N/A	G	Yes No N/A	G	Yes No N/A	
Was adjacent compartment above/ below compartment observed?	H	Yes No N/A	H	Yes No N/A	H	Yes No N/A	

Step 6: Monitor and Improve the Medical Equipment Management Program

The goals of the medical equipment management program are to provide safe and reliable equipment, train care providers in the safe and effective use of the equipment, and ensure that the equipment is maintained by qualified individuals.

The written medical equipment management plan includes provisions for the following functions:

- Establishes criteria for including equipment, regardless of ownership, on the facility inventory list. Criteria do not need to be established if the facility decides to include all equipment on the inventory. Equipment not owned by the facility may need to be examined and a safety check performed. Examples of situations in which equipment is not owned by the facility might include the following:
  - Providers may bring or purchase their own equipment to use in surgery or during other procedures.
  - Patients may bring electronic devices, such as laptop computers or tablets, for work or entertainment purposes.
- Defines time frames for inspecting, testing, and maintaining the equipment in the inventory. The organization maintains documentation of the inspection, testing, maintenance, and repair of each piece of equipment in the inventory.
- Defines how equipment and medical device recalls will be handled
- Provides for reporting incidents in which a medical device may have caused death, serious injury, or illness to any patient
- Identifies processes to respond to equipment malfunction or failure

- Specifies cleaning and infection control procedures for receiving and handling equipment between patients
- Facility support or clinical engineering departments should develop an inventory of clinical, life safety, and security alarms. Alarms should be evaluated to determine the frequency of inspecting, testing, and maintenance.

Step 7: Monitor and Improve the Utilities and Building Management Program

The utilities management program is designed to ensure that utilities systems throughout the EC are planned and maintained safely and comfortably; that utilities are delivered without interruption; and that mechanical systems operate safely, accurately, and reliably. A good utilities management program helps the organization minimize the risk of hospital-acquired illnesses that may be transmitted through the utility systems. Facility support personnel work closely and proactively with infection control to control dust and to test and maintain air handlers and cooling towers. Infection control procedures also require that stained ceiling tiles, carpeting, and flooring be replaced to proactively prevent contaminants from reaching the patient.

The written utilities management program describes the following:

- The processes the organization maintains to manage the safe and reliable operation of utility systems.
- The risk criteria for evaluating the operating components of the utility systems and developing an inventory. As in the medical equipment program, a facility may elect to use risk criteria but should include all utility systems in the inventory.
- The schedules for inspecting, testing, and maintaining components of the utility systems.
- The emergency procedures for responding to utility disruptions or failures.
- The location of schematics and facility maps that show the location of utility systems and controls for partial or complete shutdown in an emergency. The controls for shutdown in the facility should be labeled.
- Infection control and facility surveillance processes. Water-stained ceiling tiles may signify an infection control issue. Damp tiles are a medium for mold. When stained ceiling tiles are found, facility support personnel should determine, if possible, the cause of the stain and repair any problems above the ceiling before replacing tiles. One pediatric facility noted that ceiling tiles appeared to be water stained, but the cause of the problem could not be found until the infection control practitioner and the safety manager discovered that the toys used to distract the children in the care environment included squirt guns.

The EC integrates closely with the Joint Commission Patient Safety Initiatives. A safe and secure environment supports the provision of care and treatment in a healthcare organization. Important patient safety goals to be managed in the EC program are infection control, fire safety, emergency management, medical equipment, and alarms. The infection control practitioner and the safety committee inspection team are important allies.

The EC infection control focus is in the areas of airborne contaminants, waterborne pathogens, housekeeping procedures, and building construction issues. Figure 13.6 shows an example of an audit worksheet used to survey for issues related to the EC plans and infection control surveillance. Physical plant changes may affect infection control for immunosuppressed or immunocompromised patients. Preconstruction risk assessments are conducted with the infection control practitioner, safety manager, facility support staff, and construction supervisory personnel.

Figure 13.6A. Environmental tour and facility audit—clinical departments

Environmental Tour/Facility Audit
Clinical Departments

Location: _____
Date: _____
Survey Team _____
Director/Mgr: _____

	Needs Correction	Surveyor Comments	Management Response
Safety			
Exit lights lit and visible			
All fire doors close and latch			
Propped doors found			
Crash Cart checked daily			
No unapproved space heaters in the area			
No items stored under sinks/ no water/spots/mold			
Sharps containers are no more than 2/3 full			
No tripping hazards			
Staff food/drinks not in work area			
Emergency Flip Chart posted			
Linen cart covered, has solid bottom shelf			
No outdated supplies were found			
Hazardous Material			
Current Haz Mat Inventory Available			
SDS on Demand number posted and visible			
Chemicals in secondary containers are appropriately labeled			
Separation of biohazardous from regular medical trash			
Appropriate labeling of trash			
Appropriate lids on waste containers			
Spill Kit available			

Figure 13.6B. Environmental tour and facility audit—clinical departments (Continued)

	Needs Correction	Surveyor Comments	Management Response
Fire			
Extinguishers have current inspection tag			
Hallways clear of storage/or equipment on one side of hall			
Fire exits, pull stations, fire doors, and extinguishers not blocked			
Waste paper disposed properly			
All items 18" below sprinkler heads			
All items 4" off of the floor			
Nothing stored in any stairwell			
Furniture, Wheelchairs, Beds, Gurneys, IV Poles			
Wheels and brakes in good condition			
Broken furniture found			
Wagons clean			
Beds/cribs in good condition			
General Maintenance			
Ceiling tiles free from cracks, holes, breaks and stains/mold ● Causation? What is above the tiles? Bathroom? Shower?, etc			
Flooring free from tears, bulges, holes, etc			
Random check for fire penetrations			
Seams on splash boards of sinks			
Under counter refrigerators – no dust/water			
Potential hazards – Countertops laminate chipped or lifting Ceramic tile			
Guard rails secure			
Patient restroom grab bars are secure			
Patient Care Equipment inspections up to date			

Figure 13.6C. Environmental tour and facility audit—clinical departments (*Continued*)

	Needs Correction	Surveyor Comments	Management Response
Electrical			
Outlet covers are attached and in good condition			
All electrical cords in good condition			
Electric panels are secured unobstructed and no storage in closets			
Nurse call buttons functioning			
Child proof/tamper proof outlets (GFI) in appropriate areas			
Limited use of extension cords – cords are stickered			
Housekeeping			
No unlocked housekeeping closets or unattended carts in the area			
No unlabeled bottles on the cart			
Approved trash/shredding/recycling receptacles			
General cleanliness			
Refrigerator Protocol			
Refrigerator/freezer temperature checks documented appropriately			
Thermometers in place freezer and refrigerator			
All food is covered, dated			
Food and medication kept in separate refrigerators			
Medication			
Open multi-use bottles/vials dated, timed			
No outdate IV solutions or medications			
Outdated formula, baby food, and supplemental feedings disposed			
All medication kept in locked or controlled area, includes refrigerators			
All controlled substances are in double locked cabinets			
Unattended, drawn syringes found in the area			
Medication in syringes marked with name and strength			

Figure 13.6D. Environmental tour and facility audit—clinical departments (*Continued*)

	Needs Correction	Surveyor Comments	Management Response
Oxygen and other medical gases			
All medical gas cylinders secured in upright position in approved holders or chained			
Secured during transport/use			
All medical gas shut-off valves clearly marked and accessible			
Additional Comments:			

_____ _____
Management Signature   Date

Facility support services should work closely with infection control to report water system or air handling issues or concerns with drains, ice machines, carpeting, flooring, ceiling tiles and the space above the tiles, and garbage handling and storage areas.

A facility must conduct an infection control risk assessment prior to construction and have a plan in place to mitigate the effects of airborne contaminants and other infection control concerns on patients and others. The infection control professional, facility support staff, and construction personnel should routinely inspect areas affected or potentially affected by construction. The team will ensure that designated routes for construction workers are enforced and cleaned when removing garbage or bringing materials into the building and that dust barriers between construction and the rest of the facility are intact.

Check Your Understanding 13.1

1. Rick recently began working at a local hospital as the environmental services director. As part of his role at the hospital he has been tasked with conducting an analysis to not only meet accreditation requirements, but also to determine the types of disasters the hospital may face. What can you conclude about the type of analysis Rick is conducting based on this information?
   a. Hazard vulnerability analysis
   b. Emergency analysis
   c. Safety analysis
   d. Life safety analysis

2. Paul is returning to his unit after his dinner break while working the graveyard shift. After entering the unit, he notices a fire has started in one of the vacant patient rooms. It appears to have started in the garbage can, but is quickly spreading. Apply the acronym used to train healthcare employees on the proper methods for responding to this situation.

3. The Joint Commission requires a varying number of safety functions and plans depending on the license or services provided by an organization. The standards require the assessment of safety features for patients, staff, and visitors. Which of the following lists are required safety standard plans for the environment of care?
   a. Emergency management, security management, and patient management
   b. Medical equipment management, life safety management, and safety management
   c. Utilities management, employment management, and medical equipment management
   d. Employment management, hazardous materials and waste management, and life safety management

Criteria for an Annual Evaluation

Each of the seven safety plans is to be evaluated annually, taking into consideration the objectives, scope, performance, and effectiveness of the individual program. Depending on functions performed, the policies and procedures in place, and regulatory requirements, the safety officer or the individual responsible for the plan can prepare questions that will solicit responses from evaluators on the efficacy of the program. (See table 13.5 for an example of an emergency management annual evaluation.)

Table 13.5A. Example of an emergency management annual evaluation

HOSPITAL/MEDICAL CENTER ANNUAL EVALUATION OF THE EMERGENCY MANAGEMENT PROGRAM				
Criteria	Yes	No	Partial	Findings Page 1
Reviewed scope and objectives of the Emergency Management Plan				
Reviewed current accreditation standards				
Has the hospital conducted a Hazard Vulnerability Analysis?				
Disaster drills were conducted at least 2 times per year, 4 months apart.				
Has the hospital identified specific procedures to mitigate, prepare for, respond to, and recover from the identified procedures?				

Table 13.5B. Example of an emergency management annual evaluation (*Continued*)

HOSPITAL/MEDICAL CENTER ANNUAL EVALUATION OF THE EMERGENCY MANAGEMENT PROGRAM				
Criteria	Yes	No	Partial	Findings Page 2
Has the hospital defined a common command structure that links and integrates with the community?				
Does the hospital have representation in the community in regard to emergency management and preparation?				
Does the hospital have a means to notify external authorities of a possible community emergency, such as a bioterrorist attack?				
Does the hospital have procedures to • Notify personnel when emergency response measures are initiated? • Identify care providers during an emergency?				
Assign personnel to necessary staff positions during an emergency?				
Does the hospital have the ability to manage the following under emergency conditions? • Patient care–related activities • Staff support activities • Family support activities • Logistics in relation to critical supplies • Security				
Communication with the news media				
Does the hospital have a plan for evacuation if needed?				
Does the hospital have alternate care sites and agreements with other hospitals in the event of an evacuation or other emergency?				
Does the hospital have a plan to reestablish operations following an emergency?				
Does the plan identify • Alternate means of meeting essential building needs? • Backup communications? • Facilities for isolation? • Alternate roles for personnel during an emergency				
Does the plan provide for orientation and education of personnel who participate in emergencies?				
Does the hospital have the ability to provide decontamination in the event of an emergency?				
Does the hospital have the appropriate facilities, equipment, and supplies for decontamination procedures?				
Does the hospital conduct emergency drills at least twice a year?				
Were problems/concerns identified during drills or actual events?				
What actions were taken to resolve them?				
Does the hospital "fit test" those who will use respirators during decontamination procedures?				
Are hospital schematics available to those who may need them during an emergency?				
Does the hospital coordinate emergency management activities with its satellite facilities?				

Objectives, as stated in each of the EC management plans, are evaluated for current relevance to the organization. The evaluation should state that objectives have been reviewed and considered. If a plan's objectives have not changed, it is acceptable to note "no change."

The scope of each plan is reviewed and changes within the organization are noted, such as new security department hours, added or expanded services, or additional facilities that have been acquired (for instance, a new clinic that will require safety inspections, hazardous material inventory, and so forth).

Performance measurement is the foundation of the annual evaluation. Data relative to the performance improvement (PI) goals provide information for the involved staff to assess their accomplishments and compliance with regulatory standards. The data collection supports the findings of the annual evaluation. For example, if security events show an increase in lost patient belongings (as monitored under safety inspections in table 13.1), a PI goal to address the lost belongings should be included in the annual evaluation of the security plan.

The effectiveness of a plan is determined by what went well during the year, what accomplishments were achieved, whether the organization was in compliance with regulatory requirements, what procedures or policies need to be updated or implemented, and what functions need to be improved. This information, along with the data collected for performance measurement, may be the basis for determining performance goals or quality improvement projects for the following year.

Information Collection and Evaluation System

The information collection and evaluation system (ICES) shown in table 13.1 comprises many documents, facts, reports, and performance monitoring. Information collected and evaluated may include patient reports of unusual occurrence, security incident reports, employee injuries or illness reports, and the number of hazardous materials spills. Most accrediting bodies require monitoring, investigation, and reporting of the following items:

- Patient or visitor injuries
- Incidents of property damage
- Occupational injuries or illnesses
- Security incidents
- Hazardous materials and waste spills and exposures
- Fire prevention problems, deficiencies, and failures
- Equipment problems, deficiencies, and failures
- Utility systems problems, deficiencies, and failures

Information collection may be the responsibility of one designated individual, such as the quality department director, the risk manager, or the safety officer. A reasonable expectation is that data collection and transmission are the responsibility of each safety plan leader. The safety committee, a multidisciplinary group, reviews the information and makes recommendations to the individual responsible for the safety plans. The safety committee ensures that the information is circulated to the administration, the medical staff, and the board of trustees.

At a minimum, data should be collected on the pertinent functions or performance standards of each safety plan and submitted to the safety committee quarterly for comment and recommendations.

QI Toolbox Technique: Postprogram Assessment

Postprogram assessments are the most common method used to evaluate employee knowledge of care environment and safety area issues. The assessments are given to employees after each training session. At a minimum, every employee must attend training in each of the areas annually. Human resources systems track each employee's training attendance and record it in the employee's personnel file. (Employee training attendance may be the function of the education department, with files maintained separately. However the function is designated, training files must be available for surveyors.) Figure 13.7 shows an example of a posttraining assessment tool used at Community Hospital of the West.

Figure 13.7. Posttraining assessment tool used at Community Hospital of the West

---

INTERVIEW OF STAFF (circle questions asked)

1. What orientation did you receive on the following?
    a. General safety [ ]
    b. Department safety [ ]
    c. Job-specific hazards [ ]
2. What continuing safety education have you received? [ ]
3. What are the emergency procedures for:
    a. Bomb threat [ ]
    b. Hostage crises [ ]
4. How are security incidents reported? [ ]
5. Give an example of the safe use of a hazardous chemical and waste in your department. [ ]
6. What is the procedure for reporting a hazardous materials spill? [ ]
7. What is appropriate personal protective equipment to handle hazardous materials in your department? [ ]
8. What is your role in the disaster plan? [ ]
9. Describe the emergency communication system (red phones). [ ]
10. What are your role and responsibilities at the site of a fire? [ ]
11. What are your role and responsibilities away from the fire site? [ ]
12. Describe your role in evacuation of patients and staff. [ ]
13. Describe how to report equipment problems. [ ]
14. Where are the SDS kept? [ ]
15. Describe how to report utility failures. [ ]

Some organizations have safety fairs. They set up carnival games or similar activities in which staff are asked EC questions. Staff members who answer the questions correctly are entered into drawings or awarded small prizes. Many kinds of activities can be developed to keep safety issues in the forefront, such as participating in a community-wide mock disaster drill.

Many organizations have developed a safety response flip chart that is posted in a prominent area in each department of the facility for rapid access by personnel. Each page has emergency response information to assist employees in the first 15 to 45 minutes of an emergency.

Check Your Understanding 13.2

1. Explain how postprogram assessments are used to evaluate employee knowledge of care environment and safety area issues.
2. A hospital employee is transporting a patient to the imaging department for a CT scan. After pushing the gurney into the elevator, the employee drops an item and bends down to pick it up as the elevator doors are closing. The employee's head is struck by the elevator and the employee is injured. Evaluate whether or not this incident needs to be reported and investigated and justify your answer.

Real-Life Example

On a hot Saturday afternoon in July, a construction company was laying cable under the street about a quarter mile north of Community Hospital. The workers were using an auger to drill under the roadway so they would not need to tear up the street. Although the gas and electric lines in the area had been marked with blue stakes, the construction crew inadvertently damaged the main electrical line under the street. The hospital and other businesses in the area were without electrical power.

The hospital did have a backup generator; however, this generator did not automatically turn on when the main power was lost. Facilities management went to investigate and discovered that the generator was no longer operable. At this point, the facility management director attempted to contact hospital administration, only to learn that all executive leadership was on vacation. An acting manager contacted a neighboring hospital that allowed Community Hospital to borrow their backup generator. When the borrowed generator was connected, power was restored to the hospital. Upon further investigation, the administration determined that the backup generator had not been tested per policy for over a year.

Because the organization had not been prepared for this type of emergency, the hospital's safety council met later to initiate the following steps:

- Tighten all policies and procedures related to testing of backup utility equipment to include an annual audit of all related documentation
- Implement a policy that at least one member of the executive leadership team is always in town and available for emergency purposes
- Practice emergency procedures related to loss of utilities with staff twice a year

Case Study

 During remodeling and renovation of two patient care areas at a hospital, a new nurse call system was installed. A Code Blue alarm specific to each room was a component of the new system. The other patient care areas in the hospital were to receive the new nurse call system later in the year. After installation of the new system, the nurses were instructed to begin using the Code Blue button in the patient rooms, and they were assured that the alarm and room number would automatically appear on the hospital operator's computer. The new system made it unnecessary to call the operator to request a Code Blue and for the operator to announce the room number because it was done automatically.

Unfortunately, this was a case in which patient safety was overlooked in the excitement of receiving new technology. It was soon discovered that the room number that appeared on the console did not correspond to the room number in which the button was being pushed. The discrepancy was noted with the first Code Blue in one of the renovated areas when the room number that appeared on the console was not a recognized room number in the hospital. Use of the Code Blue button was suspended immediately. The procedure of calling the operator was reinstituted and remained in effect until all clinical areas received the new nurse call system. This gave the clinical engineering personnel time to make sure the new system was functioning properly, and it prevented the confusion that would have resulted from maintaining two different methods of alerting the hospital operator of a Code Blue.

> **Case Study Questions**
> 1. How could this patient safety issue have been avoided?
> 2. Which of the required written safety standards or plans for the environment of care should have been used to avoid this situation?

Review Questions

1. Which program is designed to manage the physical and personal safeguard of patients, staff, and other individuals coming to the facility?
   a. Safety management
   b. Security management
   c. Hazardous materials and waste management
   d. Emergency management

2. Safety data sheets are provided by the chemical manufacturer, distributor, or importer to any user to provide details about any hazards of their products. Explain why healthcare organizations must have processes in place to educate employees to mitigate safety issues related to hazardous substances.

3. Bonnie's estranged husband has threatened to harm her and states he "will get her after work." What action can Bonnie take to reduce the threat of violence to her on hospital property?
   a. Ask for a security escort to/from her vehicle and to/from her unit.
   b. Call her attorney and inform her of the situation and the threat.
   c. Walk out to the parking lot with a coworker.
   d. Call the hospital risk manager and ask for their assistance.

4. The hazard communication standard is based on the premise that employees who may be exposed to hazardous chemicals in the workplace have a right to know about the hazards and how to protect themselves. This standard sets forth guidelines and requirements. What areas are covered by this standard?

5. Which program is designed to ensure that electricity, water, sewer, and natural gas systems throughout the environment of care are planned and maintained safely and comfortably, that services are delivered without interruption, and that mechanical systems operate safely?
   a. Safety management
   b. Security management
   c. Emergency management
   d. Utilities management

References

Joint Commission. 2024a. "Environment of Care." In *Hospital Accreditation Standards*. Oakbrook Terrace, IL: Joint Commission Resources.

Joint Commission. 2024b. "Emergency Management." In *Hospital Accreditation Standards*. Oakbrook Terrace, IL: Joint Commission Resources.

Joint Commission. 2024c. "Glossary." In *Hospital Accreditation Standards*. Oakbrook Terrace, IL: Joint Commission Resources.

Joint Commission. 2024d. "Life Safety." In *Hospital Accreditation Standards*. Oakbrook Terrace, IL: Joint Commission Resources.

Kaiser Permanente. 2021. "Updated HVA Tool." https://www.calhospitalprepare.org/post/updated-hva-tool-kaiser-permanente.

OSHA (Occupational Safety and Health Administration). n.d. "Hazard Communication Standard." Accessed July 1, 2024. https://www.osha.gov/dsg/hazcom/ghs-final-rule.html.

Resources

ANSI (American National Standards Institute). 2024. https://www.ansi.org/.

CDC (Centers for Disease Control and Prevention). 2024. https://www.cdc.gov/index.htm.

NIMS (National Incident Management System). 2024. https://www.fema.gov/emergency-managers/nims#:~:text=The%20National%20Incident%20Management%20System,to%20and%20recover%20from%20incidents.

Developing Staff and Human Resources

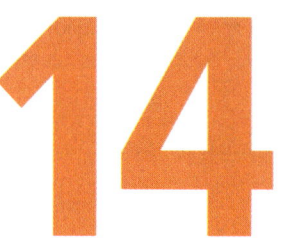

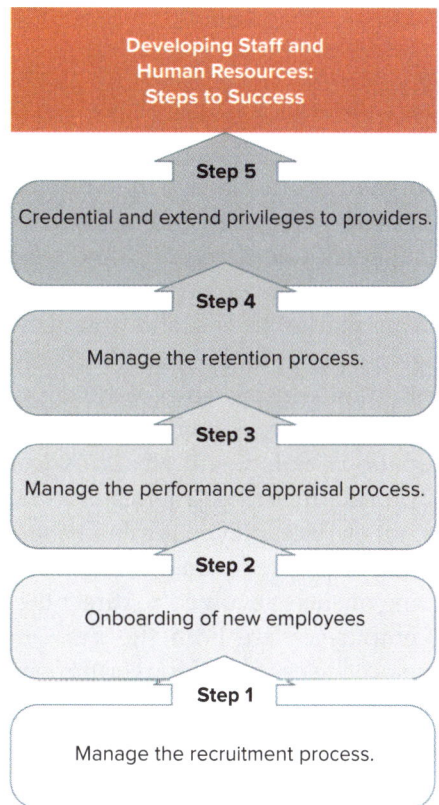

Learning Objectives

- Assess the need to integrate performance improvement and patient safety data into management of the human resources function in healthcare
- Apply the tools and processes commonly used to manage the recruitment and retention of human resources
- Use the credentialing process to develop provider profiles

Key Terms

Clinical privileges
Credentialing process
Credentials
Due process

Licensed provider
Licenses
National Practitioner Data Bank (NPDB)

The environment in which healthcare organizations manage their human resources is dictated in large part by state and federal employment laws, regulatory agencies, and market trends. Variations in the way healthcare is delivered also affect the organization's recruitment, training, and retention practices. Potential legal action undertaken by employees against healthcare organizations must also be considered. This chapter introduces information on laws, regulations, shifting market trends, and organizational policy to demonstrate some of the processes and tools used to manage people in today's healthcare environment.

During the 20th century, inequitable and unsafe employment practices were a driving force in the passage of legislation intended to improve the work environment. Legislation that addressed issues such as safe working conditions (the Occupational Safety and Health Act of 1970), wages and hours (the Equal Employment Opportunity Act of 1972), disabilities (the Americans with Disabilities Act of 1990), and medical leave (the Family and Medical Leave Act of 1993) played a role in shaping the workplace environment and standardizing employment practices. Other employment guidelines and standards of practice in the areas of state licensure and outside accrediting agencies evolved to direct the employer-employee relationship.

For any healthcare organization, employees are both the most important resource and the greatest potential liability. Developing effective processes related to recruitment, retention, competence, orientation, and continuing education of all staff members is a critical function of an organization's leadership, which must ensure that it employs highly skilled staff.

Effective leadership is defined as how well an organization's leaders plan, direct, integrate, and coordinate services, and how well they create a culture that focuses on continual performance improvement (PI) while maintaining a balanced budget and fiscal viability in the market. These key leadership functions are demonstrated through human resources management in the following ways:

- Defining the qualifications, competencies, and performance expectations for all staff positions
- Providing competent staff
- Ensuring orientation and other ongoing training and education
- Assessing, maintaining, and improving staff competence
- Promoting self-development and learning

Today's work environment encourages and empowers employees to take responsibility for improving the environment in which they work, no matter their position in the organizational structure. PI can be a powerful concept when woven into the culture of an organization. Organizations that embrace ongoing PI do so because their leaders foster a culture of competence through staff self-development and lifelong learning. The competitive advantage for healthcare organizations lies in their intellectual capital and organizational effectiveness. This style of motivating and developing employees is grounded in the ability of leaders to create, communicate, and model the organization's mission, vision, and values.

Steps to Success: Developing Staff and Human Resources

Historically, healthcare organizations have used a number of different criteria to determine the actual number of full-time equivalent (FTE) staff, including the patient census, the acuity of the patients being treated, licensing regulations that may specify the staff-to-patient ratio, and the qualifications of the type of staff required. In planning its budget, an organization must take into account the revenue that needs to be generated and the number of FTEs required to run a facility that meets licensing agreements, addresses patient safety issues, and maintains fiscal viability.

Accreditation requirements include the need for measurable standards related to staffing effectiveness in an attempt to make maintaining prescribed staffing levels a more realistic, dynamic process. Effective staffing is complex, dynamic, and unique to each individual organization. At the core of staffing effectiveness are the competence and skill mix of staff members currently assigned to care for a particular set of patients, as well as the associated acuity ratios (how sick the particular set of patients is) for the population in question. Staffing has a direct impact on the quality and safety of patient care. An aging workforce, which points to potential shortages of key staff, will continue to challenge and impact staffing effectiveness.

The standard approach to evaluation of effective hospital staffing includes the use of multiple hospital-specific clinical and service measures and human resources indicators as screening tools to identify potential staffing issues. Many organizations have clinical measures and human resources indicators for each patient population, defined by internal PI activities. Identified performance measures relate to processes appropriate to the care and services provided and to problem-prone areas experienced in the past (for example, infection rates or incidences of patient falls). The rationale for indicator selection is based on relevance and sensitivity to each patient area where staffing is planned. The intent is that multiple indicators examined together may provide information related to staffing effectiveness. Because staffing effectiveness is considered a critical process in healthcare, accrediting bodies require a thorough analysis to be initiated whenever an organization detects or suspects significant undesirable performance or variation in performance due to staffing issues.

Most organizations define their clinical staffing needs in two categories: direct and indirect caregivers. Examples of direct caregivers include nursing staff, physical therapists, chaplains, and social services staff. Indirect caregivers include clinical support professionals from the pharmacy, laboratory, housekeeping, dietary, and other departments. Both direct and indirect caregivers may be included in human resources screening indicators.

Step 1: Manage the Recruitment Process

A well-defined recruitment process provides both the organization and the applicant with an opportunity to evaluate and determine their potential compatibility. The recruitment process is usually initiated to fill a vacant position, to fill a newly created position, to staff a newly instituted service, or to support increases in patient acuity or census. Organizations sometimes retain the services of an outside recruitment agency when there are shortages of qualified applicants or because of an organization's remote geographic location.

Position requisitions, position descriptions (also called job descriptions), and employment applications are the primary tools used in the recruitment process. A position requisition begins the formal communication between the human resources staff and the department or service area initiating the recruitment process. (See figure 14.1.)

Figure 14.1. Sample position requisition

PERSONNEL REQUISITION		
JOB TITLE	DATE OF REQUEST	DATE REQUIRED

DEPARTMENT
☐ Replacement for:

☐ Additional Personnel:	Budgeted: ☐ Yes ☐ No			
☐ Temporary: End Date _____	☐ Full Time	☐ Part Time	☐ Exempt ☐ PRN	☐ Per Diem
Shift: Hours per week:	Suggested Pay Grade:			
Qualifications needed: education, experience, training, duties, physical fitness		Actual:	Budgeted:	Prior Year:
	YTD FTEs			
	MH/STAT			
	SAL $/STAT			
	Reason for additional personnel or new position:			

APPROVALS (must be obtained prior to offering position)	

DIRECTOR/MANAGER:
               DATE:
	CEO:
	               DATE:

CFO:
               DATE:
	HUMAN RESOURCES:
	               DATE:

NEW PERSONNEL			
To be completed by human resources			Date Required:
Employee's Name:		Department:	Employee Number:
Address:		Social Security Number:	
Telephone Number:		Birth date:	
Date of Hire:		Temporary Date of Termination:	
☐ New Hire ☐ Rehire ☐ Full Time ☐ Part Time ☐ PRN ☐ Per Diem ☐ Exempt ☐ Temp.			
RATE/HOUR	BIWEEKLY RATE	RACE EEO CAT. TAX EXEMP.	POS CODE
COMMENTS OR SPECIAL INSTRUCTIONS:			

A detailed position requisition provides human resources staff with the information needed to advertise the open position, including the position title, qualifications and experience required, work schedule, and salary. Position requisitions also can be used to monitor the appropriateness of personnel requests. For example, a nonbudgeted position or a new position request may require additional documentation and administrative approval before recruitment can begin.

Job descriptions define the responsibilities of the position and the qualifications needed to fulfill those responsibilities. Qualifications may define education; licensure, certification, or registration status; and experience required. Qualifications also may include previous experience requirements, such as a pediatric nurse position requiring training and experience working with children and adolescents in particular pediatric settings.

In healthcare organizations, credentials, certifications, and licenses are qualifications of foremost importance. Clinical professionals, such as physicians, nurses, occupational therapists, physical therapists, respiratory therapists, psychologists, and social workers, as well as some ancillary services professionals, such as radiology, laboratory, and pharmacy technicians, are required to hold a credential or license to practice their profession.

Credentials are the recognition by healthcare organizations of previous professional practice responsibilities and experiences commonly accorded to licensed providers. A **licensed provider** is any individual permitted by law to provide healthcare services without direction or supervision, within the scope of the individual's license as conferred by state regulatory agencies and consistent with individually granted clinical privileges. **Licenses** are conferred by state regulatory agencies and allow an individual to provide healthcare services within a specific scope of service and geographical location. Certifications are usually conferred by a national professional organization dedicated to a specific area of healthcare practice. Certification and licensing processes usually require an applicant to pass an examination to initially obtain the license or certification and then to maintain the certification or license through continuing education activities.

Job responsibilities describe the major tasks of the position. Responsibilities should be stated in measurable terms, which is the standard in healthcare today. A clinical position, for example, may describe a responsibility as "completing a nursing assessment on each admission within the time frame defined by policy."

In general, position descriptions provide guidance to human resources staff by defining the initial selection criteria for potential candidates. Position descriptions also provide the applicant or new employee with information about position expectations. With the support of human resources specialists, managers maintain job descriptions that reflect local market and current position requirements.

Open positions are typically advertised on the healthcare organization's website and may also be promoted on job boards or other third-party employment websites. Interested candidates may complete an employment application using the organization's online system. A review of the completed application and the applicant's resumé provides human resources and the recruiting department or service area manager with enough information to determine whether the applicant meets the minimum position requirements. Applicants who meet the initial position requirements and who are the most qualified are invited to interview for the position.

The interview gives the applicant and the organization an opportunity to exchange information not listed on the employment application or in the position advertisement. The organization may have additional questions specific to experience, skills, and qualifications that are not addressed in the application. The candidate, in turn, may have questions related to salary, benefits, working conditions, or the organization's history. The interview provides the opportunity for the interviewer to evaluate the applicant's communication skills, general personality, and demeanor.

During the interview process, the interviewee may be asked to sign a release for information on a background check. Most states offer this service as a risk-reduction and patient safety strategy for facilities that provide physical and emotional care to vulnerable patient populations. This regulation was put into place to safeguard clients and facilities from individuals with documented histories of abuse. Potential employees in these settings must pass a criminal background check before being offered a position.

Several types of interviews can be used to screen applicants, such as structured, unstructured, and stress interviews. A *structured interview* is conducted using a set of standard questions that are asked of all job applicants to gather comparative data. The *unstructured interview* uses general questions from which other questions are developed over the course of the conversation. The purpose of this type of interview is to prompt the interviewee to speak openly.

The following are examples of unstructured questions that may be used during an interview:

- Tell us about your previous position. In general, what kinds of duties did you perform?
- Tell us about your personal understanding of the need for maintaining the patient's rights to confidentiality.

The *stress* interview uses specific questions to determine how the interviewee responds under pressure. Questions in this type of interview set up specific scenarios and ask the interviewee how they would handle the situation. The following are examples of questions that might be asked in a stress interview:

- If a news reporter came to you and wanted you to reveal information from a prominent person's health record, how would you respond?
- If an attorney came to your nursing unit and wanted to review a client's health record, what would you do?

Certain types of questions should be avoided during an interview. Questions that might be interpreted as attempts to learn personal information about the applicant (such as the applicant's age, marital status, or family status) are prohibited by federal regulations. Figure 14.2 includes examples of appropriate, job-related, questions and inappropriate questions that are not related to employment, which would be considered discriminatory.

Figure 14.2. Appropriate and inappropriate interview questions

Examples of Appropriate Job-Related Questions	Examples of Inappropriate, Non–Job-Related Questions
• How does your education and work experience relate to the position we are discussing?	• Where were you born?
• What courses did you take in school?	• What race are you?
• Are you willing to work weekends?	• What is your height and weight?
• Are you willing to work overtime?	• What is your religious faith?
• What kind of work did you do in your previous positions?	• Do you own or rent your residence?
• What kind of work do you enjoy the most? The least?	• What is your current marital status?
• What areas of your work skills would you like to improve?	• What is your spouse's full name?
• How do you perform under pressure?	• Do you anticipate having children in the next few years?
• How many people were you responsible for supervising in your previous position?	• Have you ever been arrested?
• Why did you leave your position?	• Do you have any physical or mental disabilities or handicaps?
• How do you explain the gaps in your employment history?	• When was the date of your last physical exam?
• What are your career goals?	• Which clubs and organizations do you belong to?
• Tell us about a time you dealt with a difficult customer; how did you handle it?	• Who cares for your children while you are at work?
	• Is your spouse likely to be transferred?

Some facilities add a skills-testing or competency review segment such as a coding test, medication exam, developmental age exam, or a computer literacy test to their interview process. This testing adds additional information of a concrete nature to the screening for possible candidates.

Whichever approach or combination of approaches is used, the information collected at this point in the recruitment process should be enough to determine who will advance to the next stage of the selection process. Reference checks; criminal background checks; and verifications of licensure, training, and educational requirements should be documented before any applicant is offered a position. In the past, checking past employment references sometimes yielded important new information about a candidate. Today, however, most organizations release only general information regarding an employee's past work performance, such as dates of employment and whether the applicant is eligible for rehire. While the information received from these contacts may be minimal in terms of a potential employee's skills, they do speak to the veracity of documentation in the resumé in general and may be critical in a legal defense situation for a facility.

Some facilities use a point-scoring process for interviews that awards points for education, knowledge at time of interview, and experience with the specific population of patients. This system helps ensure that the top-qualified individuals will be in the running for a position.

Step 2: Onboarding of New Employees

Onboarding should be provided to every new hire, including contracted staff, agency personnel, and volunteers. New staff members receive an overview of the organization as well as details about their specific job responsibilities. The organization's leaders are expected to develop an onboarding process to ensure that all new staff members are informed of performance expectations and specific responsibilities. When these issues are addressed before new staff members are allowed to perform independently, this process promotes safe and effective job performance. In general, staff should be oriented to the organization's mission; vision; values; PI program; life safety procedures; infection control practices; privacy practices; policies toward patient, client, or resident abuse; specific job duties; and safety issues specific to their job assignments. Introducing a new employee to these key policies and practices will help to develop a culture of teamwork and collaboration among diverse staff members. Additional orientation and training may be specific to a type of healthcare organization, such as age-specific training for staff working with neonatal or pediatric age groups for which skills at interpreting nonverbal communication are essential.

New staff members should not work independently until they have completed the onboarding process and demonstrated competence. Testing to assess the competence of a clinical staff member may include having the employee insert a catheter, draw blood, or use a piece of medical equipment. This type of training and orientation may include having the new employee shadow a seasoned employee for a specified period of time, complete a self-directed study course, or attend classroom instruction and then demonstrate their competence by performing a particular job skill a set number of times for a certified trainer.

As part of the onboarding process, orientation and demonstrated job competencies must be documented. Some organizations use a training checklist to document employee orientation. The checklist documents the names of the trainee and trainer(s), orientation dates, tasks, and demonstrated competencies. The orientation checklist should be maintained in the employee's personnel file so that it can be used in the performance appraisal process to monitor whether training and competency requirements have been met.

Aggregate data also can be compiled from training checklists to monitor organization-wide and care- or service-specific competency requirements. In hospitals, aggregate data on the levels of staff competence, relevant patterns and trends in training needs, and competence in maintenance activities should be reported to the governing body at least annually. Gathering data for the competency assessment process can be accomplished through observations, demonstrations, and PI reports such as occurrence report findings, peer review findings, and staffing effectiveness and satisfaction surveys.

Policies and procedures facilitate the onboarding of staff and form the basis for individual accountability. Policies and procedures should clearly represent and communicate the required functions and tasks the employee is expected to perform as well as the procedures to initiate when an unacceptable incident occurs in the facility, such as a medication error. It is critical that all employees be trained in the areas of risk identification and reduction and incident reporting. Data collected from this process become the basis for much PI in healthcare facilities.

Step 3: Manage the Performance Appraisal Process

Every healthcare organization should have a process in place to periodically reassess each staff member's ability to meet the performance expectations and competencies described in the job description. Healthcare organizations determine how often these reassessments should occur. For example, competence can be assessed at hire; by the end of the onboarding process; at regular intervals (such as once per year); when job responsibilities change; or when new or updated technologies, products, procedures, or services are introduced.

The employee performance appraisal process should be specific to the staff member's assigned responsibilities and assessed competencies. Ideally, the appraisal should include a one-on-one discussion between the employee and the supervisor or manager along with a written appraisal that provides room for employee response. The employee and the supervisor or manager should work together to develop new performance goals and to modify or enhance performance standards. The manager or supervisor should follow up with the employee to monitor their progress in meeting goals and performance standards through frequent, informal assessments as well as periodic formal appraisals. At a minimum, the periodic assessment should address each of the following areas of the employee's performance:

- Degree of compliance with written standards of performance as stated in the staff member's job description
- Participation in ongoing PI and patient safety activities
- Findings from competency assessment activities

Other areas, such as a staff member's strengths, weaknesses, working relationships, morale, motivation, and attendance, also may be addressed during the appraisal process.

The performance criteria used in the appraisal process should be directly linked to the employee's current position description and to the organization's mission. This process should also verify that the employee has maintained their credentials or license(s), as appropriate.

Organizations that have successfully implemented a PI culture have expanded the appraisal process to include team performance in tandem with individual performance. Teams may include a clinical treatment team, an administrative or leadership team, or a single department team. The appraisal process includes the team's definition of performance expectations and goals and a periodic assessment of its performance as a team rather than as individuals.

Ideally, organization-wide performance measures should be referenced and incorporated into the employee and team appraisal process. Provider- or employee-specific PI and patient safety monitoring activities may identify staff development needs. This same information reported in aggregate may identify trends in care that support the need for changes in staffing patterns, skill sets, or the care environment. Other clinical service and human resources screening criteria used to monitor staffing effectiveness are also reviewed in preparation for the organization's annual strategic planning process.

Step 4: Manage the Retention Process

Commitment to the development and retention of human resources is of strategic importance to every healthcare organization. High retention rates communicate a strong message about the organization's values to existing and potential employees. Many organizations offer tuition and professional education reimbursement as an incentive for ongoing staff development and retention. Maintaining a competitive salary and benefits package continues to be a primary leverage point in recruitment and retention programs. Organizations that go beyond traditional incentives use employee input to create reward structures to promote employee retention. Incentives such as profit sharing, job sharing, sign-on bonuses, shared leadership, and cutting-edge technological resources are a few of the trends.

Certainly, the most compelling link to employee retention is the creation of a work environment in which organizational and personal values mesh, creating a natural synergy. Teams working together with a common vision begin with a self-directed, motivated workforce. Many times, this team factor directly influences employee retention even more than salary issues do. Employees who have been prepared for their jobs through education and who believe that they are part of a vital team that provides excellent care are willing to stay, even if their salary is not top in the field.

Another important aspect of managing employee retention in healthcare is the maintenance of employee competence. Healthcare professionals must follow many standard processes and procedures to provide quality care, while at the same time protecting patient safety. Maintaining professional knowledge and competence to perform these processes becomes of paramount importance. To accomplish this, many organizations require all employees to obtain recertification in areas specific to their clinical license, such as CPR and basic life-support skills, or in areas specific to the organization's safety issues, such as fire safety, infection control, and so forth. Clinical and nonclinical staff must demonstrate their applicable competencies on an annual basis.

Managing the curriculum content, posttraining assessments, and calendar of annual updates for thousands of employees who are required to perform annual competence recertification can be a daunting task. Many healthcare organizations use a training platform to provide learning modules, track employee completion, and aggregate data on employee training.

Step 5: Credential and Extend Privileges to Providers

The medical staff who work in healthcare organizations may include employed providers, licensed independent providers, physician assistants, and nurse practitioners. These individuals are permitted by law and the organization to provide patient-care services without direction or supervision, within the scope of their license and individually granted **clinical privileges** (permission given by a healthcare organization to practice in a specific area of specialty within that organization). Physicians, dentists, and podiatrists are the most commonly credentialed providers working in healthcare organizations. However, certified nurse-anesthetists, physician assistants, nurse practitioners, registered nurse-midwives, speech pathologists, dietitians, clinical psychologists, and clinical social workers are also privileged and credentialed by the healthcare organization, as either supervised employees or contract workers.

The credentialing and privileging process for the initial appointment and reappointment of providers should be defined in the healthcare organization's medical staff bylaws and should be uniformly applied. The **credentialing process** includes obtaining, verifying, and assessing qualifications of a licensed healthcare provider. The primary sources of state licenses, postgraduate degrees, residency and fellowship training, specialty board status, and other healthcare affiliations should all be verified. Primary source verification involves contacting the original source of a specific credential to affirm qualifications reported by an individual healthcare provider. The primary source verification process is sometimes contracted out by the healthcare organization to a credentials verification organization, such as the American Medical Association Physician Master File, which verifies a physician's medical school graduation and residency completion, or the American Board of Medical Specialties, which verifies a physician's board certification. Although using such agencies may relieve the organization of the process of gathering the information, the organization is still responsible for having complete and accurate information on the applicant to substantiate its privileging decisions.

Each provider who practices under the auspices of a healthcare organization must do so in accordance with delineated clinical privileges based on the provider's training, experience, and proven clinical competence. The privilege lists sent to applicants at initial appointment and at reappointment should be associated with the applicant's type of practice and limited to hospital-specific privileges.

The initial appointment process includes the provider requesting, completing, and submitting an application to the medical staff along with a request for delineated clinical privileges. The credentialing and privileging process is generally initiated upon completion and approval of an application for membership and request for privileges. The applicant should submit the following information:

- Education, both undergraduate and postgraduate, with names of institutions
- Training, including residencies, fellowships, and any continuing medical education or training for new skills or privileges

- Previous and current healthcare affiliations (hospitals practiced in, private office locations)
- Specialty board certifications
- Current state licenses
- Drug Enforcement Administration (DEA) registration number with expiration date(s)
- Professional (peer) references who have personal knowledge of the applicant's recent professional performance and experience
- Information on current health status
- Professional liability insurance coverage
- Past and present professional litigation and liability history
- Clinical privileges being requested

Requests for references are generally sent to at least two peer references and one healthcare organization where the applicant currently holds privileges, requesting specific information about the applicant's qualifications and competencies in relation to the privileges requested, health status, and professional working relationships as observed by the reference source.

Healthcare organizations are required by law to query the **National Practitioner Data Bank (NPDB)** for information on applicants requesting clinical privileges. The NPDB is a national database that maintains reports on medical malpractice settlements, clinical privilege actions, and professional society membership actions against licensed healthcare providers, as well as reports on civil judgments, criminal convictions, federal and state licensing and certification actions, and exclusions from participation in federal or state healthcare programs.

Once applicant information has been source verified and references and data bank queries have been returned, the application and supporting documentation are reviewed by the organization's credentials or medical executive committee(s). Individual appointment and privilege delineation recommendations are then forwarded to the organization's governing body for final determination. When the application is approved, the appointment period must not exceed two years. A provisional period is generally required (the medical staff bylaws should specify a time limit) for all new staff members. The performance of new staff members should be observed and monitored by an assigned proctor during the provisional period.

Accrediting agencies require hospital medical staffs to initiate a process to identify and manage issues of individual provider health. This must be done separately from the disciplinary function of the medical staff. The purpose is to help facilities address the physical health of providers who are at risk in their industry for such job-related illnesses as addiction, stress-related physical illness, and emotional illness. Regular staff education regarding these potential illnesses is also required. Healthcare organizations must facilitate the process for confidential diagnosis, treatment, and rehabilitation for any potentially impairing conditions such as the ones defined. These procedures must be done in compliance with any state or federal reporting regulations.

The reappraisal and reappointment process generally occurs every two years and includes a review of current licenses, DEA registration, professional liability coverage, national data bank queries, continuing medical education (as required by the state or for competency training), peer references, information related to claims and litigation, health, and changes in outside affiliations. Training, education, and certification, as well as the frequency with which a clinical privilege has been exercised, should show evidence of continuing proficiency for the privileges requested. An assessment of the provider's profile since the last staff appointment to verify peer review activities provides the final basis for supporting reappointment or reprivileging. Due to the nature of unannounced surveys by accrediting bodies and government regulators (such as the Joint Commission and the Centers for Medicare and Medicaid Services [CMS]), these files should be kept up to date and monitored continuously.

An ongoing professional practice evaluation includes both administrative aspects of staff membership (for example, meeting attendance statistics, health record delinquency status, medical staff committee appointments, and practice volume statistics) and clinical performance data (for example, clinical outcome statistics, committee or department citations, peer review, and performance-monitoring reviews and actions). The evaluation allows the organization to identify professional practice trends that affect quality of care and patient safety. Such identification may require intervention by the organized medical staff. The criteria used in the ongoing professional practice evaluation includes key performance metrics such as procedures performed and their outcomes, blood use, and complications. (See figure 14.3 in the Case Study section later in this chapter for an example.)

Following review of the reappointment application information and provider profile information, the chief of staff or clinical department chairperson provides a written recommendation on reappointment and reprivileging to the credentials or executive committee(s) of the medical staff. These bodies then make their own recommendations and forward them to the governing body for a final decision. When a recommendation for continuing privileges is not made, or a restriction in privileges is requested, the provider must be offered due process. **Due process** provides for fair treatment through a hearing procedure that is usually outlined in the healthcare organization's medical staff bylaws. The procedure stipulates the means by which the provider's application and supporting materials will be reviewed by an impartial panel to ensure objective assessment.

QI Toolbox Technique: Provider Profile Summary

Summary profiles of provider performance supply the credentials committee with significant data about providers scheduled for reappointment to the medical staff. The summary provides the credentials committee with the information needed to make sound decisions on the performance of members of the hospital's medical staff.

The type of data captured on a provider profile summary should be unique to the healthcare organization's specific needs. The sample form in figure 14.3 is designed for a physician in the specialty area of obstetrics/gynecology (OB/GYN). It includes data about the physician's cesarean section (C-section) rate, the number of vaginal births after a cesarean section (VBACs), types of medications used, transfusion usage, record completion delinquency rates, risk management issues, and attendance at medical staff meetings. It also includes documentation of any disciplinary action against the physician that has taken place since the last credentialing process.

Check Your Understanding 14.1

1. During the onboarding process for new employees in a hospital setting, what is an important objective that contributes to both enhanced patient care and organizational success?
   a. Implementing state-of-the-art medical technologies to streamline diagnostics
   b. Establishing a culture of teamwork and collaboration among diverse staff members
   c. Restructuring traditional workflows by maximizing the use of digital tools
   d. Balancing individual achievements with collective success to foster a dynamic work environment

2. Landmark Hospital is a rural facility that has been struggling to recruit new physicians. In an effort to meet the needs of the community, the hospital recently hired two new physician assistants (PAs). Although the new PAs are able to provide much of the care the hospital is in need of, the PAs are governed by a scope of practice determined by their:
   a. Clinical knowledge
   b. Credentials
   c. Position on the staff
   d. Clinical privileges

Real-Life Example

University Hospital recently completed a national search and recruitment effort to fill its chief clinical officer (CCO) position. The position had been vacant for six months and had experienced rapid turnover of two previous CCOs within the past two years. The members of the search team invited to participate in the recruitment effort included the chief executive medical director, the chief financial officer, the human resources director, the medical staff president, and the nurse managers from each clinical care area.

The search team followed internal policy requirements related to the recruitment process. The position description was reviewed and updated, and from it, minimum position requirements were identified and included in the job posting. The search team also retained the services of a national recruitment firm in an effort to fast-track the recruitment process because the organization was less than a year away from its accreditation on-site survey.

The search generated 15 applicants. The team screened the applicants and narrowed the list down to six who seemed to meet the minimum position requirements. These applicants (five of whom were out-of-state candidates) were interviewed remotely. The selection was then narrowed to two candidates, who were invited to fly in and meet with the search team.

Of primary importance to this search team's recruitment charge was finding a CCO who had a clinical background and experience that paralleled the services provided at the hospital. Experience, strong knowledge of accreditation and licensure requirements, educational background with a master's degree, past employment patterns, personal demeanor, communication style, leadership philosophy, and availability were important factors in the selection. The final candidate selected by the search team met the important criteria and minimum position requirements. Reference checks and source documents verifying the applicant's credentials confirmed the search team's decision to hire the final candidate as the CCO.

Five months into the new CCO's tenure, and six weeks before the accreditation survey, The hospital's director of risk and quality management resigned. Because the risk and quality position reported to the CCO, the new CCO was asked to facilitate survey preparations. Within days of this decision, the CCO requested that the leadership team recruit a local consulting group to assist in survey coordination efforts. Just two weeks before the anticipated survey, the CCO resigned.

Two main factors contributed to the CCO's resignation. First, the source documents confirming the CCO's graduate education were not in the CCO's human resources file. As personnel files were being reviewed in preparation for survey inspection, it was noted that the primary source verification of the CCO's graduate degree was incomplete. When the graduate program was contacted, it was revealed that the CCO had never completed the master's program. Second, although the CCO's curriculum vitae and references confirmed that the CCO had 20-plus years' experience in nursing administration and accreditation survey work, the CCO was unable to assume a leadership role in facilitating the nursing component of the accreditation survey preparation process.

University Hospital has since defined what information it primary source verifies (verbal and written) when confirming education, experience, and licensure. The hospital has also implemented a checklist for human resources to use to ensure that key action items are completed in the recruitment process. They also developed sets of interview questions that better evaluate applicants' key competencies and skill sets.

Case Study

The provider performance data for the Obstetric Service at Community Hospital are provided in figure 14.3. Figure 14.4 gives an example of a physician profile for an individual physician, Dr. Jones. The physician index summary for Dr. Doe, an OB/GYN physician on the medical staff, is provided in figure 14.5. (Electronic versions of figures 14.5 and 14.6 are located in the student resources.)

Using the physician index summary, complete the utilization and outcome sections of the profile in figure 14.6. Data for Dr. Doe are provided for the performance review, data quality, risk and safety management, and meeting attendance sections of the profile. After completing the physician profile for Dr. Doe, answer the following questions:

Figure 14.3. Provider profile for OB/GYN group

COMMUNITY HOSPITAL				
PROVIDER PERFORMANCE REVIEW SUMMARY FOR REAPPOINTMENT				
PROVIDER	OB/GYN GROUP		**Profile Time Frame:**	
SERVICE	OB/GYN		From:	1/1/yyyy
CATEGORY	Active		To:	12/31/yyyy
UTILIZATION:				
Discharges	1,400	Procedures	598	
Patient Days	5,143	Pts with prev C-Sections	346	
Deliveries	1,187	VBACs	89	
C-Sections	137	Blood Given	25	
OUTCOMES:				
Category	#	%	Comments:	
C-Section Rate	137	11.5%		
VBAC Rate	89	25.7%		
Hospital-acquired Inf Rate	21	1.5%		
Surgical Wound Inf Rate	5	0.84%		
Mortality Rate	1	0.07%		
PERFORMANCE REVIEW:				
Category	# Reviewed	# Appropriate/%	Comments:	
Surgical/Inv/Noninvasive Procedures	60	58/96.7%		
Medication Use	140	139/99.3%		
Blood Use	25	25/100%		
Utilization Management	140	135/95.7%		
Other Peer Review	140	130/92.8%	Clinical Pert.	
DATA QUALITY:				
Data Quality Monitoring			Comments:	
Delinquency (>21 days)	15	7.70%		
Suspensions	5	2.60%		
RISK/SAFETY MANAGEMENT:				
Incidents reported by other professionals or Administration	2	2/100%	Comments:	
Litigation	1	0.07%		
MEETING ATTENDANCE:				
Medical Staff Meetings	26	93%	Comments:	
Committee Meetings	40	85%		

Figure 14.4A. Physician profile for Dr. Jones

COMMUNITY HOSPITAL				
PROVIDER PERFORMANCE REVIEW SUMMARY FOR REAPPOINTMENT				
PROVIDER	*Bob Jones, M.D.*		**Profile Time Frame:**	
SERVICE	*OB/GYN*		From:	1/1/yyyy
CATEGORY	*Active*		To:	12/31/yyyy
UTILIZATION:				
Discharges	175	Procedures	53	
Patient Days	540	Pts with prev C-Sections	75	
Deliveries	145	VBACs	15	
C-Sections	22	Blood Given	2	
OUTCOMES:				
Category	#	%		Comments:
C-Section Rate	22	15.2%		
VBAC Rate	15	20.0%		
Hospital-acquired inf Rate	3	1.71%		
Surgical Wound Inf Rate	2	3.8%		
Mortality Rate	1	0.57%		
PERFORMANCE REVIEW:				
Category	# Reviewed	# Appropriate/%		Comments:
Surgical/Inv/Noninvasive Procedures	6	5/83.3%		
Medication Use	10	8/80%		
Blood Use	2	2/100%		
Utilization Management	18	18/100%		
Other Peer Review	N/A			
DATA QUALITY:				
Data Quality Monitoring				Comments:
Delinquency (>21 days)	3	12.5%		
Suspensions	5	2.60%		
RISK/SAFETY MANAGEMENT:				
Incidents reported by other professionals or Administration	2	2/100%		Comments:
Litigation	1	4.20%		
MEETING ATTENDANCE:				
Medical Staff Meetings	4	100%		Comments:
Committee Meetings	10	80%		

Figure 14.4B. Physician profile for Dr. Jones (*Continued*)

For Completion by Service Chair or Credentials Committee Chair			
CATEGORY	YES	NO	Comments:
Has the applicant been considered for or subject to disciplinary action since last reappointment?		√	
Have the applicant's privileges or staff appointment been suspended, revoked, or diminished in any way, either voluntary or involuntary, since last reappointment?	√		
Are there any currently pending challenges to any licensure or registration or the voluntary relinquishment of such?		√	
Are there any physical or behavioral conditions or limitations?		√	
Has the applicant exhibited satisfactory professional performance?	√		

APPROVALS:		APPROVED?		
REVIEWER	SIGNATURE	YES	NO	DATE
Service Chair				
Credentials Chair				

Figure 14.5A. Provider index summary for Dr. Doe

Patient Age	LOS	Discharge Status	Final Diagnosis	Diagnosis Text	Final Procedure	Procedure Text
52	3	Home	N920	Excessive and frequent menstruation with regular cycle	0UT90ZZ	Resection of uterus, open approach
			I428	Other cardiomyopathies	0UTC0ZZ	Resection of cervix, open approach
			I10	Essential (primary) hypertension	0UT20ZZ	Resection of bilateral ovaries, open approach
			E119	Type 2 diabetes mellitus without complication	0UT70ZZ	Resection of bilateral fallopian tubes, open approach
			D251	Intramural leiomyoma of the uterus		
29	4	Home	O334XX0	Maternal care for disproportion of mixed maternal and fetal origin, not applicable or unspecified	10D00Z1	Extraction of products of conception, low cervical, open approach
			O621	Secondary uterine inertia	0U7C7ZZ	Dilation of cervix, via natural or artificial opening
			O411030	Infection of amniotic sac and membranes, unspecified, third trimester, not applicable or unspecified	10907ZC	Drainage of amniotic fluid, therapeutic from products of conception, via natural or artificial opening
			O481	Prolonged pregnancy		
			Z370	Single live birth		
27	2	Home	O34211	Maternal care for low transverse scar from previous cesarean delivery	0W8NXZZ	Division of female perineum, external approach
			Z370	Single live birth	10E0XZZ	Delivery of products of conception, external approach
					10907ZC	Drainage of amniotic fluid, therapeutic from products of conception, via natural or artificial opening
79	4	Home	N993	Prolapse of vaginal vault after hysterectomy	0USG0ZZ	Reposition vagina, open approach
			N9989	Other postprocedural complications and disorders of the genitourinary system	0DNG0ZZ	Release left large intestine, open approach
			N390	Urinary tract infection, site not specified		
			J9589	Other postprocedural complications and disorders of respiratory system, not elsewhere classified		
			J9811	Atelectasis		
			N3941	Urge incontinence		
			Y838	Other surgical procedures as the cause of abnormal reaction of the patient, or of later complication, without mention of misadventure at the time of the procedure		
			I10	Essential (primary) hypertension		
			N994	Postprocedural pelvic peritoneal adhesions		
25	4	Home	O321XX0	Maternal care for breech presentation, not applicable or unspecified	10D00Z1	Extraction of products of conception, low, open approach

Figure 14.5B. Provider index summary for Dr. Doe (*Continued*)

Patient Age	LOS	Discharge Status	Final Diagnosis	Diagnosis Text	Final Procedure	Procedure Text
			O23593	Infection of other part of genital tract in pregnancy, third trimester		
			N739	Female pelvic inflammatory disease, unspecified		
			O691XX0	Labor and delivery complicated by cord around neck, with compression, not applicable or unspecified		
			Z370	Single live birth		
39	1	Home	O6981X0	Labor and delivery complicated by cord around neck, without compression, not applicable or unspecified	10E0XZZ	Delivery of products of conception, external approach
			O10013	Pre-existing essential hypertension complicating pregnancy, third trimester		
			Z370	Single live birth		
			I10	Essential (primary) hypertension		
34	2	Home	O99810	Abnormal glucose complicating pregnancy	10E0XZZ	Delivery of products of conception, external approach
			Z370	Single live birth	0HQ9XZZ	Repair perineum skin, external approach
			O700	First-degree perineal laceration during delivery	10907ZC	Drainage of amniotic fluid, therapeutic from products of conception, via natural or artificial opening
20	1	Home	O80	Encounter for full-term uncomplicated delivery	10E0XZZ	Delivery of products of conception, external approach
			Z370	Single live birth	0W8NXZZ	Division of female perineum, external approach
36	3	Home	O0889	Other complications following an ectopic and molar pregnancy	0UT90ZZ	Resection of uterus, open approach
			N9489	Other specified conditions associated with female genital organs and menstrual cycle	0UTC0ZZ	Resection of cervix, open approach
			F329	Major depressive disorder, single episode, unspecified		
			N920	Excessive and frequent menstruation with regular cycle		
			D252	Subserosal leiomyoma of uterus		
			D251	Intramural leiomyoma of the uterus		
			R112	Nausea with vomiting, unspecified		
48	3	Home	D251	Intramural leiomyoma of the uterus	0UT90ZZ	Resection of uterus, open approach
					0UTC0ZZ	Resection of cervix, open approach
			K8018	Calculus of gallbladder with other cholecystitis without obstruction	0UT20ZZ	Resection of bilateral ovaries, open approach
					0UT70ZZ	Resection of bilateral fallopian tubes, open approach

Figure 14.5C. Provider index summary for Dr. Doe (*Continued*)

Patient Age	LOS	Discharge Status	Final Diagnosis	Diagnosis Text	Final Procedure	Procedure Text
			N8001	Superficial endometriosis of the uterus	0TSD0ZZ	Reposition urethra, open approach
			D259	Leiomyoma of uterus, unspecified	0UQG0ZZ	Repair vagina, open approach
			N393	Stress incontinence (female)(male)	0FT44ZZ	Resection of gallbladder, percutaneous endoscopic approach
			N816	Rectocele		
42	2	Home	O34211	Maternal care for low transverse scar from previous cesarean delivery;antenatal care for scar from previous cesarean delivery	3E033VJ	Introduction of other hormone into peripheral vein, percutaneous approach
			Z370	Single live birth	10903ZC	Drainage of amniotic fluid, therapeutic from products of conception, percutaneous approach
			O6981X0	Labor and delivery complicated by cord around neck, without compression, not applicable or unspecified	10E0XZZ	Delivery of products of conception, external approach
			O99810	Abnormal glucose complicating pregnancy		
			O329XX0	Maternal care for malpresentation of fetus, unspecified, not applicable or unspecified		
22	2	Home	O7020	Third-degree perineal laceration during delivery	0KQM0ZZ	Repair perineum muscle, open approach
			O368930	Maternal care for other specified fetal problems, third trimester, not applicable or unspecified	0DQR0ZZ	Repair anal sphincter, open approach
			Z370	Single live birth	10E0XZZ	Delivery of products of conception, external approach
37	14	Home	O76	Abnormality in fetal heart rate and rhythm complicating labor and delivery	10D00Z1	Extraction of products of conception, low cervical, open approach
			O2233	Deep phlebothrombosis in pregnancy, third trimester	0UL73ZZ	Occlusion of bilateral fallopian tubes, percutaneous approach
			O99013	Anemia complicating pregnancy, third trimester		
			O42113	Preterm premature rupture of membranes, onset of labor more than 24 hours following rupture, third trimester		
			O321XX0	Maternal care for breech presentation, not applicable or unspecified		
			O6014X0	Preterm labor third trimester with preterm delivery third trimester, not applicable or unspecified		
			O09523	Supervision of elderly multigravida, third trimester		
			O26893	Other specified pregnancy related conditions, third trimester		

Steps to Success: Developing Staff and Human Resources **279**

Figure 14.5D. Provider index summary for Dr. Doe (*Continued*)

Patient Age	LOS	Discharge Status	Final Diagnosis	Diagnosis Text	Final Procedure	Procedure Text
			D7589	Other specified diseases of blood and blood-forming organs		
			R21	Rash and other nonspecific skin eruption		
			Z370	Single live birth		
			Z302	Encounter for sterilization		
28	1	Home	O6981X0	Labor and delivery complicated by cord around neck, without compression, not applicable or unspecified	0W8NXZZ	Division of female perineum, external approach
			O752	Pyrexia during labor, not elsewhere classified	3E033VJ	Introduction of other hormone into peripheral vein, percutaneous approach
			Z370	Single live birth	10903ZC	Drainage of amniotic fluid, therapeutic from products of conception, percutaneous approach
22	2	Home	O6981X0	Labor and delivery complicated by cord around neck, without compression, not applicable or unspecified	10907ZC	Drainage of amniotic fluid, therapeutic from products of conception, via natural or artificial opening
			O752	Pyrexia during labor, not elsewhere classified	10E0XZZ	Delivery of products of conception, external approach
			O701	Second-degree perineal laceration during delivery	0JQB0ZZ	Repair perineum subcutaneous tissue and fascia, open approach
			Z370	Single live birth		
42	2	Home	O09523	Supervision of elderly multigravida, third trimester	0U7C7ZZ	Dilation of cervix, via natural or artificial opening
			Z370	Single live birth	10E0XZZ	Delivery of products of conception, external approach
			O701	Second-degree perineal laceration during delivery	0JQB0ZZ	Repair perineum subcutaneous tissue and fascia, open approach
67	3	Home	N950	Postmenopausal bleeding	0UT90ZZ	Resection of uterus, open approach
			M316	Other giant cell arteritis	0UTC0ZZ	Resection of cervix, open approach
			E860	Dehydration	0UT20ZZ	Resection of bilateral ovaries, open approach
			D251	Intramural leiomyoma of the uterus	0UT70ZZ	Resection of bilateral fallopian tubes, open approach
			N840	Polyp of corpus uteri	0DNE0ZZ	Release large intestine, ope approach
			N994	Postprocedural pelvic peritoneal adhesions		
			Z86718	Personal history of venous thrombosis and embolism		
			J45909	Unspecified asthma, uncomplicated		
51	3	Home	N924	Excessive bleeding in the premenopausal period	0UT90ZZ	Resection of uterus, open approach
			D500	Iron deficiency anemia secondary to blood loss (chronic)	0UTC0ZZ	Resection of cervix, open approach
			D251	Intramural leiomyoma of the uterus	0UT20ZZ	Resection of bilateral ovaries, open approach

Figure 14.5E. Provider index summary for Dr. Doe (*Continued*)

Patient Age	LOS	Discharge Status	Final Diagnosis	Diagnosis Text	Final Procedure	Procedure Text
			N838	Other noninflammatory disorders of ovary, fallopian tube and broad ligament	0UT70ZZ	Resection of bilateral fallopian tubes, open approach
			N8301	Follicular cyst of ovary		
			N9489	Other specified conditions associated with female genital organs and menstrual cycle		
33	1	Home	O328XX0	Maternal care for other malpresentation of fetus, not applicable or unspecified	10907ZC	Drainage of amniotic fluid, therapeutic from products of conception, via natural or artificial opening
			Z370	Single live birth	10E0XZZ	Delivery of products of conception, external approach
			O730	Retained placenta without hemorrhage	0W8NXZZ	Division of female perineum, external approach
			O481	Prolonged pregnancy	10D17Z9	Manual extraction of products of conception, retained, via natural or artificial opening
22	2	Home	O6981X0	Labor and delivery complicated by cord around neck, without compression, not applicable or unspecified	10E0XZZ	Delivery of products of conception, external approach
			Z370	Single live birth	10907ZC	Drainage of amniotic fluid, therapeutic from products of conception, via natural or artificial opening
					0W8NXZZ	Division of female perineum, external approach
25	2	Home	O328XX0	Maternal care for other malpresentation of fetus, not applicable or unspecified	0W8NXZZ	Division of female perineum, external approach
			Z370	Single live birth	10E0XZZ	Delivery of products of conception, external approach
					3E033VJ	Introduction of other hormone into peripheral vein, percutaneous approach
					10907ZC	Drainage of amniotic fluid, therapeutic from products of conception, via natural or artificial opening
31	2	Home	O701	Second-degree perineal laceration during delivery	10E0XZZ	Delivery of products of conception, external approach
			Z370	Single live birth	0JQB0ZZ	Repair perineum subcutaneous tissue and fascia, open approach
					10903ZC	Drainage of amniotic fluid, therapeutic from products of conception, percutaneous approach
40	3	Home	N80203	Endometriosis of bilateral fallopian tubes, unspecified depth	0UT90ZZ	Resection of uterus, open approach
			D259	Leiomyoma of uterus, unspecified	0UTC0ZZ	Resection of cervix, open approach
			E119	Type 2 diabetes mellitus without complication	0UT20ZZ	Resection of bilateral ovaries, open approach

Figure 14.5F. Provider index summary for Dr. Doe (Continued)

Patient Age	LOS	Discharge Status	Final Diagnosis	Diagnosis Text	Final Procedure	Procedure Text
32	3	Home	N736	Female pelvic peritoneal adhesions (postinfective)	0UT70ZZ	Resection of bilateral fallopian tubes, open approach
			O321XX0	Maternal care for breech presentation, not applicable or unspecified	10D00Z1	Extraction of products of conception, low, open approach
			O745	Spinal and epidural anesthesia-induced headache during labor and delivery	3E0S3GC	Introduction of other therapeutic substance into epidural space, percutaneous approach
			O99283	Endocrine, nutritional and metabolic diseases complicating pregnancy, third trimester		
			E039	Hypothyroidism, unspecified		
			Z370	Single live birth		
81	4	Home	N993	Prolapse of vaginal vault after hysterectomy	0UQG0ZZ	Repair vagina, open approach
			J9811	Atelectasis	0JQC0ZZ	Repair pelvic region subcutaneous tissue and fascia, open approach
			N393	Stress incontinence (female)(male)	0TSD0ZZ	Reposition urethra, open approach
			I10	Essential (primary) hypertension		
			E039	Hypothyroidism, unspecified		
			M129	Arthropathy, unspecified		
			R112	Nausea with vomiting, unspecified		
			K5900	Constipation, unspecified		
28	2	Home	O322XX0	Maternal care for transverse and oblique lie, not applicable or unspecified	10907ZC	Drainage of amniotic fluid, therapeutic from products of conception, via natural or artificial opening
			O722	Delayed and secondary postpartum hemorrhage	10E0XZZ	Delivery of products of conception, external approach
			O7182	Other specified trauma to perineum and vulva	0UQMXZZ	Repair vulva, external approach
			Z370	Single live birth	0W8NXZZ	Division of female perineum, external approach
					10D07Z6	Extraction of products of conception, vacuum, via natural or artificial opening
54	3	Home	C541	Malignant neoplasm of endometrium	0UT90ZZ	Resection of uterus, open approach
			I340	Nonrheumatic mitral (valve) insufficiency	0UTC0ZZ	Resection of cervix, open approach
			N812	Incomplete uterovaginal prolapse	0UT20ZZ	Resection of bilateral ovaries, open approach
			N393	Stress incontinence (female)(male)	0UT70ZZ	Resection of bilateral fallopian tubes, open approach
			N950	Postmenopausal bleeding	0UQG0ZZ	Repair vagina, open approach
			N8011	Superficial endometriosis of the ovary	0TSD0ZZ	Reposition urethra, open approach

Figure 14.5G. Provider index summary for Dr. Doe (Continued)

Patient Age	LOS	Discharge Status	Final Diagnosis	Diagnosis Text	Final Procedure	Procedure Text
			N8001	Superficial endometriosis of the uterus	0TSD0ZZ	Reposition urethra, open approach
			E669	Obesity, unspecified		
			T502X5S	Adverse effect of carbonic-anhydrase inhibitors, benzothiadiazides and other diuretics, sequela		
19	1	Home	O6014X0	Preterm labor third trimester with preterm delivery third trimester, not applicable or unspecified	10907ZC	Drainage of amniotic fluid, therapeutic from products of conception, via natural or artificial opening
			Z370	Single live birth	10E0XZZ	Delivery of products of conception, external approach
			O411030	Infection of amniotic sac and membranes, unspecified, third trimester, not applicable or unspecified	0W8NXZZ	Division of female perineum, external approach
37	3	Home	O321XX0	Maternal care for breech presentation, not applicable or unspecified	10D00Z1	Extraction of products of conception, low, open approach
			Z370	Single live birth		
24	2	Home	O702	Third-degree perineal laceration during delivery	0KQM0ZZ	Repair perineum muscle, open approach
			O6981X0	Labor and delivery complicated by cord around neck, without compression, not applicable or unspecified	0DQR0ZZ	Repair anal sphincter, open approach
			Z370	Single live birth		
21	2	Home	O80	Encounter for full-term uncomplicated delivery	0W8NXZZ	Division of female perineum, external approach
			Z370	Single live birth	10E0XZZ	Delivery of products of conception, external approach
					10907ZC	Drainage of amniotic fluid, therapeutic from products of conception, via natural or artificial opening
					3E033VJ	Introduction of other hormone into peripheral vein, percutaneous approach
39	2	Home	O0943	Supervision of pregnancy with grand multiparity, third trimester	10E0XZZ	Delivery of products of conception, external approach
			O09523	Supervision of elderly multigravida, third trimester		
			O700	First-degree perineal laceration during delivery		
			Z370	Single live birth		
			Z302	Encounter for sterilization		
33	1	Home	O80	Encounter for full-term uncomplicated delivery	0W8NXZZ	Division of female perineum, external approach
			Z370	Single live birth	10E0XZZ	Delivery of products of conception, external approach
					10907ZC	Drainage of amniotic fluid, therapeutic from products of conception, via natural or artificial opening

Figure 14.5H. Provider index summary for Dr. Doe (*Continued*)

Patient Age	LOS	Discharge Status	Final Diagnosis	Diagnosis Text	Final Procedure	Procedure Text
22	1	Home	O6981X0	Labor and delivery complicated by cord around neck, without compression, not applicable or unspecified	10E0XZZ	Delivery of products of conception, external approach
			Z370	Single live birth	10907ZC	Drainage of amniotic fluid, therapeutic from products of conception, via natural or artificial opening
			O99824	Streptococcus B carrier state complicating childbirth	0W8NXZZ	Division of female perineum, external approach
20	1	Home	O42913	Preterm premature rupture of membranes, unspecified as to length of time between rupture and onset of labor, third trimester	0W8NXZZ	Division of female perineum, external approach
			O76	Abnormality in fetal heart rate and rhythm complicating labor and delivery	10E0XZZ	Delivery of products of conception, external approach
			O6014X0	Preterm labor third trimester with preterm delivery third trimester, not applicable or unspecified		
			O691XX0	Labor and delivery complicated by cord around neck, with compression, not applicable or unspecified		
			O99824	Streptococcus B carrier state complicating childbirth		
			Z370	Single live birth		
34	3	Home	O321XX0	Maternal care for breech presentation, not applicable or unspecified	10D00Z1	Extraction of products of conception, low cervical, open approach
			O4292	Full-term premature rupture of membranes, unspecified as to length of time between rupture and onset of labor	0UL73ZZ	Occlusion of bilateral fallopian tubes, percutaneous approach
			O99333	Smoking (tobacco) complicating pregnancy, third trimester		
			Z370	Single live birth		
			Z302	Encounter for sterilization		
22	1	Home	O328XX0	Maternal care for other malpresentation of fetus, not applicable or unspecified	10E0XZZ	Delivery of products of conception, external approach
			O76	Abnormality in fetal heart rate and rhythm complicating labor and delivery	0HQ9XZZ	Repair perineum skin, external approach
			O6981X0	Labor and delivery complicated by cord around the neck without compression, not applicable or unspecified	10907ZC	Drainage of amniotic fluid, therapeutic from products of conception, via natural or artificial opening
			O700	First-degree perineal laceration during delivery	0UJD7ZZ	Inspection of uterus and cervix, via natural or artificial opening
			Z370	Single live birth		

Figure 14.5I. Provider index summary for Dr. Doe (Continued)

Patient Age	LOS	Discharge Status	Final Diagnosis	Diagnosis Text	Final Procedure	Procedure Text
41	2	Home	O9981O	Abnormal glucose complicating pregnancy	10907ZC	Drainage of amniotic fluid, therapeutic from products of conception, via natural or artificial opening
			Z370	Single live birth	10E0XZZ	Delivery of products of conception, external approach
			O6014X0	Preterm labor third trimester with preterm delivery third trimester, not applicable or unspecified	0W8NXZZ	Division of female perineum, external approach
			O403XX0	Polyhydramnios, third trimester, not applicable or unspecified	10D07Z3	Extraction of products of conception, low forceps, via natural or artificial opening
			O09513	Supervision of elderly primigravida, third trimester		
			O7589	Other specified complications of labor and delivery		
			R1110	Vomiting, unspecified		
			O621	Secondary uterine inertia		
			O4393	Unspecified placental disorder, third trimester		
59	3	Home	N812	Incomplete uterovaginal prolapse	0UT97ZZ	Resection of uterus, via natural or articial opening
			D252	Subserosal leiomyoma of uterus	0UQG0ZZ	Repair vagina, open approach
			N840	Polyp of corpus uteri	0JQC0ZZ	Repair pelvic region subcutaneous tissue and fascia, open approach
			E049	Nontoxic goiter, unspecified	0T9B00Z	Drainage of bladder with drainage device, open approach
33	1	Home	O640XX0	Obstructed labor due to incomplete rotation of fetal head, not applicable or unspecified	10907ZC	Drainage of amniotic fluid, therapeutic from products of conception, via natural or artificial opening
			O700	First-degree perineal laceration during delivery	0HQ9XZZ	Repair perineum skin, external approach
			Z370	Single live birth	10E0XZZ	Delivery of products of conception, external approach
30	2	Home	O328XX0	Maternal care for other malpresentation of fetus, not applicable or unspecified	0W8NXZZ	Division of female perineum, external approach
					10D07Z3	Extraction of products of conception, low forceps via natural or artificial opening
			O752	Pyrexia during labor, not elsewhere classified	10E0XZZ	Delivery of products of conception, external approach
			O34211	Maternal care for low transverse scar from previous cesarean delivery	0UJD7ZZ	Inspection of uterus and cervix, via natural or artificial opening
			Z370	Single live birth		
67	3	Home	N8110	Cystocele unspecified	0UQG0ZZ	Repair vagina, open approach
			N816	Rectocele	0JQC0ZZ	Repair pelvic region subcutaneous tissue and fascia, open approach

Figure 14.5J. Provider index summary for Dr. Doe (*Continued*)

Patient Age	LOS	Discharge Status	Final Diagnosis	Diagnosis Text	Final Procedure	Procedure Text
			N393	Stress incontinence (female) (male)	0TSD0ZZ	Reposition urethra, open approach
			N815	Vaginal enterocele		
81	3	Home	N814	Uterovaginal prolapse, unspecified	0UT90ZZ	Resection of uterus, open approach
			N841	Polyp of cervix uteri	0UTC0ZZ	Resection of cervix, open approach
			N840	Polyp of corpus uteri	0UT20ZZ	Resection of bilateral ovaries, open approach
			D251	Intramural leiomyoma of the uterus	0UT70ZZ	Resection of bilateral fallopian tubes, open approach
			E119	Type 2 diabetes mellitus without complication	0UQG0ZZ	Repair vagina, open approach
			I10	Essential (primary) hypertension		
			E785	Hyperlipidemia, unspecified		
26	2	Home	O80	Encounter for full-term uncomplicated delivery	10E0XZZ	Delivery of products of conception, external approach
			Z370	Single live birth	3E033VJ	Introduction of other hormone into peripheral vein, percutaneous approach
					0W8NXZZ	Division of female perineum, external approach
18	1	Home	O701	Second-degree perineal laceration during delivery	0JQB0ZZ	Repair perineum subcutaneous tissue and fascia, open approach
			O99333	Smoking (tobacco) complicating pregnancy, third trimester	10E0XZZ	Delivery of products of conception, external approach
			Z370	Single live birth		
72	3	Home	C541	Malignant neoplasm of endometrium	0UT90ZZ	Resection of uterus, open approach
			E039	Hypothyroidism, unspecified	0UTC0ZZ	Resection of cervix, open approach
			N83202	Unspecified ovarian cyst, left side	0UT20ZZ	Resection of bilateral ovaries, open approach
			R823	Hemoglobinuria	0UT70ZZ	Resection of bilateral fallopian tubes, open approach
					07BC0ZZ	Excision of pelvis lymphatic, open approach
38	3	Home	N993	Prolapse of vaginal vault after hysterectomy	0USG0ZZ	Reposition vagina, open approach
50	3	Home	N8001	Superficial endometriosis of the uterus	0UT90ZZ	Resection of uterus, open approach
			D500	Iron deficiency anemia secondary to blood loss (chronic)	0UTC0ZZ	Resection of cervix, open approach
			N80203	Endometriosis of bilateral fallopian tubes, unspecified depth	0UT20ZZ	Resection of bilateral ovaries, open approach
			N8011	Superficial endometriosis of the ovary	0UT70ZZ	Resection of bilateral fallopian tubes, open approach
			N393	Stress incontinence (female) (male)	0TSD0ZZ	Reposition urethra, open approach
			N920	Excessive and frequent menstruation with regular cycle		
			D251	Intramural leiomyoma of the uterus		
			N72	Inflammatory disease of cervix uteri		
			N8030	Endometriosis of pelvic peritoneum, unspecified		

Figure 14.5K. Provider index summary for Dr. Doe (*Continued*)

Patient Age	LOS	Discharge Status	Final Diagnosis	Diagnosis Text	Final Procedure	Procedure Text
			R102	Pelvic and perineal pain		
			E119	Type 2 diabetes mellitus without complication		
			K449	Diaphragmatic hernia without obstruction of gangrene		
28	1	Home	O4103X0	Oligohydramnios, third trimester, not applicable or unspecified	0W8NXZZ	Division of female perineum, external approach
			O752	Pyrexia during labor, not elsewhere classified	10D07Z3	Extraction of products of conception, low forceps, via natural or artificial opening
			O328XX0	Maternal care for other malpresentation of fetus, not applicable or unspecified	10E0XZZ	Delivery of products of conception, external approach
			O665	Attempted application of vacuum extractor and forceps	0HQ9XZZ	Repair perineum subcutaneous tissue and fascia, open approach
			O701	Second-degree perineal laceration during delivery	10D17Z9	Manual Extraction of Products of Conception, Retained, Via Natural or Artificial Opening
			O6981X0	Labor and delivery complicated by cord around neck, without compression, not applicable or unspecified	3E033VJ	Introduction of other hormone into peripheral vein, percutaneous approach
			Z370	Single live birth		
24	2	Home	O365930	Maternal care for other known or suspected poor fetal growth, third trimester, not applicable or unspecified	3E033VJ	Introduction of other hormone into peripheral vein, percutaneous approach
			O752	Pyrexia during labor, not elsewhere classified	10903ZC	Drainage of amniotic fluid, therapeutic from products of conception, percutaneous approach
			Z302	Encounter for sterilization	10E0XZZ	Delivery of products of conception, external approach
			O328XX0	Maternal care for other malpresentation of fetus, not applicable or unspecified	0W8NXZZ	Division of female perineum, external approach
			Z23	Encounter for immunization	0UJD7ZZ	Inspection of uterus and cervix, via natural or artificial opening
39	2	Home	O6981X0	Labor and delivery complicated by cord around neck, without compression, not applicable or unspecified	0W8NXZZ	Division of female perineum, external approach
			Z370	Single live birth	3E033VJ	Introduction of other hormone into peripheral vein, percutaneous approach
					10E0XZZ	Delivery of products of conception, external approach
					10903ZC	Drainage of amniotic fluid, therapeutic from products of conception, percutaneous approach
30	1	Home	O6981X0	Labor and delivery complicated by cord around neck, without compression, not applicable or unspecified	3E033VJ	Introduction of other hormone into peripheral vein, percutaneous approach
			Z370	Single live birth	10E0XZZ	Delivery of products of conception, external approach
					0W8NXZZ	Division of female perineum, external approach

Figure 14.6A. Incomplete provider profile for case study

COMMUNITY HOSPITAL OF THE WEST			
PROVIDER PERFORMANCE REVIEW SUMMARY FOR REAPPOINTMENT			
PROVIDER	Dr. Doe	**Profile Time Frame:**	
SERVICE	OB/Gyn	From:	
CATEGORY	Active	To:	
UTILIZATION:			
Discharges		Procedures	
Patient Days		Pts with prev C-Sections	
Deliveries		VBACs	
C-Sections		Blood Given	
OUTCOMES:			
Category	#	%	Comments:
C-Section Rate			
VBAC Rate			
Hospital-acquired inf Rate	0	N/A	
Surgical Wound Inf Rate	0	0.0%	
Mortality Rate	0	0.0%	
PERFORMANCE REVIEW:			
Category	**# Reviewed**	**# Appropriate/%**	Comments:
Surgical/Inv/Noninvasive	3	3/100%	
Medication Use	5	4/80.0%	
Blood Use	0	N/A	
Utilization Management	10	9/90.0%	
Other Peer Review	N/A		
DATA QUALITY:			
Data Quality Monitoring			Comments:
Delinquency (>21 days)	0	N/A	
Suspensions	0	N/A	
RISK/SAFETY MANAGEMENT:			
Incidents reported by other professionals or Administration	0	N/A	Comments:
Litigation	0	N/A	
MEETING ATTENDANCE:			
Medical Staff Meetings	4	100%	Comments:
Committee Meetings	10	80%	

Figure 14.6B. Incomplete provider profile for case study (*Continued*)

For Completion by Service Chair or Credentials Committee Chair			
CATEGORY	YES	NO	Comments:
Has the applicant been considered for or subject to disciplinary action since last reappointment?		√	
Have the applicant's privileges or staff appointment been suspended, revoked, or diminished in any way, either voluntary or involuntary, since last reappointment?		√	
Are there any currently pending challenges to any licensure or registration or the voluntary relinquishment of such?		√	
Are there any physical or behavioral conditions or limitations?		√	
Has the applicant exhibited satisfactory professional performance?	√		

APPROVALS:		APPROVED?		
REVIEWER	SIGNATURE	YES	NO	DATE
Service Chair				
Credentials Chair				

Case Study Questions

Using the provider profile created for Dr. Doe:

1. How did Dr. Doe perform compared to Dr. Jones??
2. How did Dr. Doe perform compared to the rest of the Obstetric service?
3. Do you have any concerns regarding Dr. Doe's performance as documented in the provider profile?

Review Questions

1. Providing additional benefits to employees such as tuition and professional education reimbursement, a competitive salary and benefits package, and incentives such as profit sharing can assist a healthcare organization in increasing their:
   a. Employee credentialing process
   b. Employee retention
   c. Employee performance appraisal process
   d. Employee performance profile.

2. This status is conferred by a state regulatory agency giving an individual permission to practice their trade or profession.
   a. Credential
   b. Certificate
   c. License
   d. Degree

3. The credentialing process of providers within a healthcare organization must be defined in:
   a. Hospital policies and procedures
   b. Medical staff bylaws
   c. Accreditation regulations
   d. Hospital licensure rules

4. This database maintains reports on medical malpractice settlements, clinical privilege actions, and professional society membership actions against licensed healthcare providers.
   a. National Practitioners Data Bank
   b. National Physician Database
   c. Healthcare Integrity and Protection Data Bank
   d. Healthcare Security of Physicians Database

5. Explain why the steps in the initial credentialing process for medical staff help ensure that healthcare organizations are hiring and retaining competent care providers.

Resources

Americans with Disabilities Act of 1990. Public Law 101-336.

Becker, K. and A. Bish. 2021. A framework for understanding the role of unlearning in onboarding. *Human Resource Management Review* 31(1), https://doi.org/10.1016/j.hrmr.2019.100730.

Equal Employment Opportunity Act of 1972. Public Law 92-261.

Family and Medical Leave Act of 1993. Public Law 103-3.

Gomez-Mejia, L. R., D. B. Balkin, R. L. Cardy, and K. P. Carson. 2020. *Managing Human Resources*, 9th ed. Upper Saddle River, NJ: Pearson.

Joint Commission. 2024. *2024 Hospital Accreditation Standards*. Oakbrook Terrace, IL: Joint Commission Resources.

Occupational Safety and Health Act of 1970. 29 CFR Parts 1900 to 2400.

Simpson, C. J. and B. J. Fried. 2021. *Human Resources in Healthcare: Managing for Success*, 5th ed. Chicago: Health Administration Press.

PART III
Management of Performance Improvement Programs

Organizing and Evaluating Performance Improvement

15

Learning Objectives

- Identify the role of an organization's leaders in performance improvement activities
- Examine the committee and reporting structures that integrate performance improvement within the organization
- Describe how healthcare organizations train and orient their governance, leaders, and employed staff in performance improvement strategies and methods
- Delineate the best ways to organize performance improvement data for effective review by a board of directors
- List the areas that should be addressed in the development of a healthcare organization's performance improvement plan
- Explain various ways performance improvement activities are implemented and findings are communicated throughout the organization
- Apply evaluation processes to performance improvement programs
- Determine what organizations should do with information gathered from the performance improvement program evaluation

Key Terms

Dashboard
Decision matrix
Peer review

Strategic plan
SWOT analysis

Performance improvement (PI) does not happen effortlessly. The term *continuous* is often attached to improvement efforts (as in *continuous quality improvement*) for a reason: It serves to remind healthcare workers that PI activities require organizational and individual commitment and need to be incorporated into daily operations.

Given that PI requires commitment and continuity, which types of management environments make this happen? Many employees come from a traditional management environment, in which managers direct subordinates in exactly what to do and when to do it. However, the guiding principle of quality improvement in the Deming, Juran, Crosby, and Donabedian models is that all members of an organization must be empowered by its leadership to contribute to PI activities if the program is to be successful.

Today, those working in the healthcare industry commonly recognize that unless leaders are committed to maintaining PI activities in the organization and motivating employees to do the same, PI that reaps genuine benefits for the organization cannot take place. Leadership endorsement of PI is a crucial and integral contribution to an organization's continuous development.

Leading PI Activities

Healthcare organizations must put formal structures in place for meaningful PI to occur. The leaders of a healthcare organization set expectations, develop plans, and hire employees to implement procedures that assess and improve the quality of important functions. Leaders include the members of the governing body (most often termed board of "directors" or "trustees" but sometimes configured from other entities such as "public commissioners"), the chief executive officer (CEO), the director of nursing, the medical director, and other senior directors or managers, as well as the leaders of the medical staff.

The board of directors has ultimate responsibility for maintaining the quality and safety of patient care provided by the organization. Because the board is responsible for patient care, quality, and safety, it must ensure the competence and integrity of the providers and other staff. There is a link between the governing board's focus and commitment to quality and patient safety activities and the overall organization's quality performance (Leonhardt 2023). The "board should spend more than 25 percent of their time in activities related to quality and safety, overseeing the effective execution of a plan to achieve their aims to reduce harm, just as they oversee finance" (Conway 2008, 218). The board establishes policies and directs appropriate actions to monitor and assess all services and to detect variations from acceptable standards of care or service. The board operates under a set of bylaws that provides guidance and establishes the framework for supporting quality of patient care, treatment, and services.

As in any other corporation, the board designates an executive to be its agent or managing partner. The CEO, sometimes known as the administrator or executive director, is responsible for implementing board directives and for acting as board representative in managing the operations of the organization. Although proper functioning of the organization remains the responsibility of the board, the CEO is a partial or full voting member of the board and is responsible for ensuring that the board is knowledgeable about its governing responsibilities. These responsibilities include understanding the structure and composition of the governing board; understanding the functioning, participation, and involvement in the oversight and operation of the organization; being aware of all federal and state laws, regulations, and standards pertinent to board member roles; and understanding the organization's approach to PI.

There are three main components of a healthcare organization: governance (board of directors and organized medical staff), management (leaders), and the employed staff. The key to a healthcare organization's success is the coordination and cooperation of these three groups as they work together to identify community needs and pursue organizational goals. Although responsibilities vary from group to group, all groups share common interests and must work together on planning, budgeting, capital development, expenditures, PI, and patient satisfaction. Figure 15.1 shows an example of a hospital organization chart.

Figure 15.1. Example of a hospital organization chart

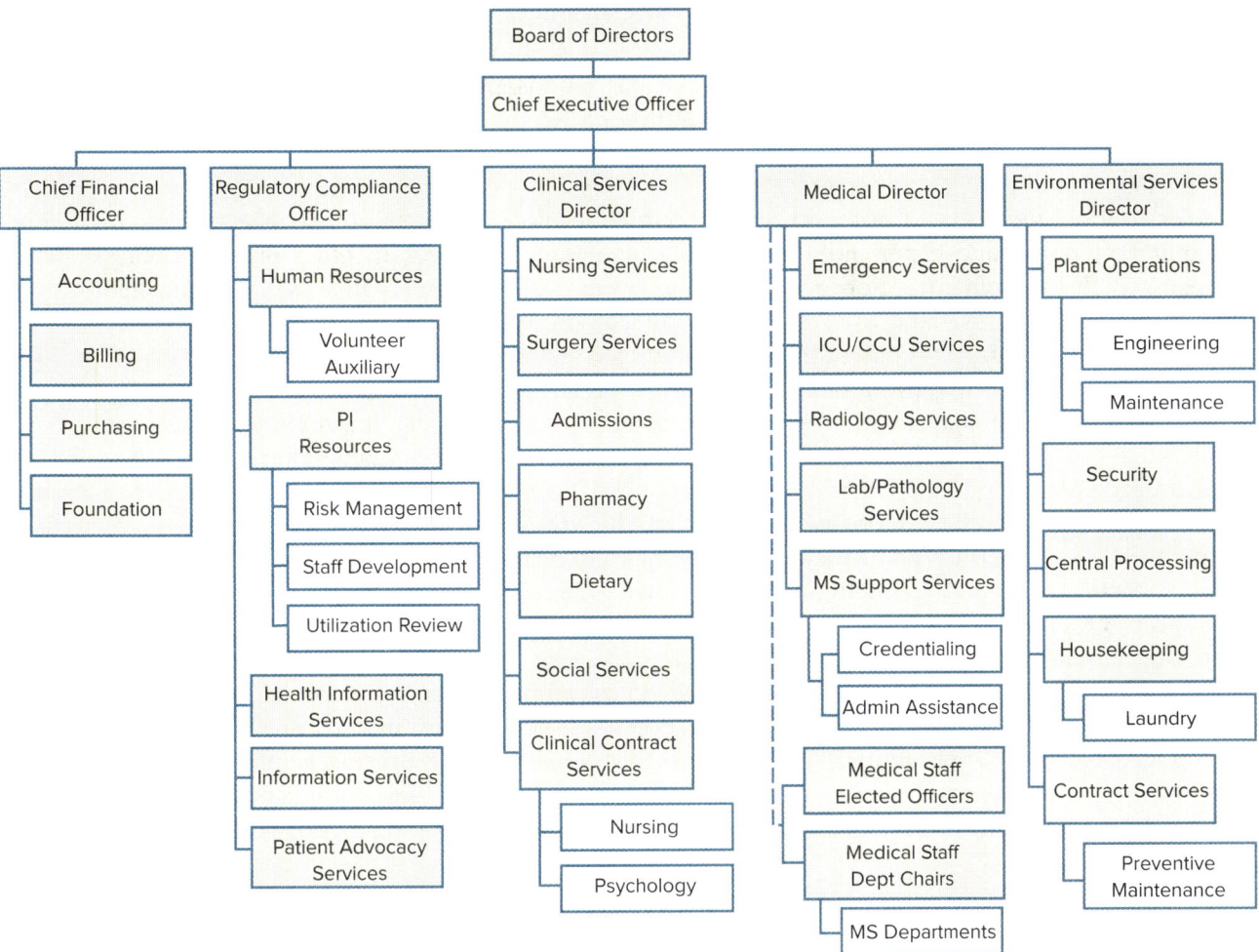

The medical staff elects its own officers and, through its bylaws, sets up an effective governing structure to accomplish its tasks. The medical staff is, in effect, an organization operating within a larger organization. (See figure 15.1.) Providers assembled as a medical staff give clinical oversight to the healthcare organization on care, treatment, and services they provide through established channels. However, the medical staff is accountable to the organization's board of directors. Neither the board nor the medical staff can unilaterally change the medical staff bylaws; both groups must approve any changes. Planning for the provision of an organization's healthcare services, on the other hand, is a function of the organization's leaders.

The leaders of the healthcare organization must carefully consider the needs of the community the organization serves, the technologies available to it, the expectations of customers, and the expertise of personnel and medical staff when crafting the mission, vision, and organizational goals. Organizational leaders are responsible for planning and creating the environment within the organization in which the mission, vision, and organizational goals can be achieved. A **strategic plan** is a document in which the leadership of a healthcare organization identifies the organization's overall mission, vision, and goals to help set the long-term direction of the organization as a business entity. Leaders are responsible for ensuring that a process is in place to measure, assess, and improve the hospital's governance, management, clinical, and support functions. Further reading on leadership is recommended for any student of PI in healthcare. A summary of the expectations of the leadership in healthcare organizations can be found in accrediting bodies' specific standards.

Ideally, every individual in the organization understands the PI principles and can contribute to PI activities when they recognize the need. In some organizations, defining PI initiatives and goals around the organization's strategic plan is one approach; identifying initiatives of frontline employees—those responsible for providing products and services directly to healthcare consumers—is another approach. However, in other organizations, commitment to the PI philosophy and activities is not as widespread. In such organizations, leaders actively promote PI philosophies and encourage healthcare workers at all levels to participate in improvement efforts. The leaders are usually department managers or administrators.

Some organizations develop an interdisciplinary PI council. The council may include representation from the board of directors, medical staff, administration, committee chairs from the organization's standing committees, and other interested and experienced individuals who lead PI efforts. In other organizations, a quality management department is developed to coordinate, oversee, and document PI activities. Some organizations retain the services of consultants to assist in developing an infrastructure that supports PI activities.

Finally, some organizations place the responsibility for PI activities in the hands of top management. This is the most conservative and traditional PI management approach. Because improvements come by mandate from higher levels of management, this is often referred to as a "top-down improvement initiative."

Regardless of the approach, the community and the populations the organization serves expect that the organization will provide the highest-quality products and services possible. Accreditors and regulators want to see evidence of PI activities and the ways in which those activities have benefited the organization's customers. Ultimately, the organization's performance will be judged against that expectation.

PI in healthcare is most effective when it is well-planned, systematic, and organization-wide and when all appropriate individuals and professions work collaboratively to plan and implement activities. When individuals from different departments representing the scope of care, treatment, and services across the organization are included in PI activities, complex problems and processes can be improved. Collaboration on PI activities enables an organization to create a culture that focuses on PI and to plan and provide improvements that endure. When planning PI activities, the organization should identify those areas needing improvement based on data collection and analysis and the desired changes that will lead to sustained improvements. This chapter introduces the process of developing a PI plan.

Strategic Planning

Planning for PI activities in healthcare organizations is an outgrowth of the organization's overall strategic planning process. The strategic plan, which contains the organization's overall mission, vision, and goals, is developed by the organization's senior leaders and board of directors, whom the public holds accountable for the quality of the organization's products and services. Strategic planning may include a process called **SWOT analysis**, in which the leaders complete an assessment of the organization's *S*trengths, *W*eaknesses, *O*pportunities, and *T*hreats. Findings from SWOT analyses are used to validate the mission of the organization as a whole and determine the direction the organization is going as a business entity during the coming year. The organization's leaders carefully consider input from the community it serves, its scope of services, the available technologies, staff expertise, the needs and expectations of its customers, and outcome information from PI activities during the past year.

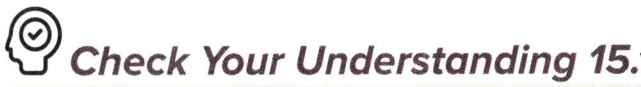

Check Your Understanding 15.1

1. Compare and contrast the role of the board of the directors and the role of the chief executive officer in a hospital.
2. The board of directors and hospital administrators at Community Hospital are working on a document that will include the long-term direction for the future of the facility. As part of this process, the board and administrators are not only determining the goals of the hospital, but are also including performance initiatives that will be conducted during the time frame of the plan. Based on this scenario, this plan is a(n):
   a. Operational plan
   b. Organizational plan
   c. Safety plan
   d. Strategic plan

PI Plan Design

Key to the implementation of an effective PI program is a formal plan that systematically describes the structure and approach the organization will follow in the continuous assessment and improvement of its important systems, processes, and outcomes of care. This plan should represent the various patient types and services of the healthcare organization and include provisions for the systematic collection, analysis, aggregation, and reporting of PI activities. Figure 15.2 shows an example of an organization-wide PI plan.

Figure 15.2A. PI and patient safety plan, Community Hospital

Community Hospital is a 350-bed tertiary medical center with an inpatient and outpatient continuum of care that provides medical and surgical services to a community of approximately 250,000. The facility's scope of services includes cardiology, orthopedics, obstetrics/gynecology, oncology, and psychiatry. The Community Hospital board of directors is committed to continually improving the delivery and effectiveness of the care and services provided and to proactively monitoring and assessing care delivery, patient safety, and customer satisfaction. The board supports an environment that encourages the identification of improvement opportunities from all sources throughout the organization and community and the provision of care and service that is reflective of the organization's mission and vision.

Mission
Community Hospital is the preeminent regionally integrated healthcare delivery system in the Intermountain West dedicated to providing compassionate, quality, high-value healthcare services to the residents of our communities.

Vision
Community Hospital seeks to provide leadership in patient-centered care that is built on a foundation of knowledge, innovation, and human values.

Performance Improvement Approach and Model
An interdisciplinary, continuous performance improvement approach is recognized across our continuum of care and service areas utilizing a Plan-Do-Check-Act (PDCA) model. Patient care and safety, and all other important organizational functions, are continually monitored, analyzed, and improved.

Organizational Performance Improvement Structure and Expectations
The leaders of Community Hospital (the board of directors, the medical staff officers, and the senior hospital administrators) are committed to the integration of performance improvement activities. All staff are educated in the principles of performance improvement and participate in identifying opportunities for improvement, data collection, and reporting activities, performance improvement team activities, and ongoing education. The board of directors has overall responsibility for ensuring the quality of care and services provided to the community. The board has delegated implementation responsibility for the organization-wide continuous performance improvement activities to the Performance Improvement and Patient Safety Council.

Performance Improvement and Patient Safety Council
The Performance Improvement and Patient Safety Council is an interdisciplinary senior leadership committee that provides oversight and direction for the design and implementation of the organization-wide continuous performance improvement and patient safety program

Figure 15.2B. PI and patient safety plan, Community Hospital (*Continued*)

The council annually reviews outcome data and survey information as part of its strategic planning and prioritization processes. The council reports monthly to the medical executive committee and quarterly to the board of directors any adverse outcomes, significant process variations, and actions taken to improve care and address patient safety issues, both proactively and reactively. Standing committees of the medical staff, clinical and department discipline meetings, and this council are responsible for managing and improving patient care and safety issues within their particular high-risk areas. Prioritized measures that include high-risk and problem-prone areas identified throughout the organization are trended, analyzed, and reported to the council by assigned committees/staff on a preestablished schedule. The performance improvement department coordinates the implementation of the performance improvement and patient safety plan. The department provides organization-wide support in the design of data collection tools, data display, statistical analysis, benchmark data research, and the preparation of council reports. The council is responsible for receiving findings and acting on recommendations from the board and all committees, departments, and performance improvement teams, as well as customer survey data, sentinel events, near misses, and other identified trends in areas such as risk management and infection control. The council also is responsible for the design of the organization-wide staff development program related to continuous performance improvement and patient safety, and for the assessment and assignment of an annual proactive risk-reduction activity. At least annually, the council reviews the activities of the performance improvement program and makes recommendations for the continuous improvement of the performance improvement and patient safety plan to the board of directors. The council membership is composed of a physician chairperson, the chief executive officer, the medical director, clinical and administrative service directors, performance improvement team members, and other invited staff and guests as appropriate. The council meets at least every other month and as needs indicate.

Standing Committees of the Medical Staff

All standing committees of the medical staff are chaired by a physician with representation, as appropriate, from hospital leadership, department directors, and frontline staff. Reports are submitted to the Performance Improvement and Patient Safety Council, which in turn forwards critical events and findings to the executive committee and to the board of directors. Communication throughout the organization among the board, committees, councils, hospital departments, medical staff, employed and contract staff, and patients and families is open and flows in all directions, as appropriate and as allowed by regulations.

Medical Executive Committee

An elected official from the medical staff, medical staff committee chairs, the medical director, the chief executive officer, the clinical service director, the compliance officer, and the chief financial officer are standing members of this committee. This committee meets monthly and coordinates the business of the medical staff (recommending changes to their bylaws, rules, and regulations; reviewing appointment and reappointment recommendations; and election of officers) and the integration of patient care and hospital support services. Significant issues related to performance improvement and patient safety forwarded from the Performance Improvement and Patient Safety Council are reviewed, discussed, acted upon, and forwarded to the board and, as appropriate, to other departments, committees, and staff.

Medical Staff and Specialty Department Meetings

Each clinical staff specialty department meets at least quarterly to review and discuss performance improvement activities, staff development issues, and other related planning and directing activities. The medical staff at large meets at least annually for the election of officers, bylaws review, and general staff education.

Ethics Committee

This committee is responsible for serving as a resource regarding medical and ethical issues that surface for patients, their families, and the organization's clinical care providers.

Credentials Committee

This committee is responsible for the design and implementation of the organization's credentialing process and includes reviewing applications for appointment and reappointment, defining privilege delineation criteria, and evaluating physical health issues. Recommendations on all credentialing-related issues are reported to the executive committee and forwarded to the board of directors for final approval.

Utilization and Documentation Standards Committee

This committee is responsible for the review of findings from the monitoring activities on patient-specific data and information, timeliness of clinical record entries, and appropriateness of admissions and continued stays. Significant findings and recommendations are reported to the Performance Improvement and Patient Safety Council, the executive committee, provider quality profiles, other committees, and departments and individuals, as appropriate.

Pharmacy and Therapeutics Committee

This committee is responsible for formulary review and development, policy setting, procedure development, medication-related safety education, and monitoring the safety and efficacy of medication use throughout the organization. Medication monitoring includes a systematic, ongoing process of reviewing prescribing/ordering, procurement and storage, preparation and dispensing, administration, and adverse drug reactions. This committee performs data collection, analysis of aggregate data for patterns and trends, recommendations for process/system changes, and reporting of significant findings and actions to the Performance Improvement and Patient Safety Council.

Figure 15.2C. PI and patient safety plan, Community Hospital (*Continued*)

Environmental Safety Committee

This committee is responsible for planning and directing environmental services within all environments of care. It also is responsible for educating staff on environmental safety issues and performance monitoring, data analysis, and continuous improvement efforts. This committee meets monthly and reports data collection, analysis, and improvement initiatives to the Performance Improvement and Patient Safety Council at least quarterly. The committee submits an environmental safety report identifying and reviewing improvement goals to the board of directors annually. Committee representation includes individuals from hospital and medical staff leadership, engineering and maintenance, housekeeping, central processing, security, and employee health.

Strategic Planning Process

The strategic planning process occurs annually prior to the start of the fiscal year and coincides with organization-wide plan/program reviews and the budgeting process. Performance improvement and patient safety program review is initiated by the council using findings from the leaders' strategic goals, the council's self-assessment, and staff survey data on the program's effectiveness. Additional information, such as aggregate outcome data from performance measures, effectiveness of corrective actions implemented as a result of process variations and adverse outcomes, input from customer surveys, status on past year's goals, findings and actions from the annual proactive risk assessment/reduction activity, and regulatory and hospital process changes, is reviewed and considered in the planning process and in the prioritization of performance initiatives and measures for the upcoming year.

Criteria for Prioritization of Improvement Goals, Performance Measures, and Data Collection

- Does the improvement opportunity/measure support the organization's mission, scope of care, and service provided and/or population(s) served?
- Is the performance measure a required regulatory measure, and does it provide performance information on an important function?
- Does the opportunity improve patient safety?
- Does the opportunity relate to an event that resulted in a sentinel event or near miss?
- Does the opportunity reflect patient feedback on needs or expectations?
- What degree of adverse impact on patient care can be expected if the improvement opportunity remains unresolved?
- Does the opportunity reflect a high-volume, problem-prone, or high-risk process?
- Are resources available to conduct the improvement process?
- Does the opportunity involve changing regulatory requirements?

Performance Measurement

This organization collects data on key systems, processes, and outcomes to monitor its performance. Data collection is prioritized based on this organization's mission, scope of care, services provided, and populations served. Data collection is systematic and may be used to establish a performance baseline, describe process performance stability, identify areas for more focused data collection, and determine whether improvement has been sustained. Available benchmark information for established performance measures is drawn from internal and external databases. Data collection, responsibilities, and reporting schedules are defined in an appendix to this plan. Data collected to monitor performance include the following:

- Performance measures related to accreditation requirements
- Patient safety issues, including the following error-prone areas: medication events, falls, blood events, procedure/treatment/surgical events, behavioral events, equipment events, and laboratory events
- High-risk processes that may have the potential to result in a sentinel event, including operative or other invasive procedures that place patients at risk, medication management, restraint use, seclusion use, blood and blood product use, and outcomes related to resuscitation
- Relevant clinical practice guidelines
- Adverse drug events (ADEs)
- Needs, safety concerns, expectations, and satisfaction of patients and their families
- Failed processes related to the National Patient Safety Goals
- Readmission rates
- Utilization management activities
- Performance of new and modified processes
- Quality control activities in the clinical laboratory, diagnostic radiology, nutritional services, nuclear medicine, radiation oncology, and pharmacy
- Infection control surveillance and reporting
- Medical record documentation for quality of care and timeliness
- Risk management information, including sentinel events, near misses, complaints, findings from inspections by regulatory agencies, and compensable events
- Environmental safety
- Efficacy of services provided through contract or written agreement
- Appropriateness and effectiveness of pain management
- Appropriateness of behavior management procedures
- Autopsy results, when performed
- Customer demographics and diagnoses
- Financial data

Figure 15.2D. PI and patient safety plan, Community Hospital (*Continued*)

- Staff opinions and needs
- Measures established when performance improvement and patient safety teams are chartered to design/redesign a process
- Other measures that may warrant targeted study

Measurement Process and Tools

When clinical conditions or systems are evaluated, measurement includes the following components:

- Design and assessment of new processes
- Assessment of data from customer satisfaction surveys, financial analysis, clinical outcomes of care, and functional outcomes of care
- Development of indicators of care or service that are measurable and focus on processes or outcomes
- Utilization of benchmarks or thresholds for performance
- Identification of data sources
- Development of a method of data collection and organization of data measures
- Measurement of the level of performance and stability of important existing processes
- Aggregation and trending of data
- Use of established clinical practice guidelines as a framework for standards of care and practice, when applicable
- Evaluation of individual cases that have potential or actual risk to the patient (adverse event/sentinel event review)
- Benchmarks/thresholds are based on current professional literature, national standards, clinical practice guidelines, or internal benchmarks for improvement. Thresholds are derived from retrospective data relative to previous measurements within the organization or from comparable organization data. A benchmark is a quantitative goal embraced by the organization and is reflective of best practices within the internal and/or external environment. These goals serve as a mechanism for acceleration of performance curves through the process of continuous improvement.

Data Sources and Sampling

Data sources include health records, encounter data, satisfaction surveys, complaint information, and internal clinical databases. Sampling methodology shall be relevant to the performance measures or study being conducted.

Aggregation and Analysis of Performance Data

The results of systematic, ongoing measures are aggregated and analyzed to identify trends, variances, and opportunities to improve patient care and safety. Data analysis should answer the following questions:

- What is our current level of performance?
- How stable are current processes?
- Do any steps in the process have undesirable variation(s)?
- Have strategies to stabilize or improve performance been effective?
- Are there areas that could be improved?
- What should the improvement priorities be?
- Was there sustained improvement in the processes that were changed?

Data Review

Trended data are reviewed when

- Trended performance measures significantly and undesirably vary from those of other organizations, requiring a more detailed review.
- Trended performance measures significantly and undesirably vary from recognized standards, benchmarks, or statistical process controls.
- The occurrence of an event is questionable or too infrequent to make judgments about patterns in care or to analyze statistical significance.

Intensive review of an incident requires the review of health records or other data elements to determine whether process problems exist and if an ongoing performance measure should be established to monitor process stability. An intensive review is undertaken when

- A significant adverse drug reaction or medication error occurs
- An external regulatory agency requests the review
- The Performance Improvement and Patient Safety Council requests the review
- An organization is performing proactive risk-reduction activities

Root-cause analysis is conducted when a significant negative deviation from expected outcomes occurs or when a near miss occurs and further study is recommended by the council.

Peer Review Process

Cases are referred to peer review when they meet criteria as defined in the medical staff peer review plan. Findings are referred to appropriate committees for review and action, as warranted, and to individual provider practice profiles and are reviewed as part of the reappointment process.

Figure 15.2E. PI and patient safety plan, Community Hospital (*Continued*)

Performance Improvement Model

The model for performance improvement is plan-do-check-act (PDCA) and is defined as the following:

- **Plan** is based on the results of data collection or the assessment of a process. The plan should include how the process will be improved and what will be measured to evaluate the effectiveness of the proposed process change(s).
- **Do** includes the implementation of process changes. These changes may be tested before changing policies and procedures or conducting extensive education.
- **Check** evaluates the effect of the action taken at a given point in time.
- **Act** is to hold the gain and to continue to improve the process.

Evaluation

The measurement, assessment, and evaluation processes will continue to provide the necessary information about the effectiveness of the improvement. If the identified problem continues to persist despite the planned improvements, the PDCA model will continue until sustained improvement is achieved. Any findings, conclusions, recommendations, actions taken, and results of the actions taken based on the performance improvement process are documented and reported to the appropriate individuals, departments, or committees. This information is used in the reappointment of providers, recontracting with agencies providing outsourced patient care services, and the employee evaluation process.

Patient Safety Risk-Reduction Model

The model used to conduct the annual proactive risk assessment and reduction activity is the failure mode effects analysis (FMEA).

Communication

Performance improvement and patient safety activities are communicated through the established committee structure as well as through regular clinical, discipline, and staff meetings; emails; and the organization's website. Members of the council are responsible for maintaining communication related to performance improvement and patient safety initiatives. The treating provider is responsible for informing patients and their families (when appropriate) about the outcomes of the patients' care, including unanticipated outcomes such as sentinel events, and for documenting such communication in the patients' clinical records.

Education

The organization's leaders and council members are responsible for ongoing educational activities related to the performance improvement and patient safety program. This includes onboarding of new employees at hire, onboarding of new board members, and annual education of all employees at the annual employee fair and through participation in performance improvement teams.

Staff Support

The employee assistance program (EAP) is a resource to support staff involved in a sentinel event and other work-related performance issues. The EAP is a confidential employee service. The clinical leadership also is responsible for meeting with staff involved in sentinel events to provide a means for communication and support.

Confidentiality

All performance improvement and patient safety activities set forth in this plan, including minutes, reports, and associated work products, are confidential and may not be released or discussed with any person or agency except those mandated by hospital policy or state or federal law.

Annual Review

The performance improvement and patient safety plan is reviewed annually as part of the organization-wide strategic planning process. The plan review is based on the organization's mission, evaluation of goals from the previous year, data collection results, and external regulatory changes.

APPENDIX A: PERFORMANCE IMPROVEMENT INITIATIVES

Goal 1: To improve patient, provider, and employee satisfaction

A. Patient Satisfaction: Improve patient satisfaction as measured by the Patient Satisfaction Survey

   Action Plan:
   - Implement the caring model of nursing.
   - Refine and improve the centralized scheduling process.
   - Improve patient education and communication in the area of advance directives.

   Measurement:
   - Patient responses on the Patient Satisfaction Survey will shift from satisfied or dissatisfied to increase the very satisfied category by 5 percent.
   - The number of positive comments will increase by at least 5 percent.
   - The number of billing complaints will decrease by at least 5 percent.

B. Provider Satisfaction: Improve provider satisfaction as measured by the biannual survey

   Action Plan:
   - Implement the caring model of nursing.
   - Refine/improve the centralized scheduling process.
   - Evaluate and downsize committee structure as appropriate.

Figure 15.2F. PI and patient safety plan, Community Hospital (*Continued*)

Measurement:
- The results of the biannual survey will shift from satisfied or dissatisfied to increase the very satisfied category by 5 percent.

C. Employee Satisfaction: Improve employee satisfaction

Action Plan:
- Implement the caring model of nursing.
- Award/recognize employees for years of service.
- Review/improve the employee evaluation process.
- Implement a system of merit raises.
- Develop department-specific action plans based on employee survey results and exit interview feedback.

Measurement:
- The annual employee turnover rate will decrease by 5 percent.
- All employees will be surveyed in June/July at department meetings using Patient Satisfaction Survey questions.
- A system of performing exit interviews will be implemented.

Goal 2: To improve the infrastructure and systems used to collect, measure, and assess information so that information will be secure, accurate, appropriately accessible, useful, timely, and effective

Action Plan:
- Provide education in basic information management principles and provide tools for leaders and other staff as needed.
- Develop standing agendas for meetings to support appropriate flow of information throughout the organization.
- Develop standardized documentation measurement
- Improve communication pathways to provide information to, and encourage feedback from, patients, trustees, providers, employees, and other customers.

Measurement:
- Performance improvement/risk and safety reports will be complete, accurate, and timely.
- Compliance with documentation requirements as measured by data quality monitoring program will increase.
- Communication as measured by employee, providers, and patient survey results and through unsolicited comments will improve.

Goal 3: To improve leadership orientation, education, and performance

Action Plan:
- Revise/develop executive team and manager onboarding and reference manual.
- Provide/attend at least two leadership education programs focusing on assessed needs for trustees, medical executive staff, executive team, and managers.
- Establish protocols for development, implementation, and review of standing provider orders.

Measurement:
- Educational program feedback surveys from participants will demonstrate program effectiveness.
- Trustee self-evaluation results will improve.
- Trustee evaluations of the CEO will improve.
- Survey results and self-evaluations will improve
- Use and annual review of standing provider order protocols will be monitored.

Goal 4: To develop and improve employee competence and performance

Action Plan:
- Develop and administer an organization-wide educational needs assessment program, including feedback from providers and
- employees as well as patient satisfaction surveys.
- Develop and implement educational programming to address prioritized needs.

Measurement:
- Results of mandatory staff education posttests will demonstrate that competencies have been achieved.
- Employee perception that needs have been met will be measured by participant evaluations of the educational offerings and employee satisfaction surveys.

The leaders are expected to select an organization-wide PI approach and clearly define how all levels of the organization will monitor and address improvement issues. Accrediting and licensure bodies provide guidance regarding many of the measures for which hospitals should collect data. The following areas are some examples (the full list can be found in the appropriate accreditation standards or licensure requirements):

- Medication management
- Blood and blood product use
- Behavior management and treatment
- Operative and other invasive procedures
- Resuscitation and its outcomes

Because most organizations identify more improvement opportunities than they can act on, priorities must be set. Criteria are helpful in setting priorities and may include the following:

- High-risk, high-volume, or problem-prone processes
- The degree of adverse impact on patient care that can be expected if an improvement opportunity remains unresolved
- The degree to which patient safety is improved

For example, at Community Hospital, the managers and employees participate in organization-wide strategic planning. One year, as part of strategic planning, they identified a list of their organization's important functions and processes in which they thought improvement opportunities existed. (See figure 15.3.) The participants used brainstorming techniques and nominal group techniques to identify and prioritize improvement opportunities. The prioritized ranking shows the number of points assigned to the various opportunities for improvement upon review by the entire organization. The prioritized opportunities were then reevaluated and regrouped by the hospital's board of directors and senior leaders in light of other available survey and outcome data. Using preestablished prioritization criteria, the leaders finalized the hospital's improvement goals, the results of which can be found in figure 15.2.

Figure 15.3A. Example of a strategic planning document showing potential PI opportunities

Community Hospital—Important Functions and Opportunities, Annual Strategic Planning	
Functions and Opportunities	**Priority Points**
Provision of care, treatment, and services	
Define restraint protocol	22
Provide physical therapy services on weekends	1
Change menu service	4
Improve patient transport process	10
Develop community awareness program	12
Expand patient and family education	48
Improve discharge instruction and documentation procedures	25
Improve education for surgical patients	16
Expand blood donor program	9
Define assessment process	34
Code status on admission	55
Do more complete assessment on preop patients	11
Address regional psychiatric services support	12
Target high-risk patients for preventive care	17
Respond to changing regulations on authorized procedures	15
Define proper follow-up call from hospital to patient	10
Define proper protocol for standing orders	27
Ethics, rights, and responsibilities	
Include discussion of patient rights as part of admissions process	23
Educate staff, families, and patients about the function of the ethics committee	21
Respect patient's right to privacy and treatment with dignity	22
Surveillance, prevention, and control of infection	
Enforce universal precautions	58
Develop infection control program for home care	14
Ensure that patient rooms are clean before assigning new patients to rooms	19
Improve traffic control in patient care areas	18

Figure 15.3B. Example of a strategic planning document showing potential PI opportunities (Continued)

Community Hospital of the West—Important Functions and Opportunities, Annual Strategic Planning	
Functions and Opportunities	Priority Points
Management of the environment of care	
Develop master plan for remodeling patient care areas	22
Refine role of housekeeping	26
Look at complaints about waiting areas	22
Develop a system for providing hazardous-spill carts	2
Address after-hours and weekend security issues	25
Remodel the operating room transitional area	3
Upgrade operating room furniture and equipment	8
Improving organization performance	
Develop plan to reduce medication errors	21
Explore concurrent data collection and reporting processes	13
Improve operating room scheduling process	18
Improve teamwork for PI activities	16
Leadership	
Develop a provider–hospital organization to work with managed care	13
Conduct a community needs assessment	7
Build feedback from employee and providers satisfaction surveys into the strategic planning process	7
Develop mission, vision, and organizational goals for each department/service	5
Downsize the number of committees	9
Clarify leadership's role in all important organization-wide functions	8
Introduce staff to board of trustees and define board's expectations of staff	2
Define protocol for charity care	1
Define hospital's system for acknowledging patient deaths	2
Clarify role of administrator on call	1
Update and maintain all departmental policies and procedures	8
Management of human resources	
Provide identity badges for all providers	4
Improve communications with key customers (patients, employees, providers)	14
Improve mandatory staff education process	20
Develop and implement competencies/skills checklists for every department	18
Improve system for designating PRN staff—whom to call, how many, and so forth	1
Update provider directory	1
Utilize intranet training	3
Develop policy on lab testing for employees and providers	2
Develop staff cross-training program	10
Decrease staff turnover	1
Management of information	
Standardize organization of policies and procedures among departments	18
Raise awareness of confidentiality issues	41
Inventory the information the organization collects and determine what is necessary for quality control and leadership/governance needs	9
Provide internet access in the library	6
Provide training and policy development on CMS coding rules	6

Many of the items in the strategic planning process document are related to patient care (see Provision of care, treatment, and services section in figure 15.3). Before using strategic brainstorming, the organization had been collecting data using a patient satisfaction survey. An in-depth analysis of the data revealed a negative trend in multiple indicators related to nursing care. The measures included the following:

- Overall quality of nursing care
- Staff showed concern toward patient
- Nurses anticipated patient needs
- Nurses explained procedures to patient
- Nurses demonstrated skill in providing care
- Nurses helped calm patients' fears
- Staff communicated effectively with patients
- Nurses and staff responded to patient requests

After considerable discussion of the brainstormed opportunities and of the patient satisfaction survey data, the leadership decided to increase their focus on nursing care in response to issues affecting that area. Implementation of this care model became a PI initiative for improving patients' perceptions of nursing care. All other opportunities were aligned to this major initiative. The organization's intent was that changing the strategy for nursing care in this dramatic way would be evidenced in subsequent measures of nursing effectiveness by the Patient Satisfaction Survey.

The first part of the PI initiative document was organized to reflect the needs of the organization's mission, vision, and most important customers—patients, providers, and employees. Opportunities were then listed beneath the customers to whom they pertained. A component of the organization's PI approach was to focus on, and maintain visibility of, the customer.

The rest of the PI initiative document focused on the important processes and functions of the organization that are most likely to affect high-risk, high-volume, and problem-prone outcomes. Each section identified an action plan and how the efforts at improvement will be measured. These measurements should provide good data for the organization to assess itself and plan the following year's PI initiatives, thus maintaining a continuous PI philosophy and cycle in the organization.

Other important areas that should be addressed in an organization's PI plan include the following:

- Initial and ongoing education of the board, medical staff, and employed staff members on the PI process and annual improvement initiatives
- The expectations of all members of the organization in PI activities
- Annual review of the effectiveness of the organization's PI program

Decision Matrix

Another tool that is helpful in setting priorities is a **decision matrix**. A decision matrix assists in evaluating and prioritizing a list of potential improvement opportunities (ASQ 2023). Healthcare organizations have many competing opportunities for improvement and must determine which opportunity will yield the greatest overall benefit to the organization and customers. For example, Community Hospital plans to focus on improving organization performance in some key areas:

- Develop a plan to reduce medication errors
- Explore concurrent data collection and reporting processes
- Improve operating room scheduling process
- Improve teamwork for process improvement activities

Figure 15.4. Example of a decision matrix

Criteria ➡ Target Areas ⬇	Resource Needs	Patient Safety Impact	Organization Ability to Implement	Staff Readiness/ Potential Buy-in	Total
	1 = Great 2 = Some 3 = Minimal	1 = Slight extent 2 = Some extent 3 = Great extent	1 = Low 2 = Medium 3 = High	1 = Low 2 = Medium 3 = High	
Reduce medication errors	2	3	2	3	10
Concurrent data collection and reporting processes	1	2	2	2	7
Operating room scheduling	2	2	3	1	8
Teamwork for PI activities	1	2	1	1	5

With the use of the decision matrix, Community Hospital can determine that the highest priority improvement opportunity is to reduce medication errors throughout the organization. Reduction of medication errors received the most points in the decision matrix and is identified as the top priority PI project for the organization (see figure 15.4).

Implementing the PI Plan

The organization's leaders have a central role in initiating and maintaining the organization's PI priorities. Implementation of the organization-wide plan for PI is a challenge at best. The plan should clearly delineate how members of the organization are educated on the PI process and what their roles and responsibilities are in carrying out the organization's plan. Often, top organizational leaders' compensation and performance reviews are tied directly to successful implementation and execution of the PI plan initiatives (Daley et.al. 2018). As seen in figure 15.2, Community Hospital's PI and patient safety plan describes how the board of directors delegates plan implementation responsibility to the Performance Improvement and Patient Safety Council. The council, in turn, defines which committees, departments, and staff members are responsible for collecting data, assessing and reporting findings, and performing other PI activities.

The scope and focus of what will be measured, which data will be collected and by whom, and the frequency and intensity with which the data will be collected and reported should be clearly defined by the healthcare organization. Although healthcare organizations have some control over the types of data they collect, healthcare regulations mandate some of what must be collected. For example, the organization collects data on patients' perceptions of care, treatment, and services, including their specific needs and expectations, how well the organization meets these needs and expectations, and how the organization can improve patient safety.

PI priorities should be data driven. That is, the data the organization collects about its own performance should be analyzed and considered when setting improvement priorities. Data should be aggregated and displayed in a way that supports easy assessment of the findings. Establishing benchmarks for each measure for which data is collected and displaying the benchmark information alongside the aggregate data measures are ways to quickly identify less-than-desirable outcomes in performance. Historically, healthcare organizations have been referred to as "data rich" and "information poor," meaning that they spent too much time collecting data and failed to turn the data into meaningful information or use it in setting performance priorities. Setting measurement and data collection priorities are newer standards that have evolved over the past few years to help organizations better identify, manage, and act on collected data.

In demonstrating the effectiveness of its PI model, a healthcare organization must show evidence that the entire cycle has been completed for each of its prioritized improvements. Often, organizations fail to complete the cycle. Data can be collected, aggregated, and analyzed, and an improvement priority can be established, but without providing evidence of an effective and sustained improvement, the cycle remains incomplete. It is not unusual for process changes to initially result in variations in performance or for an organization to find that a process change may not be the correct "fix" to an identified problem. The ongoing, systematic review of measurements identified to confirm process stability is the "check" step in the improvement cycle. Monitoring a process change for up to six months, with ongoing data checks (sampling at regular intervals) once stability is achieved, validates the improvement or the need for continued improvements (the "act" step) and completes the PI cycle.

Check Your Understanding 15.2

1. A hospital is selecting a new electronic health record (EHR) system. To make an informed decision, the organization decides to use a decision matrix. Which of the following criteria is most likely to be included in the decision matrix for evaluating different EHR systems?
   a. Number of hospital beds
   b. User interface color scheme
   c. Data security and compliance
   d. Distance from the administrator's office to the server room

2. As part of the PI process, healthcare organizations use aggregated and analyzed data to determine if quality initiatives are improving care and treatment for patients. Trended data is reviewed when:
   a. Trended performance measures are not designated by the governing board
   b. Trended performance measures vary significantly and unfavorably from the standards, benchmarks, or statistical process controls
   c. Trended performance measures are not designated by the PI team
   d. Trended performance measures are unrelated to the PI process, but are organizational data that can be analyzed for review

Evaluating the Performance Improvement Program

The processes of planning and evaluating a performance improvement program should mirror each other. Taken together, they are a cyclical activity: planning leads to evaluation, and evaluation provides the impetus for new planning. The task of appraising the PI program is generally completed on an annual basis, and the results should be reported to the healthcare organization's board, management, employees, and medical staff.

PI programs are evaluated for four reasons:

1. *To determine whether the organization's approach to designing, measuring, assessing, and improving its performance is planned, systematic, and organization-wide.* Forethought and deliberation help the organization focus on important issues and lead to better results of program activities. Systematizing the PI program makes it possible for participants to understand what is expected and enables them to anticipate program requirements. Committing to the organization-wide nature of the program ensures that everyone in the organization is in concert with the program's objectives and understands what they are expected to contribute. The PI evaluation process includes the participation of all employees, medical staff, and organizational leaders, from frontline staff to the board of directors. Involvement of the organization's staff in the evaluation process can be demonstrated through team or committee input, questionnaires and surveys, self-evaluation, suggestion boxes, and so forth. For example, each department can assess the educational competency of individual staff as it relates to PI knowledge. Department competency then can be compared with an established organization-wide PI competency goal.

2. *To determine whether the organization's approach and activities are carried out collaboratively.* PI activities should be interprofessional or multidisciplinary and should improve performance across department lines; in other words, they should be cross-functional or interdepartmental. Another expectation is that all factors that contribute to a problem will be remedied. For example, PI teams should be assessed in an annual evaluation of frontline staff, interprofessional or multidisciplinary team participation through documentation of regular attendance at meetings, data collection, and overall success of the team's improvement efforts.

3. *To determine whether the organization's approach needs redesigning in light of changes in the strategic plan or organizational objectives.* If the organization's mission, vision, organizational structure, or strategic initiatives have changed since the PI program was planned, then new measures and assessment activities may have to be undertaken. For example, if an organization has a strategic initiative to add a new service, all relevant departments, organization leaders, and the board of directors would be included in defining measures and assessment activities for the new service. Modifications should be implemented as soon as possible after major changes in organization objectives have been made. In addition, the organization needs to assess the adequacy of the human, information, physical, and financial resources allocated to support PI and safety activities.

4. *To determine whether the program was effective in improving overall organizational performance.* It is important to identify whether the PI program was responsible for important improvements in organizational performance or whether those improvements were due to other factors. It is also important to identify whether improvements were achieved and maintained. Review of program performance should identify whether program processes are efficient, effective, timely, and appropriately supported with personnel, budget, and other resources. Figure 15.5 shows survey questions used in one organization to assess the effectiveness of various departments' PI programs. The results from the survey can be used to assess and then recommend changes to the organization's PI program.

Figure 15.5. Example of PI staff survey questions

- How is PI used in your department/service?
- Are you asked for suggestions/ideas for processes that need to be improved in your area?
- Are you asked for suggestions/ideas for processes that need to be improved in your organization-wide?
- Have you been involved in any PI activities in the past year?
- Have the results of PI activities been communicated to you on a regular basis? If yes, how have they been communicated?
- Have you used the results of any PI activities in the delivery of patient care/service in the past year?
- Have PI activities improved patient care or service in your area in the past year?
- What PIs need to be made to improve the safety of patient care delivery?
- Do the staff in your work area understand PI activities?
- Which patient care process is strongest in your work area?
- Which process related to patient care is weakest in your work area?
- If you could improve only one patient process or outcome, which would you choose?
- Do you feel that your area has adequate resources to support PI and patient safety activities?

Components of Program Review

PI review is performed on an annual basis. The results from this evaluation are reported to the board of directors, medical staff, and leaders of the organization. During program review, each area in which clinical and nonclinical services are provided should be examined for continued focus and relevance. Each area should document opportunities for improvement that were identified and PI goals that were met. Each area should document which problems remain unresolved from prior evaluation periods and which have not shown significant improvement. Each area should identify issues in the PI program that, if changed, would better support the organization's overall mission and PI efforts.

Executive Summary

The executive summary section of the PI review summarizes the main points of the annual report. This section highlights the results of key PI initiatives undertaken by the organization in the previous year.

Overview

This section highlights the organization's philosophy and strategy related to all quality and PI activities. It includes how these PI activities relate to the organization's mission, vision, values, and strategic plan, and how organization leaders use this information to prioritize operations for the future.

PI Structure

The leaders and staff responsible for the organization's quality and PI activities are described here. How PI teams are developed and guided toward improvement activities are outlined, as well as how this information is communicated throughout the organization and among leaders. The process for ongoing monitoring and the identification of critical data collection activities are provided. Responses from the annual staff PI survey might include answers to the following questions:

- Does the organization's current PI methodology continue to support its PI activities and management style?
- Could some activities in the model be made more efficient or be simplified?
- Do all members of the organization understand the model and how it can help structure PI activities?

Improvement Opportunities

Trends from aggregate data analysis, interventions, corrective actions or improvements, or changes in policies and procedures may be highlighted in the improvement opportunities section using graphic presentation of findings rather than detailed reports. Data should show evidence of continued and sustained improvement. System improvements may be broken into four areas: patient-focused improvements, organizational improvements, ongoing measurements, and quality data reporting (see figure 15.6).

Figure 15.6. Key system improvement areas

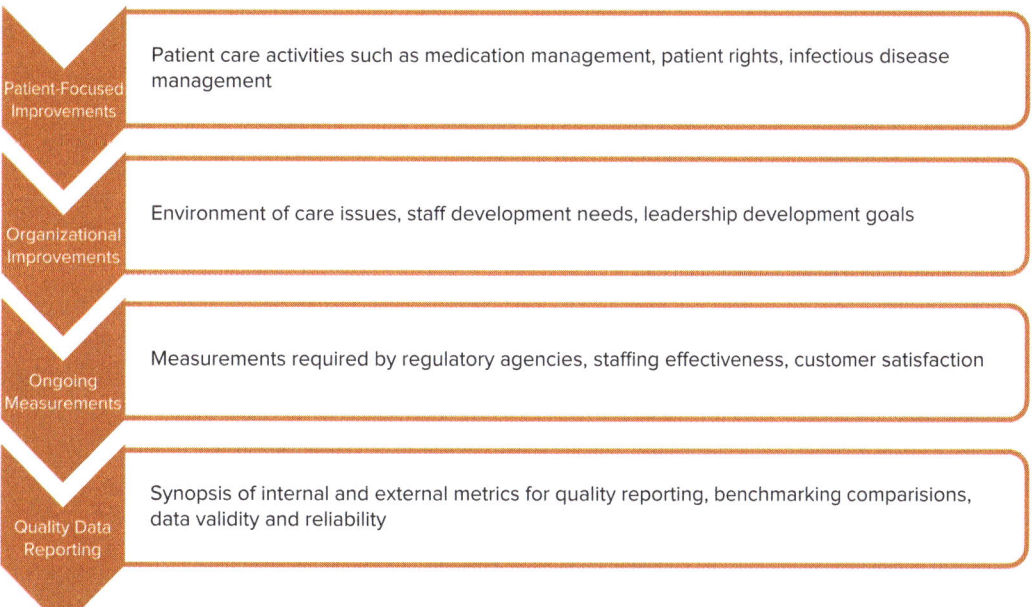

PI Team Activities

The PI team activities section of the report highlights the work of PI teams sanctioned by the organization's PI council and should provide answers to the following questions:

- Has the team's work resulted in measurable and sustained improvements?
- What process changes and training occurred to support and sustain the improvement(s)?
- Has the organization's staff assigned to PI team projects been effectively trained to work on PI teams?
- Is staff willing and able to take on the important roles in team activities?
- Does staff participate and interact well at team meetings to work through PI processes?
- Can they document important team milestones with appropriate tools?
- Have they implemented the organization's PI model appropriately?
- Have they learned to listen and question effectively in interpersonal communication?
- Can they effectively communicate the team's process and outcomes to the rest of the organization?

Other PI Review Topics

Other topics that may be addressed in the organization's PI plan review may include areas of focused change or improvement. See figure 15.7 for important questions to ask as part of this review.

Figure 15.7. Key questions to evaluate PI processes

Customer Satisfaction
- Have internal and external customers been identified for all PI projects?
- Have customers' requirements been identified in detail?
- Has customer satisfaction been measured objectively and with appropriate tools?

Risk Exposure and Patient Safety Assessment
- Is adherence to procedures monitored and appropriate education undertaken when necessary?
- Are the right services always rendered to the right patient, at the right time, with the right procedure?
- Are adverse events always reported per policy and procedure?
- Are care processes modified when necessary to prevent injury to patients, visitors, and employees?

Human Resources
- Are appropriate hiring, staffing, training, and competency assessment activities occurring in all departments?
- Are employees being screened for disease as required by state health regulations?
- Are required documents being maintained on all employees?
- Are required credentials and licenses being verified on all employed staff and providers?
- Are appropriate competency reviews being performed on all staff?
- Are performance appraisal activities incorporated into the PI process?

Accreditation and Licensure
- Is the annual periodic performance review being documented and are corrective actions implemented?
- Is the organization always ready for review by accrediting and licensing agencies?
- Have adverse outcomes from past regulatory surveys been corrected?
- Have new standards and changes to standards been implemented?

PI Program Effectiveness and Recommendations

The PI program effectiveness and recommendations section outlines the areas identified and prioritized for improvement, measurement, and data collection during the next year. In large part, these recommendations are based on the findings outlined in the annual report, as well as goals identified in the organization's strategic planning process.

Check Your Understanding 15.3

1. Identify the necessary components for a complete performance improvement program review and provide examples of the basic content of each.
2. Formulate a key question that should be answered in the performance improvement program evaluation process.

Managing the Board of Directors' PI Activities

Most members of healthcare boards of directors are appointed from the community at large. It is unlikely that the directors will have specific knowledge of healthcare operations or organizations when they are first appointed, but they should be recruited based on a specific set of competencies that will help them be successful directors (Joint Commission 2016, 118). Even after serving for several years, most directors will not have expertise in clinical processes. Therefore, it is important that the individuals leading PI activities in healthcare organizations know how to optimally manage the board of directors' PI oversight responsibility.

The board's oversight responsibility is a difficult task. Most directors feel awkward judging the work of providers and other clinical staff. Coordinated systems of review are imperative to assist them in making decisions about the organization's quality of care and in taking appropriate action when necessary. The board of directors is ultimately responsible for the quality and safety of the care received by patients at their organization. This responsibility can be accomplished in a variety of ways but the following are keys to successful oversight:

- Emphasize quality and patient safety goals.
- Leverage National Quality Forum–endorsed measures.
- Use benchmarking and risk adjustment to select targets.
- Access data beyond the EHR.
- Provide data and information for multiple organizational levels.
- Develop a board-specific measurement and presentation strategy (Grossbart 2019). Figure 15.8 demonstrates one way that the results of PI monitoring can be reported.

Thus, the board's ability to perform its responsibilities is of paramount importance. As individuals are appointed to serve on the board, an orientation session should occur at the beginning of their tenure. This orientation should include initiatives and activities that the organization is participating in to improve patient care quality and safety. In addition, attention on current industry issues (such as hospital readmissions and medication errors) regarding quality of care and patient safety should be covered. Ongoing board education should occur regularly on these issues.

Regular presentation of monitoring data for boards of directors is often referred to as a **dashboard**. A dashboard report (see figure 15.9 for an example) provides minute-to-minute data on the myriad functions that various systems perform. This report "provides valuable information that is in an easily readable format and can be used as a guide for making management decisions. Dashboards are oftentimes the method used to communicate findings of the benchmarking process and ongoing performance" (White 2020, 185).

Figure 15.8. Defined, specific accountabilities related to PI throughout the hospital organization

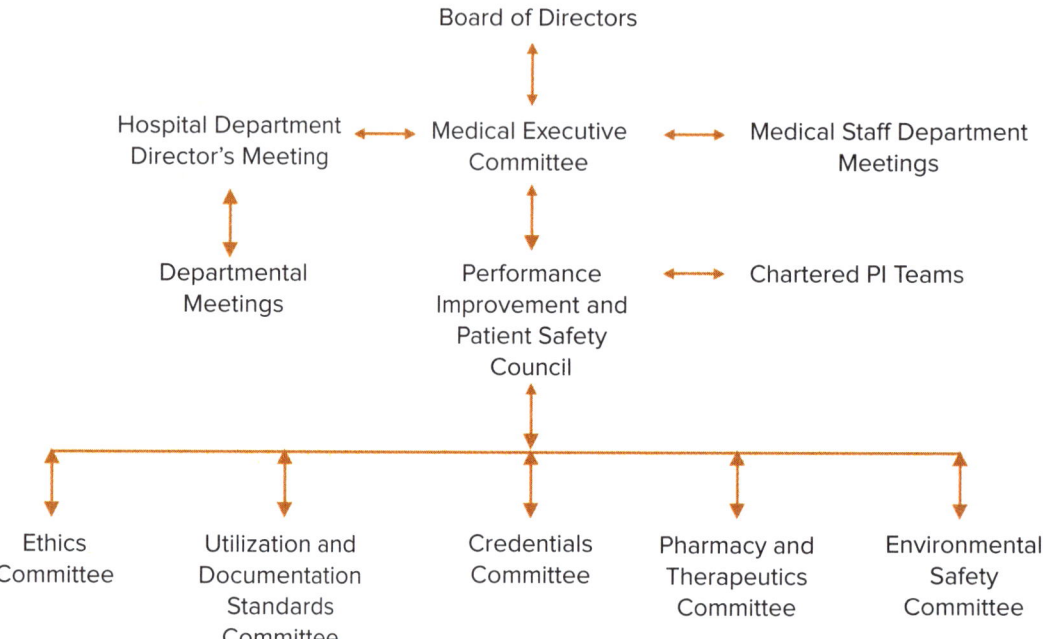

Experts recommend the following questions to boards of directors as a way to keep them focused on quality of care and patient safety:

- What is the organization's system of improvement, in terms of evaluating performance and prioritizing areas for improvement?
- How were major quality improvement efforts selected in the last two years? What criteria were used and evaluated to measure their impact?
- How does quality improvement cover the entire health system versus in-hospital improvement only?
- What analytic methods do leaders use to gather insight from the entire system to inform improvement initiatives? What are the gaps in the information and analytics?
- Recognizing that quality improvement is most sustainable when frontline staff members are engaged, how do senior leaders ensure that frontline staff lead quality improvement work, are actively providing ideas for improvement, and are willing and encouraged to speak up (Daley et al. 2018, 27)?

Ordinarily, boards of directors meet at least quarterly, whereas subcommittees of the board may meet more frequently. From the preceding discussion, it should be obvious that performance monitoring and improvement activities should be a regular subject of inquiry and decision-making at all board meetings.

Figure 15.9. Example of board of directors' dashboard report

	Goals			Prior Report	Board Goal Measurement Period
	Entry	Target	Stretch		
Implement two interventions to decrease psychiatric 30-day readmissions.	1	2	3	2	3
Optimize the treatment of heart failure patients across the continuum of care to improve care and reduce hospital readmissions.	80%	90%	95%	95%	95%
Optimize the treatment of heart failure patients across the continuum of care to improve care and reduce hospital readmissions.	1	2	3	2 of 3	3 of 3
Number of measures meeting goals: 1. Achieve 95% compliance to CBT. 2. Achieve 40% compliance to sepsis bundle. 3. Achieve 15.3% or lower mortality rate.	1 of 3	2 of 3	3 of 3	3 of 3	3 of 3
Lynch syndrome (LS) screening among colon or endometrial cancer patients	70%	80%	90%	98.2%	97.2%
Attain a reduction in the system rate of primary CAUTI for all inpatients excluding newborn and NICU patients during the third and fourth quarter. (*Note: lower is better.*)	1.967	1.833	1.699	2.00	2.29
Build a care model for children with type 1 diabetes.	75%	85%	95%	59%	87%
Improve the percentage of patients (all payers) with diabetes between age 18 and 75 seen in provider clinics who meet the 4-part bundle.	34.56%	34.56%	34.81%	37.37%	37.37%
Increase antimicrobial stewardship involvement in discharges where patient will be sent home on IV antibiotic therapy.	65%	75%	90%	97%	95%
Increase order set (pneumonia, labor induction, acute pancreatitis, and sepsis) utilization rate to 30%.	2 of 4	3 of 4	4 of 4	4 of 4	4 of 4
Increase the percentage of patients with diabetes who meet four measures of care: blood sugar control, cholesterol control, kidney function, and eye exam.	18.05%	20.05%	22.05%	18.56%	18.56%
Number of measures meeting goals: 1. Blood transfusion 2. Define clinical outcomes for development teams. 3. Decrease insta-care utilization by $25 million.	1 of 3	2 of 3	3 of 3	2 of 3	3 of 3
Improve care, cost efficiency, and resource utilization in the NICU and accurately estimate the number of babies with early-onset bacterial infection.	1 of 3	2 of 3	3 of 3	3 of 3	3 of 3
For each categorization of measures, attain Target-level performance by end of the fourth quarter.	2 of 6	4 of 6	5 of 6	5 of 6	3 of 6

Green = At or above Target
Orange = Between Entry and Target
Red = Less than Entry

Other Resources for PI Programs

In addition to the leadership and the board of directors, three other important organizational resources should be considered as organizations plan a PI program: standing committees of the medical staff, a new-hire and ongoing staff development program dedicated to understanding the approaches to and methods of PI, and formal quality management structures.

Standing Committees of the Medical Staff

Usually found in large healthcare organizations, standing committees of the medical staff have made significant contributions to improving quality in healthcare for many decades. Figure 15.8 provides an example of a hospital committee structure and demonstrates how important information is communicated throughout the organization.

Small organizations have small medical staffs and thus are not able to support standing committees dedicated solely to the quality of patient care. Consequently, a smaller organization frequently uses the executive committee of the medical staff as the "committee of the whole" to do the quality evaluation tasks traditionally executed by separate standing committees in larger organizations.

Commonly, standing committees are organized to review specific aspects of patient care services, such as ethical issues that may come up during the course of patient care; medication use (selecting, prescribing, preparing, administering, and monitoring); and the rate of healthcare-associated (nosocomial) infections. Standing committees are usually chaired by a physician who specializes in an area related to the purview of the committee. Committee members are usually drawn from the medical staff, nursing units, and administrative areas related to that specialty.

Routine review of care is usually undertaken by standing committees according to a preestablished protocol (peer review plan) stipulating criteria by which cases are selected for review. Special review of particular cases is undertaken when negative outcomes have been identified through administrative channels or through referrals from other organizational care review processes. The intent of the review is to identify case-specific patterns of care that could have achieved better outcomes had the care processes involved been better designed or implemented. Review also seeks to identify the need for education or the use of clinical practice guidelines among the clinicians or others involved in the particular area of care.

For example, one common area of care review currently focuses on cesarean section delivery of newborns. Contemporary obstetrical clinical practice guidelines define situations in which cesarean section delivery is appropriate because of the risk involved to infant and mother. When cesarean section is utilized in questionable circumstances, it is the responsibility of the obstetrical staff to determine appropriateness and make recommendations to the clinicians involved regarding better practice decisions. In healthcare settings, this type of review by colleagues is referred to as **peer review**. Peer review is a review by like professionals (peers) established according to an organization's medical staff bylaws, organizational policy and procedures, and/or the requirements of the state. Findings from peer reviews are aggregated and reported to the executive committee of the medical staff as well as to clinicians' professional files for consideration in the recredentialing process. Nursing and operations administrators also consider these findings when issues uncover opportunities for improving nursing or other patient care functions. Because standing committee reviews and findings are clear evidence that medical staff is involved in PI activities, it is important that the reviews and findings be documented in committee meeting minutes and reflected in the PI program documentation.

PI Education

In addition to ensuring that the mission, vision, and organizational goals are communicated throughout the organization, leaders should provide staff training in basic approaches to PI. Most healthcare organizations have a two-part training program that employees follow as part of the organization's new-hire orientation process, which is then repeated or supplemented annually for all staff. Generally, this training is a required competency. Frequently, organizations link the PI competency to the annual performance appraisal process, in which employees are rated on their participation on PI teams and completion of training.

The organization's leaders also need to meet established PI competencies. Training for leaders is frequently conducted with the expectation that the leaders understand and can conduct training themselves on the organization's established PI framework. Leaders are also expected to provide support and resources for staff involvement in PI activities.

Formal Quality Management Structures

Consideration of a formal quality management structure usually revolves around the question of whether an organization should develop a PI department. The answer to this question depends on a number of factors.

First, PI activities are data- and information-intensive. A PI department can help an organization manage PI-related information and activities. It can become the centralized repository of information from PI activities, and its staff can coordinate the preparation of reports that turn data collection into information for committee and board analysis and decision-making. Staff of this department can facilitate the PI committee's responsibilities and act as the organization's experts in facilitating PI team activities and using QI toolbox techniques. They can educate leaders and staff on PI principles, data collection, data analysis, and any regulatory changes as they occur. Finally, they can take the lead in the development of functional and cross-functional PI teams and organization-wide reporting of PI activities to quality councils and boards of directors. When used effectively within an existing PI culture, these resource departments support a healthcare organization's PI initiatives.

However, it is important to consider whether an organization is developing a PI department to deflect and perhaps hide its unwillingness to commit to a more authentic PI culture. Some organizations develop PI departments to keep from having to develop organization-wide, multidisciplinary, integrated PI processes and to avoid having to deal with issues inherent in developing a more empowered nonmanagement staff.

Creating an authentic PI culture is a daunting task for many organizations, even when the leaders are committed to the process. Commitment begins with establishing an educational process for the entire organization in the application of PI techniques. Creating a PI department allows the organization to centralize its quality efforts.

In an organization with a healthy, evolving PI culture, the PI department oversees PI efforts, ensures that individual departments complete their PI activities and meet reporting deadlines, and monitors the organizational culture to make sure that a healthy PI philosophy is developed and maintained.

Check Your Understanding 15.4

1. Kevin is a member of the PI team at a local hospital. As part of his PI team duties, he is tasked with presenting the PI team's quality data to the hospital's board of directors. He is currently presenting this information through numerous spreadsheets and graphs, but because of the volume of data the board must review, Kevin feels that the board is overwhelmed by the amount of data presented to them. He is looking for a solution to provide this information to the board in a more succinct manner. Recommend a tool for Kevin and his PI team and provide a rationale for your recommendation.

2. Explain why it is critical for hospitals to utilize a peer review process.

QI Toolbox Techniques

 Leadership teams in healthcare use dashboards, decision matrixes, and SWOT analysis to guide them in assessing the status of their current operations, making decisions for the future, developing strategy for the organization, and aligning these decisions with their mission, vision, and values.

Dashboard

A dashboard report provides minute-to-minute data on the myriad functions its various systems perform. It may also be used to communicate findings of a benchmarking process. An example is shown in figure 15.9. This report presents information in an easy to read and understandable format and can be used to guide management decision-making.

Decision Matrix

A decision matrix assists in evaluating and prioritizing a list of potential improvement opportunities (ASQ 2023). An example is shown in figure 15.4. Healthcare organizations have many competing opportunities for improvement and must determine which potential improvement will yield the greatest overall benefit to the organization and its customers.

SWOT Analysis

Strategic planning may include the use of a tool known as a SWOT analysis, which is an assessment of the organization's *Strengths*, *Weaknesses*, *Opportunities*, and *Threats*. Findings from SWOT analyses are used to validate the organizational mission and set the direction for the coming year. As part of the analysis, the organization's leaders carefully consider community input, staff input, customer needs and expectations, outcome information from PI activities, and other data.

Case Study

When a large regional medical center became part of an integrated delivery system that had a central board of directors, the medical center's board began to struggle with its revised role. The new organizational environment included several outpatient clinics, multispecialty provider practices, and an insurance entity. Many of the current board members had served the organization since the medical center was built, and board activities had always been conducted in a certain way. The administration rigidly controlled board meetings. Board members did not ask questions and routinely approved committee reports. The reports covered topics such as the organization's financial status and future financial plans, provider credentialing, care quality monitoring, new policies, and plans for a new hospital.

A new board member with a healthcare background was appointed after extensive screening and a personal interview with the executive committee. This board member was not part of the local business power structure, and the administration was concerned that her appointment might not be a wise move. During her first board meeting, two very interesting reports were given. One report detailed some reengineering projects. One of these involved redesigning nursing staffing patterns. This redesign decreased the number of registered nurses (RNs), and replaced them with licensed practical nurses (LPNs) and certified nursing assistants (CNAs). The current quality report documented a very high quality of care and positive patient satisfaction surveys. Data excerpted from this report can be seen in the "1st Quarter" column of table 15.1. Given that this was her first board meeting, the new board member remained silent and did not ask questions.

Table 15.1. Case study data

Quality Performance Measure	1st Quarter	2nd Quarter
Medication errors	3.20%	10.42%
Patient falls	4.21%	8.56%
Cesarean sections	14.21%	17.87%
Rate of vaginal births after C-section	18.27%	15.72%
Healthcare-associated infections	1.78%	4.85%
X-ray discrepancies	0.15%	0.21%
Patient Satisfaction Measure	**1st Quarter**	**2nd Quarter**
Overall service	40.52%	20.74%
Overall clinical	86.72%	70.82%
Overall quality of service	45.40%	22.34%
Food	30.56%	32.54%
Overall cleanliness	85.89%	83.26%

Within four months, the new nursing staffing pattern had been launched. Data excerpted from the quality indicators report presented to the board can be seen in the "2nd Quarter" column of table 15.1. After reviewing the data presented by the chief nursing officer (CNO), the new board member was very concerned and decided to ask if the values in the quality report, which show a negative trend, were for the nursing units with the new nursing staffing patterns. The CNO reported that there was a direct correlation. This answer-initiated discussion among other board members who were accustomed to using quality indicators in their businesses. This was the first substantive board-level discussion that the new board member had seen. One board member wanted to know whether any data had been gathered from patient focus groups. Another board member asked whether the average length-of-stay had increased, and someone else asked about a cost–benefit analysis of the new staffing patterns. Following the usual process, the chair called for approval of the report and presentation of the next item on the agenda.

Case Study Questions

1. What changes or patterns do you see in the data?
2. Has the medical center CEO carried out their responsibility for educating the board? Why or why not?
3. Has hospital leadership empowered the board to fulfill their role in the organization? Why or why not? What strategies would you recommend at this point?
4. What quality data should be reported and utilized by this board of directors?

Review Questions

1. Which group has ultimate responsibility for maintaining the quality and safety of patient care provided by the healthcare organization?
   a. Board of directors
   b. Executive team
   c. Nursing leadership
   d. State board of licensure

2. Using the four reasons why healthcare organizations evaluate their performance improvement plan, provide an example of how this evaluation might occur in regard to each reason.

3. Governance, management, and employed staff are key to a healthcare organization's success as they work together to identify community needs and pursue organizational goals. Provide an example of how each of these key groups might accomplish this.

4. Medical staff standing committees are organized to review specific aspects of patient care services. List two of these areas.

5. Why are organization-wide strategic planning and planning for performance improvement interrelated activities?
   a. Because strategic planning sets the overall direction and goals, while performance improvement focuses on optimizing processes to achieve those goals.
   b. Because both activities are mandated by regulatory bodies and must be executed simultaneously.
   c. Because performance improvement is a subset of strategic planning, addressing only short-term goals.
   d. Because strategic planning is solely concerned with financial outcomes, while performance improvement focuses on operational efficiency.

References

ASQ (American Society of Quality). 2023. "What is a Decision Matrix?" https://asq.org/quality-resources/decision-matrix.

Conway, J. 2008. Getting boards on board: Engaging governing boards in quality and safety. *The Joint Commission Journal of Quality and Patient Safety* 34:214–220.

Daley U. E., T. K. Gandhi, K. Mate, J. Whittington, M. Renton, and J. Huebner. 2018. Framework for Effective Board Governance of Health System Quality. Boston: Institute for Healthcare Improvement. https://www.ihi.org/resources/white-papers/framework-effective-board-governance-health-system-quality.

Grossbart, S. 2019. "Engaging Health System Boards of Trustees in Quality and Safety: Six Must-Know Guidelines." https://www.healthcatalyst.com/insights/healthcare-boards-quality-safety-pivotal-role.

Joint Commission. 2016. *Getting the Board on Board: What Your Board Needs to Know about Quality and Patient Safety*, 3rd ed. Oakbrook Terrace, IL: Joint Commission Resources.

Leonhardt, K. K. 2023. "Refocus Your Board's Attention on Quality and Patient Safety." The Joint Commission. https://www.jointcommission.org/resources/news-and-multimedia/blogs/dateline-tjc/2023/09/refocus-your-boards-attention-on-quality-and-patient-safety/#:~:text=Previous%20Post-,Refocus%20Your%20Board%E2%80%99s%20Attention%20on%20Quality%20and%20Patient%20Safety,-09/27/2023.

White, S. 2020. "Healthcare Data Analytics: Impact of Sampling." Chapter 16 in *Health Information Management: Concepts, Principles, and Practice*, 6th ed., edited by P. K. Oachs and A. L. Watters. Chicago: AHIMA.

Resources

Erwin, C. O., A. Y. Landry, A. C. Livingston, and A. Dias. 2019. Effective governance and hospital boards revisited: Reflections on 25 years of research. *Medical Care Research and Review* 76(2):131–166.

Gandhi, T. K. and G. R. Yates. 2024. "Boards can be safety champions." AHA Trustee Services. https://trustees.aha.org/articles/1244-hospital-boards-can-be-safety-champions.

Joint Commission. 2024. *Hospital Accreditation Manual*. Oakbrook Terrace, IL: Joint Commission Resources.

Navigating the Accreditation, Certification, and Licensure Process

16

Learning Objectives

- Explain the performance improvement perspectives of accreditation, certification, and licensure organizations
- Distinguish the various approaches of accreditation, certification, and licensure agencies to the site visit and survey
- Identify approaches that lead to success in the survey process

Key Terms

Accreditation
Accreditation standards
Certification
Compliance
Compulsory reviews
Conditions of Participation
Deemed status
Document review
Exit conference

Licensure
Opening conference
Quality improvement organizations (QIOs)
Site visit
Survey team
Tracer methodology
Triggers
Voluntary reviews

The complexities of accreditation, certification, and licensure requirements can have a significant impact on healthcare organizations. Few healthcare professionals work in the industry for long without taking part in one of these three processes. This chapter provides a basic introduction to the concepts and processes involved.

Accreditation is the act of granting approval to a healthcare organization that has demonstrated satisfactory quality of service. The approval is based on the organization voluntarily meeting a set of **accreditation standards** developed by the accreditation agency. These standards serve as the basis for comparative assessment during the review or survey process and confirm the quality of the services that the healthcare organization provides. The Joint Commission is an example of an accreditation agency. Hospitals accredited by the Joint Commission have a competitive advantage over nonaccredited hospitals in their geographical area because the Joint Commission "stamp of approval" lets the consumer know that they are receiving care from an organization that meets higher standards.

Licensure is a state's act of granting a healthcare organization or an individual healthcare practitioner permission to provide services of a defined scope in a specified geographical area. State governments issue licenses based on regulations specific to healthcare practices. For example, states issue licenses to individual hospitals, physicians, and nurses. It is illegal for organizations and professionals to provide healthcare services without a license.

Certification grants approval for a healthcare organization to provide services to a specific group of beneficiaries. For example, healthcare organizations must meet the federal *Conditions of Participation* to receive funding through the Medicare and Medicaid programs (42 CFR 482). These programs are administered by the Centers for Medicare and Medicaid Services (CMS), an agency of the Department of Health and Human Services. (The term *certification* also refers to status granted to individual healthcare practitioners by a professional association when they fulfill certain criteria, such as level of education, years of work experience, and/or passing an exam. In this chapter we use the term to refer to healthcare organization certification.)

Healthcare Accreditation, Certification, and Licensure Standards

In healthcare today, many different agencies develop and monitor standards for the quality of healthcare services. These agencies accomplish their missions through a comprehensive review process. Some of the review processes are compulsory, and others are voluntary. **Compulsory reviews** are performed to fulfill legal or licensure requirements. **Voluntary reviews** are conducted at the request of the healthcare facility seeking accreditation or certification.

Every accreditation, certification, and licensure agency develops written standards or regulations that serve as the basis for the review process. It is imperative that healthcare facilities monitor any changes and updates to the standards and regulations and keep current sets on hand at all times to help maintain compliance status. **Compliance** is the process of meeting a prescribed set of standards or regulations to maintain active accreditation, licensure, or certification status. Standards and regulations may be provided in manuals, such as the Joint Commission's *Hospital Accreditation Standards*, or in state and federal regulations, such as the CMS *Conditions of Participation*.

The Joint Commission and Its Accreditation Activities

The Joint Commission has been the most visible organization responsible for accrediting healthcare organizations since the mid-1950s. The Joint Commission describes its mission as follows:

> To continuously improve health care for the public, in collaboration with other stakeholders, by evaluating health care organizations and inspiring them to excel in providing safe and effective care of the highest quality and value (Joint Commission 2024a).

The primary focus of the Joint Commission is to determine whether organizations seeking accreditation are continually monitoring and improving the quality of care they provide. The Joint Commission requires that this continual improvement process (also called continuous improvement process) be in place throughout the entire organization, from the governing body down, as well as across all department lines.

The typical Joint Commission accreditation standards manual contains the following major chapter topics:

- Leadership
- Provision of care, treatment, and services
- Medication management
- Infection prevention and control
- Information management
- Medical staff
- Nursing
- Performance improvement
- National Patient Safety Goals
- Environment of care
- Emergency management
- Life safety
- Record of care, treatment, and services
- Rights and responsibilities of the individual
- Human resources
- Transplant safety
- Waived testing (Joint Commission 2024b)

Within each chapter, the standards associated with each topic are cited and then elaborated upon with elements of performance (EPs) that directly communicate the intent of the Joint Commission with respect to each standard. In addition, a scoring guideline is provided that allows the organization to score itself on each EP and thus get a sum total on each standard.

DNV Accreditation

The National Integrated Accreditation for Healthcare Organizations (NIAHO), offered by DNV, has attracted quite a few healthcare organizations for its accreditation processes incorporating the ISO 9001 standards (globally recognized standards for quality management). Organizations must comply or be certified as compliant with the ISO 9001 standards and the NIAHO standards for accreditation. This accrediting body has become an alternative option for healthcare organizations because of its facility-friendly yet stringent accreditation philosophy. In 2008, DNV GL, now DNV, was granted deeming authority (discussed later in this chapter) from CMS (DNV 2024).

CARF Accreditation

In 1966, the Commission on Accreditation of Rehabilitation Facilities (CARF) was established. Now known as CARF International, the private, nonprofit organization is committed to developing and maintaining practical customer-focused standards to help organizations measure and improve the quality, value, and outcomes of behavioral health and medical rehabilitation programs. CARF accreditation is based on an organization's commitment to continually enhance the quality of its services and programs and to focus on customer satisfaction (CARF 2023a). In an effort to draw greater attention to healthcare quality issues, CARF developed their Aspire to Excellence framework for quality improvement. This framework includes the following six areas: assessment of the environment, setting strategy, obtaining input from persons served and other stakeholders, implementing the plan, reviewing results, and effecting change (CARF 2023b).

National Committee for Quality Assurance

The National Committee for Quality Assurance (NCQA) began accrediting managed care organizations in 1991. Since then, the NCQA's activities have broadened to include accreditation of managed behavioral health organizations and credentials verification for physician organizations. As a private, nonprofit organization, the NCQA is dedicated to improving the quality of healthcare by assessing and reporting on the nation's managed care health insurance plans. Its efforts are focused on the development of performance measurements in key areas such as member satisfaction, quality of care, access to care, and service. The NCQA uses the Healthcare Effectiveness Data and Information Set (HEDIS) to accomplish these assessments of managed care plans. The performance measures in HEDIS are related to significant public health issues and are a basis for purchasers and consumers to compare the performance of managed care plans.

For example, University Hospital has a contractual relationship with a health plan in its region. Health plan quality management officials come to University Hospital to review cases against selected HEDIS screenings for health maintenance. This information is used in the negotiations for contract renewal, and University Hospital receives information from the health plan on how well it is meeting the required screens. In turn, HEDIS data, along with NCQA accreditation, provide organizations a method for selecting health insurance plans or providers based on demonstrated value rather than simply on cost (NCQA 2023).

Accreditation Association for Ambulatory Health Care

The Accreditation Association for Ambulatory Health Care (AAAHC) surveys and accredits ambulatory care facilities, with a primary focus on ambulatory surgery centers. In addition, AAAHC also accredits multispecialty and single-specialty group practices, dental group practices, community and student health services, independent practice associations, employer-based and retail clinics, and endoscopy, diagnostic imaging, and radiation oncology centers (AAAHC 2024).

CMS *Conditions of Participation*

Every healthcare organization that provides services to Medicare and Medicaid beneficiaries must demonstrate compliance with the CMS *Conditions of Participation* (CMS 2023). The compliance process is known as certification (discussed later in this chapter), and it is usually carried out by state departments of health. The *Conditions of Participation* for healthcare facilities cover issues related to medical necessity, level of care, and quality of care. CMS also contracts with nongovernmental agencies across the country to monitor the care provided by independent healthcare practitioners. These agencies, called **quality improvement organizations (QIOs)**, retrospectively review patient records to ensure that the care provided meets the federal standards for medical necessity, level of care, and quality of care.

State Licensure

Every healthcare facility must have a license to operate in the state in which it is located. This license grants the facility the legal authority to provide healthcare services within its scope of services. To maintain its licensed status, the organization must adhere to state regulations that govern issues related to staffing, physical facilities, services provided, documentation requirements, and quality of care. The regulations are usually monitored and evaluated on a regular basis by the licensing agencies of state departments of health. Many state health departments publish online "report cards" on the performance of the organizations they license.

Check Your Understanding 16.1

1. What is the role of quality improvement organizations in quality of care?
2. Central City Surgical Center is interested in external accreditation for their organization. They would like an accrediting body that specializes in outpatient surgical centers. Which of the following would be the most appropriate accreditation process for this surgical center?
   a. AAAHC
   b. CARF
   c. NCQA
   d. DNV

Development of Policies and Procedures to Meet Multiple Standards and Regulations

At a minimum, healthcare organizations must consider state licensure regulations when they develop policies and procedures that relate to the documentation and quality of their healthcare services. When a facility provides care to patients who are Medicare and/or Medicaid beneficiaries, it must determine which of the *Conditions of Participation* apply. When a facility is accredited by an accreditation organization, those standards must also be taken into consideration.

To ensure compliance, the healthcare organization must continually review its operating policies and procedures to make sure they reflect ongoing changes to accreditation standards and federal and state regulations that may affect the scope of care and services provided. The organization should identify the most stringent standard or regulation for each aspect of care and base its organizational policies and procedures on that standard or regulation. For example, when a healthcare facility is setting its policy on charting by exception, it must review the state licensure regulations for their requirements. Then the organization must review the *Conditions of Participation* regulations for their requirements. Finally, it must review all relevant accreditation standards. The strictest of all standards should be written into the policy and procedure for chart documentation by exception.

Surviving the Survey Process

Ongoing foresight and planning are the keys to successful completion of accreditation and licensure reviews. The leaders of the healthcare organization must stay focused on the organization's accreditation, certification, and licensure status to ensure that these issues are not overlooked in the flurry of day-to-day operations. Preparation for accreditation and licensure processes cannot be accomplished a few weeks before the organization is due for review. A solid accreditation and licensure infrastructure must be built and maintained so that the organization is ready for an inspection at any time.

Some accreditation processes are scheduled and others are unannounced. The Joint Commission's progression over the years from scheduled triennial surveys to periodic self-assessments and unannounced surveys represents a gradual paradigm shift in its attitude toward survey readiness, which has become increasingly stringent. State agencies representing state licensing or federal Medicare and Medicaid certification programs may conduct unannounced surveys. State licensing agencies make unannounced visits to healthcare organizations in response to complaints and reports of sentinel events. In order to prepare for an accreditation site visit, many hospitals conduct a mock survey that includes the same type of activities and tasks that accreditors perform when on site.

CMS accepts accreditation by organizations with deeming authority in granting what it calls **deemed status**. When granting deemed status, CMS assumes that the organization meets the *Conditions of Participation* if it is currently accredited by one of these organizations. In addition, CMS may conduct a validation survey of accredited facilities to ensure compliance with the *Conditions of Participation*. Many state licensing agencies routinely survey organizations to qualify them for deemed status.

A review process with any of these agencies is more than just an issue of appearances. The reviewing agency becomes part of, and observes, the day-to-day operations of the healthcare organization. For example, surveyors from the Joint Commission want to be assured that the facility's leadership and staff can successfully execute organizational policies and procedures. They want to confirm that the leadership and staff are continuously monitoring and improving organizational performance and that those improvements are tied to the organization's strategic plan. Therefore, surveyors will want to validate these aspects as operative in the organization when they arrive for a review.

Although state licensure surveys may be more focused on a facility's ability to meet department of health regulations, the emphasis is still on high-quality care. It is important to remember that the goal of reviewers is to help healthcare organizations consider their own performance. Members of the organization are often too close to everyday activities and events to recognize important trends or consequences of the organization's inaction.

There is no standard review process for accrediting and licensing agencies. Processes may change from year to year as philosophies change within the agencies. In general, voluntary accreditation processes, such as those of the Joint Commission and CARF, are more flexible and tailored to the type of organization being reviewed. Governmental processes tend to be more bureaucratic.

Following is an overview of the more prominent accreditation and licensure processes.

Accreditation of Acute Care and Other Facilities: The Joint Commission

Currently, the Joint Commission's accreditation survey process is an unscheduled one. This approach shifts the organization's focus from survey preparation to continuous survey readiness because Joint Commission surveyors may show up at any time during a predefined window of opportunity to perform the accreditation survey. An organization interested in becoming accredited by the Joint Commission must file an application that provides information on organization type, services provided, certain statistical characteristics, and the names of its executive officers.

Most organizations undergo a **site visit**, an in-person review conducted by an accreditation survey team. The site visit is generally unannounced and occurs 18 to 36 months after the organization's previous full survey. Accredited organizations also submit a midpoint self-assessment, the timing of which will vary. This self-assessment facilitates a more continuous, efficient accreditation process. The organization evaluates itself against applicable standards and submits a written progress report to the Joint Commission. As part of this assessment, the organization also must submit a corrective action plan. The organization's chief executive officer must attest to the accuracy of the self-assessment and corrective action plan. At the time of the triennial survey, surveyors will devote their time to validating the resolution of action plans submitted.

Hospitals must notify the state licensure organization of the occurrence of a Joint Commission site visit and must announce it to the public through postings throughout the facility. This announcement allows the public the opportunity to meet with the **survey team**, a group of individuals sent by an accrediting agency to review a healthcare organization for accreditation purposes, to discuss any issues of concern. Failure to post these notifications may impact the final accreditation decision. The Joint Commission may also preschedule the state licensing organization to accompany its survey for CMS *Conditions of Participation* validation.

Survey Team

The composition of a Joint Commission survey team will vary depending on the size of the organization. It may include a physician, an administrator, a registered nurse, and other master's-level clinicians. Representatives from state licensing agencies who have arranged to join the survey for their own examination of the organization for licensing and CMS validation purposes may bring a survey team that may include a physician, nurse, pharmacist, nutritionist, and/or life safety professional. Since 2005, most survey teams have included an expert in environment of care and life safety issues. The Joint Commission surveyors have many years of experience practicing in the healthcare industry. Every surveyor undergoes considerable training in Joint Commission accreditation processes prior to being assigned to a survey team. The Joint Commission requires surveyors to successfully complete a surveyor certification examination to participate in healthcare organization surveys.

Survey Process

Surveyors tailor review activities to the characteristics and services of the organization under review. These activities are based on information, data, and the corrective action plans provided in the midpoint self-assessment. It is important to remember that Joint Commission processes are not static from year to year because the Joint Commission institutes regular improvements in its own survey processes. Any healthcare professional preparing for a Joint Commission accreditation survey must be aware of the current requirements, constraints, and expectations of surveyors.

The survey process lasts three to five days, depending on the size and complexity of the organization. For a large and highly complex organization, such as a university medical center, the accreditation survey activities most likely will last five days.

The site visit begins with an opening preliminary planning session at which the surveyors review current documentation from the organization. Depending on the type of organization to be surveyed, they would expect to review lists of sites eligible for survey and the services provided at each site, performance improvement (PI) data from the last 12 months, infection-related data, environment of care data, patient and resident rosters, and data specifically developed for the organization's compliance with Joint Commission standards ("measure of success" data). Following the preliminary planning session, the organization's leaders are expected to provide an overview of the organization's mission and vision, strategic goals and objectives, current experiences and outcomes, and performance monitoring and improvement activities. If the organization is experiencing significant new challenges in any areas, it is expected to identify those areas for the surveyors. Information about the organization's recent achievements is very important as well, because the surveyors want an accurate picture of the status of the organization.

Surveyors are interested in seeing how members of the organization collaborate to provide healthcare services and products, how they measure the quality of those services and products, and how they identify and develop opportunities for improvement. Therefore, the **opening conference**, a meeting conducted at the beginning of the accreditation site visit during which the surveyors outline the schedule of activities and list any individuals whom they would like to interview, is an important opportunity for the organization to set the tone for the survey process.

Surveyors arrive with knowledge of the organization from its midpoint self-assessment action plan, any consumer complaints reported to the Joint Commission, previous accreditation data, core measure data, and other information related to the organization's performance. Having this knowledge allows surveyors to tailor the on-site survey process to critical areas of focus called priority focus areas (PFAs). These PFAs include processes, systems, and structures within the organization known to significantly impact patient safety and quality of care.

The on-site survey utilizes a **tracer methodology** that permits assessment of operational systems and processes in relation to the actual experiences of selected patients currently under the organization's care. Tracer methodology analyzes an organization's systems, with particular attention to identified PFAs, by following individual patients through the organization's healthcare process in the sequence experienced by its patients. Patients are selected on the basis of the current census of patients that the organization identifies as typical of its case mix. As cases are examined in relation to the actual care processes, the surveyor may identify performance issues or trends in one or more steps of the process or in the interfaces between processes. Patients selected on subsequent days may be chosen based on the issues raised.

The Joint Commission's accreditation process emphasizes a systems approach to evaluate continuous improvement in key safety and quality areas. The performance reports of accredited organizations emphasize information that demonstrates an organization's commitment to quality and safety, such as achieving the National Patient Safety Goals (NPSGs), performing well in mandated core measures, or obtaining disease-specific care certification.

Surveyors visit patient care settings and conduct interviews with selected patients, department and program staff, and the organization's leaders. During the patient-specific tracer interviews on nursing units and in clinics, the surveyors gain firsthand knowledge about how well the staff understands current treatment objectives for the patient and how well that treatment is coordinated across all the care modalities available in the organization.

During interviews with various staff members and organization leaders, surveyors gain insight into the organization's recent successes and current challenges. They expect to gain insight into the management philosophy of the organization and the means by which the organization implements change as a result of PI. As surveyors "trace" caregiving to specific patients in patient care settings, their mission is to verify at the first-line level of employees the status of the organization as conveyed in presurvey documents and in the opening conference. They want to see that staff members in direct contact with patients know and carry out policies and procedures that managers and leadership have developed for the important issues that healthcare organizations encounter. Taking the patient's care in its specific context, surveyors want staff to be able to explain how the patient came to be in the hospital, what the current diagnoses and therapies are (particularly medications), and the rationales for their use. If the patient came through the emergency department, they may want to visit the area where the patient was treated and examine its processes. If the patient required surgery in the operating suite, they may want to visit that care site and examine its processes. If the patient had a procedure in interventional radiology, they may want to visit the radiologic suite and examine its processes as they relate to the tracer patient's specific care. They will expect to see all areas adhering to policy regarding staff communication, patient rights, and patient safety in addition to the everyday processes of providing patient care.

As the tracer activities progress, general themes may begin to emerge, showing that staff may not be as well prepared or as conversant as is necessary. Table 16.1 shows aspects of the nursing process that emerged at University Hospital during the first day's tracer activities. These themes were communicated to nurse managers so that on subsequent days staff could be better prepared to discuss these aspects with surveyors.

Table 16.1A. Nursing themes and actions

Accreditation and Licensing Survey—Nursing	
Common Theme	Action
Date/time of progress notes and orders	Review all orders and notes.
Do not use abbreviations	Review all orders.
Pain assessments	Know your policy practice on when an assessment/reassessment is done and where it is documented in your area.
Admission/discharge criteria	Know your area's criteria; refer to your Statement of Conditions.
Restraints	We start with least restrictive. All four side rails up is considered a restraint!
Hand hygiene	Artificial nails are not allowed in ICU, OR, NICU, and ED units.
High-alert medications	Focus on insulin administration (especially drips).
Infant security	Articulate your role in Code Pink, 6C, and 6H; know your policy regarding ID badges, family, lists, exits, etc.
Moderate sedation	Know the policy in your area. Concentrate on preprocedure assessments (especially airway).
Staffing	Managers and charge nurses should be able to speak to your practice.

Table 16.1B. Nursing themes and actions (*Continued*)

Accreditation and Licensing Survey—Nursing	
Common Theme	**Action**
Fire extinguishers	Ensure that staff know the location of the fire extinguishers. All Behavioral Health staff should have keys to the fire extinguishers.
Communication between levels of care	Know your organization's practice of communicating pertinent clinical data to the next level of care, to the primary care provider, and to referral findings.
Assessment for falls	Ensure that patients have risk assessments for falls, and communicate information on high-risk patients to the next level of care or to their diagnostic care areas.
Infection control	Know the surveillance in your area. Specific risk assessment and monitoring for long-term care.
Medication storage	Ensure proper storage of medications.
Loose needles	All needles need to be in a locked area so staff and/or patients do not have access to them.
Infant security; rescue drills	Look into "apron" that will hold four infants for one staff member to evacuate.
Assessment and reassessment	Ensure that all data required to be collected for an assessment are completed. Reassess in appropriate time frame and document your findings.
Documentation	Ensure that all care is documented.

Table 16.2 notes themes regarding all staff that emerged on the first day of tracer activities at the hospital.

Table 16.2A. Multidisciplinary themes and actions

Accreditation and Licensing Survey—Multidisciplinary	
Common Theme	**Action**
Range orders	Articulate the process when writing and administrating a range order.
Post anesthesia notes by an attending	Notes required in chart within 48 hours.
Medication lists (outpatient)	Outpatient is to focus the surveyors on the medication list.
Problem list (outpatient)	Outpatient is to focus the surveyors on the problem list.
Dietary consults	Ensure consults are done in the time frame required by policy.
Lab results	Know your lab results, why you are treating, and when you will need to repeat a test, especially microbiology (know the organism) and the antibiotic.
Nutrition assessment	Know your practice as to when a nutrition assessment is completed and when a referral is needed.
Provider privileges	Remember to always look up a provider's privileges on the Medical Staff website prior to the procedure.
Do not resuscitate orders	Document patient or family involvement in decision making.
Staffing effectiveness	Articulate two HR indicators (hours per patient day [HPPD] and per diem staff) and two Clinical Indicators (patient falls and patient complaints). Initially, we looked at entire hospital—no correlation. Narrowed it down to areas where falls and patient complaints were common—no correlation. Now we're looking at time of day and whether overtime is a factor.
Performance improvement	Direct surveyor to PI projects and articulate the process: data before—process/intervention—data after.
Sample medications	Know your practice and the policy.
Forms	Identify short history forms in procedure areas that could/should be consistent across the organization.

Table 16.2B. Multidisciplinary themes and actions (*Continued*)

Accreditation and Licensing Survey—Multidisciplinary	
Common Theme	**Action**
Clean/dirty utility areas	If in the same room, ensure proper designation.
Oxygen containers on wheels	If possible, keep all portable O_2 in the O_2 (yellow) storage areas.
Patient identifiable information/white boards	Patient identifiable information visible. White boards have too many patient identifiers.
Respiration therapy assessments/reassessments	Articulate your practice for a full assessment, especially if level of care changes.
"Time Out"	Ensure that this is documented for all required invasive procedures.
Preventive maintenance of biomedical equipment	Ensure that equipment is up to date. Biomed will maintain records.
Functional assessment—referrals for OT/PT/speech	Know your process for how to make referrals and document referrals.
Fire extinguishers	Ensure that staff know the locations of the fire extinguishers. All Behavioral Health staff should have keys to the fire extinguishers.
Communication among levels of care	Know your practice of communicating pertinent clinical data to the next level of care, to the primary care provider, and referral findings.
Infection control	Know the surveillance in your area. Specific risk assessment and monitoring for long-term care.

Triggers are alerts to a possible or actual adverse event or patient safety issue in a healthcare organization. Trigger issues encountered during visits to care settings and tracer activities are reviewed with staff and leadership during special issue-resolution sessions at the end of each day. These discussion sessions among surveyors and leadership may resolve issues to the surveyors' satisfaction. If issues appear significant or systemic, surveyors may request to review closed patient records retrospectively to get a picture of how the organization has handled the same issues involving the same kinds of patients over time. Alternatively, they may request reports of organizational sampling around the trigger issue from the past or concurrent to the survey. Some trigger issues on which Joint Commission surveyors focus include patient rights, communication, medication use, information management, and general safety in the care environment. Whatever the trigger issues are, the organization's leaders must be aware of them and must implement a corrective action plan.

In addition to individual patient tracer activities, surveyors also conduct leadership interviews and "system tracers." Leadership interviews typically involve talking to top administration and medical staff officials about overall systems issues. For example, the medical staff leadership interview reviews in detail the credentialing activities and processes and medical staff oversight of teaching programs. The environment of care leadership interview reviews all aspects of the organization's environment of care and disaster management processes. Results of ongoing monitoring are reviewed, and PI activities are discussed.

System tracers convene responsible individuals from across the organization to examine the following organizational issues relevant to patient care:

- The medication management system tracer reviews all aspects of the appropriate and safe preparation, distribution, and administration of medications in the organization.
- The data management system tracer examines how the organization uses data and information for quality and PI activities as well as for ongoing monitoring of important functions.
- The infection control system tracer examines the infection control program, processes, interventions, and outcomes.

After completion of the tracers, system tracers, interviews, and visits to patient care areas, the survey team sequesters itself to consider its findings. The team develops a preliminary report of the on-site survey and identifies any deficiencies that it perceives are evident in the organization.

After the team develops the preliminary report, surveyors, members of the organization's leadership team, and a representative from the state licensing agency, if applicable, reconvene for an **exit conference**. During the exit conference, Joint Commission surveyors summarize their findings and explain any deficiencies identified during the site visit. Leaders have a brief opportunity to discuss the surveyors' perspectives or to provide additional information related to any deficiencies. Deficiencies are reported to the organization as requirements for improvement (RFIs). Finally, the surveyors report the probable accreditation decision of the Joint Commission on the basis of the survey findings.

The Joint Commission uses five categories to report its decisions on accreditation. These decisions are listed in figure 16.1.

Figure 16.1. Joint Commission accreditation decisions

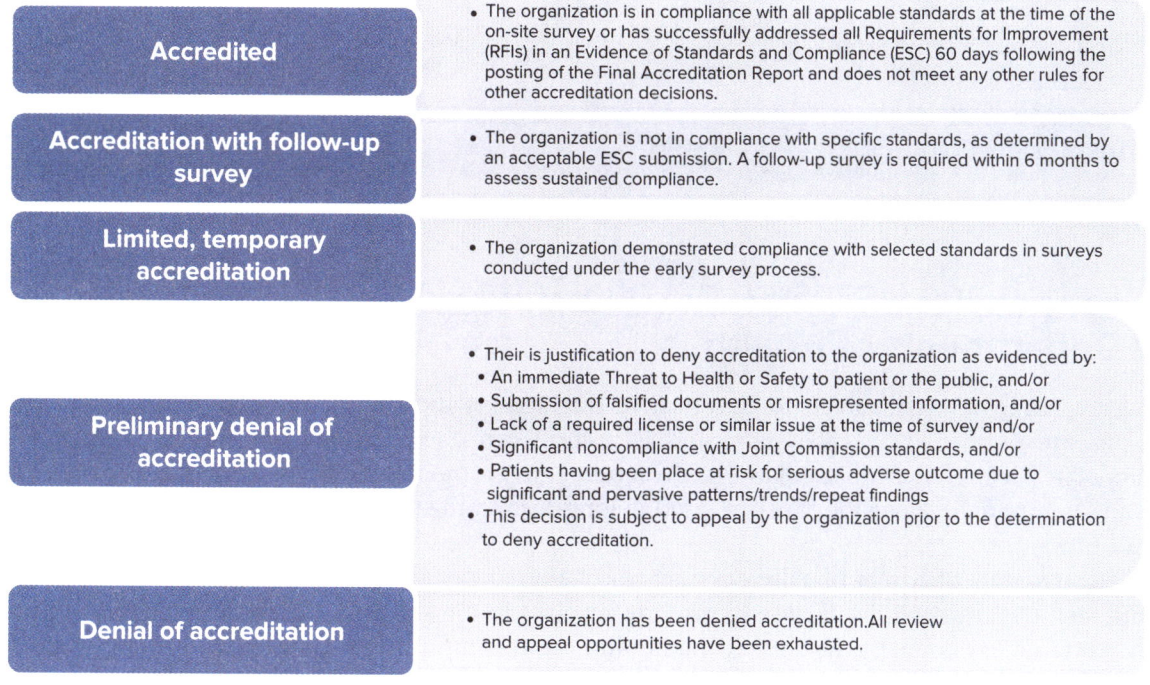

Source: Adapted from Joint Commission 2024c

All other Joint Commission–sponsored accreditations follow the same basic survey process as outlined for acute care. Site visits begin with an opening conference, proceed to care unit visits using tracer methodology (which can include a client's home in home health accreditation), and close with an exit conference.

Public Disclosure

All organizations currently accredited by the Joint Commission have quality reports published by the Commission on its website, Quality Check. Here, consumers can see how the organization has performed on implementing NPSGs and national quality improvement goals, and they can see the organization's accreditation history (Joint Commission 2023d).

Check Your Understanding 16.2

1. Community Hospital has recently been accredited by the Joint Commission for a full three-year period. Based on its accreditation status, CMS assumes that Community Hospital meets the *Conditions of Participation*. The reason CMS makes this assumption is because the Joint Commission has been granted _____.
   a. Compliance
   b. Deemed status
   c. Document review
   d. Performance improvement

2. During a recent Joint Commission survey, one of the survey team members asked a nurse in the ICU about her patient. The surveyor asked the nurse about the medications the patient was on and also asked the nurse to explain how those medications were ordered and received from the pharmacy. After the nurse explained this process, the surveyor then went to the pharmacy and asked the pharmacist to explain his role in the medication process for this specific patient. The surveyor is utilizing which process?
   a. Medication reconciliation
   b. Document review
   c. Drug diversion
   d. Tracer methodology

Certification and Licensure of Long-Term Care Facilities: State Departments of Health

Long-term care facilities are subject to government-directed certification and licensure programs. Licensure regulations are published by each state, and long-term care facilities are expected to comply with the regulations. In addition to state regulations, the federal government developed its own set of regulations in 1974 in an attempt to improve the care provided in long-term care facilities that receive federal Medicare and Medicaid funds.

State departments of health usually conduct unscheduled reviews of long-term care facilities. All long-term care facilities must have a license to provide services in the states in which they operate, and usually, licenses are renewed annually. Facility administrators understand that the state department of health will return for the next annual review within a 15-month window of the previous on-site review.

Long-term care facilities that receive Medicare and Medicaid funding must achieve certification of compliance with the *Conditions of Participation* as well. State departments of health also conduct Medicare and Medicaid certification reviews, which may or may not be performed concurrent with licensure review. The scheduling of certification reviews depends on the organizational structure of the state department of health. When there have been complaints from residents, families, or employees against a long-term care facility, department of health surveyors may visit at any time to perform a special investigation. Department of health survey teams usually consist of two surveyors who have nursing, pharmacy, nutritionist, or clinical laboratory backgrounds. If the review is not conducted in response to a complaint, the survey process encompasses all aspects of facility operations. The surveyors determine at the time of the site visit which operations will be investigated. The annual site visit begins with the posting of survey notifications on facility doors and at every nursing station. The notification requests that anyone—resident, staff member, or visitor—who has issues or perspectives to communicate to the surveyors make themselves known. An opening conference is held with the facility's administrators and the director of nursing to explain the purpose of the survey and outline the sequence of survey activities.

Long-term care site surveyors always look for evidence of three trigger issues: very high percentages of patients suffering from dehydration, decubitus ulcers in low-risk residents, and fecal impaction. Current federal regulations mandate the primary importance of these issues in the long-term care setting. Whether the facility has very high percentages is determined based on the facility Quality Indicator Survey (QIS). The report is compiled from information provided to state departments of health via the Minimum Data Set (MDS) for Long-Term Care. An MDS must be maintained for every resident of a long-term care facility. Focused review of the health records of residents with these conditions is carried out when excessive numbers are identified.

After delineating survey objectives, the surveyors begin examining facility operations. The president of the facility's residents' council is interviewed to determine whether any issues have been raised by residents since the last site review. If the facility does not have a residents' council, then individual residents may be interviewed. Surveyors visit ancillary departments, such as nutrition services, and review operations for continuing adherence to public health standards. Surveyors visit nursing units and review resident records as deemed necessary. Records are reviewed for compliance with state regulations regarding issues such as quarterly and annual care plan review by providers, authentication of providers' orders, proper administration of medication by nurses, and appropriate charting of care by nursing assistants.

When their review activities are complete, the surveyors reconvene with the facility's administrators and director of nursing to summarize their findings. Any deficiencies discovered during the survey process are then discussed with the facility's management team. Deficiencies are classified by the surveyors who determine the level of harm to the resident or residents involved, along with the scope of the problem within the facility by assigning an alphabetical score of A through L (a point system value based on whether the incident was isolated, a pattern, or widespread related to the severity levels) and a severity level of 1 through 4. The four severity levels are as follows:

- Level 1: No actual harm with potential for minimal harm
- Level 2: No actual harm with potential for more than minimal harm that is not immediate jeopardy
- Level 3: Actual harm that is not immediate jeopardy
- Level 4: Immediate jeopardy to resident health or safety.

With the determination of the scope and level of the deficiencies, the survey agency may recommend enforcement remedies that range from directed plans of correction, to civil penalties, up to the termination of the provider agreements. In most cases, a plan of correction is the first step, with the facility or organization required to submit a plan that covers four distinct elements:

- How the correction will be accomplished
- Title or position of the individual who will be responsible for correction implementation
- How the correction will be continually enforced, along with a monitoring plan to prevent the reoccurrence of the deficiency
- The date the correction will be in place or accomplished (CMS n.d.)

Accreditation of Psychiatric and Rehabilitative Care Facilities: CARF

Accreditation reviews by CARF are usually scheduled in advance. Organizations interested in CARF accreditation must file an application that provides information on organization type, services provided, statistical and textual descriptions of its characteristics, and the names of individuals who make up its leadership. Most CARF-accredited organizations undergo a site visit every three years (CARF 2023c).

The CARF survey team usually includes three members, although additional members may be added for special purposes unique to the applying organization. Typically, the team is made up of professionals from other CARF-accredited organizations. Their areas of expertise are similar to those in which the organization undergoing accreditation specializes. For example, when the organization under review is an inpatient psychiatric institution, the surveyors have experience with inpatient psychiatric care and have practiced as administrators or clinicians in that setting. Surveyors undergo considerable training in CARF accreditation processes before they are assigned to a survey team.

In contrast to the Joint Commission process, the CARF accreditation process is much more flexible and is highly tailored to the patient care services and communities of interest of the organization. Although a template review schedule is followed, within each segment of the schedule the activities pursued depend on the characteristics of the organization applying for accreditation.

The CARF accreditation site visit begins with an opening conference. CARF requires that the opening conference be accessible to all communities of interest in the organization. Interested participants may include payers, staff members, referring agencies, members of the community, and patients. The surveyors expect that these constituencies will be allowed to voice concerns and issues during the opening conference. The survey team then outlines the activities it wants to pursue over the ensuing two or three days of the site survey.

The second part of the CARF accreditation process is the document review. The **document review** is an in-depth study in which accreditation surveyors examine an organization's policies and procedures, administrative rules and regulations, administrative records, human resources records, and the case records of patients.

The third part of the survey involves interviews with program staff and patients. The surveyors seek to validate the information gathered from the document review and to determine whether staff or patients have raised any important issues regarding patient care services.

Finally, the CARF process ends with an exit interview with the organization's leaders. Surveyors identify any deficiencies that have been uncovered and present an overall summary of their findings (CARF 2023c).

Certification: Compliance with the CMS *Conditions of Participation*

Some US healthcare organizations do not undergo an accreditation process. Others have undergone accreditation with an accrediting agency but have been identified by federal Medicare officials as requiring specific review for compliance with the CMS *Conditions of Participation*.

Surveys to determine a facility's compliance with the *Conditions of Participation* are carried out by state healthcare certification and licensure agencies. As with the state certification and licensure processes discussed earlier, state department of health reviews are typically unannounced. The survey team visits the healthcare facility as necessary either on an annual basis or in response to complaints from patients or employees. In addition to the surveyors commonly used by the department of health in a given state, regional Medicare agencies may provide one or two Medicare officials.

During the opening conference, the Medicare officials make it known that the review is for the purpose of determining compliance with the *Conditions of Participation*. They then generally leave and do not participate in the on-site survey activities. Judgments about compliance are left to the state certification surveyors.

Check Your Understanding 16.3

1. Jane's mother is a resident at Apple Valley Nursing Home. Jane is concerned that her mother is developing a pressure ulcer on her hip. Jane has brought this concern to the attention of both the director of nursing and the facility administer with no resolution. Jane contacts the state department of health and files a complaint. From this scenario, predict what will occur next at Apple Valley Nursing Home.
    a. Jane will receive a letter thanking her for her concern.
    b. CMS will contact the nursing home administrator by phone.
    c. A department of health surveyor will visit the nursing home.
    d. The director of nursing will contact CMS.

2. Following a recent state licensure survey, Lakeside Care Center was cited for issues with the patient transfer documentation process. At the time of transfer, the care center was not forwarding current patient medication lists and documentation of the reason for transfer to the accepting facility. Lakeside Care Center developed the following corrective plan for this citation:

    Director of nursing or designee will collect relevant information on patient medications and the reason for transfer prior to sending the patient to the accepting facility. They will ensure that the accepting has received this information while the patient is in transit. This process will be set up and in place within the month following the citation.
    What element is missing from Lakeside Care Center's corrective plan?
    a. How the correction will be continually enforced and an ongoing monitoring plan
    b. The date the correction will be in place or accomplished
    c. Title or position of the individual who will be responsible for correction implementation
    d. How the correction will be accomplished

Real-Life Example

Table 16.3 provides an example of how applicable regulations can be reviewed as a basis for developing an organization's policies and procedures to meet multiple regulations. The rural community hospital for which this analysis was developed documents the care provided for patients at many levels of care (e.g., inpatient hospitalization, partial hospitalization, outpatient). Hospital administrators wanted to develop a policy for charting patient care in their medical records that would meet all applicable regulations for all patient types. Each regulatory body's standards were reviewed and then organized in a tabular format that allows easy viewing to determine which standard sets the strictest requirements.

Table 16.3A. Regulations pertaining to charting patient encounters in the medical record

Regulatory Body	Regulation	Interpretive Guideline	Comments
Medicare *Conditions of Participation*	§482.24 Standard: Content of record. The medical record must contain information to justify admission and continued hospitalization, support the diagnosis, and describe the patient's progress and response to medications and services.	§482.24(c) The medical record must contain information such as notes, documentation, records, reports, recordings, test results, assessments etc. to: • Justify admission; • Justify continued hospitalization; • Support the diagnosis; • Describe the patient's progress; • Describe the patient's response to medications; • Describe the patient's response to services such as interventions, care, treatments, etc. The medical record must contain complete information/documentation regarding evaluations, interventions, care provided, services, care plans, discharge plans, and the patient's response to those activities.	Regulations do not require specific documentation standards for progress notes and other information. However, the documentation must be sufficient to follow the care process.
https://aspe.hhs.gov/sites/default/files/private/pdf/76706/EHRPI-appendQ.pdf			
	482.61 The medical records maintained by a psychiatric hospital must permit the determination of the degree and intensity of the treatment provided to individuals who are furnished services in the institution.	§482.61 The clinical record should provide information that indicates the need for admission and treatment, treatment goals, changes in status of treatment, discharge planning, follow-up, and the outcomes experienced by patients. The structure and content of the individual patient's record must be an accurate functional representation of the actual experience of the individual in the facility. It must contain enough information to indicate that the facility knows the status of the patient, has adequate plans to intervene, and provides sufficient evidence of the effects of the intervention, and how their interventions served as a function of the outcomes experienced. You must be able to identify this through interviews with staff, and when possible with individuals being served, as well as through observations.	These standards are more specific to your treatment setting but still do not appear to require a specific documentation standard. They do require enough information to be sufficient to justify the care and treatment being administered.
www.cms.gov/regulations-and-guidance/guidance/manuals/downloads/som107ap_a_hospitals.pdf			
	482.13(b)(1) The patient has the right to participate in the development and implementation of his or her plan of care.	§482.13(b)(1) This regulation requires the hospital to actively include the patient in the development, implementation and revision of their plan of care. It requires the hospital to plan the patient's care, with patient participation, to meet the patient's	By regulation patients do have the right to be included in their care planning and treatment, so the documentation of care planning participation is required.

Table 16.3B. Regulations pertaining to charting patient encounters in the medical record (*Continued*)

Regulatory Body	Regulation	Interpretive Guideline	Comments
		psychological and medical needs. The patient's (or patient's representatives, as allowed by state law) right to participate in the development and implementation of their plan of care includes at a minimum, the right to: participate in the development and implementation of their inpatient treatment/care plan, outpatient treatment/care plan, participate in the development and implementation of his/her discharge plan, and participate in the development and implementation of their pain management plan.	
https://www.cms.gov/regulations-and-guidance/guidance/manuals/downloads/som107ap_a_hospitals.pdf			
	482.61(c)(2) The treatment received by the patient must be documented in such a way to assure that all active therapeutic efforts are included.	Active treatment is an essential requirement for inpatient psychiatric care. Active treatment is a clinical process involving ongoing assessment, diagnosis, intervention, evaluation of care and treatment, and planning for discharge and aftercare, under the direction of a psychiatrist. The patient is in the hospital because it has been determined that the patient requires intensive, 24-hour, specialized psychiatric intervention that cannot be provided outside the psychiatric hospital. The medical record must indicate that the hospital adheres to the patient's right to be counseled about medication, its intended effects, and the potential side effects. If the patient requires, because of danger to self or others, a more restrictive environment, the hospital must indicate that the staff attempted to care for the patient in the least restrictive setting before progressing to a more restrictive setting.	Ancillary departments also have to document services provided in the medical record
	482.61(c)(2) The treatment received by the patient must be documented in such a way to assure that all active therapeutic efforts are included. telemedicine entity is a contractor of services to the hospital and as such, in accordance with §482.12(e), furnishes the contracted services in a manner that permits the hospital to comply with all applicable conditions of participation for the contracted services, including, but not limited	§482.12(a)(8) & §482.12(a)(9) "Telemedicine," as the term is used in this regulation, means the provision of clinical services to patients by physicians and practitioners from a distance via electronic communications. The distant-site telemedicine physician or practitioner provides clinical services to the hospital patient either simultaneously, as is often the case with teleICU services, or non-simultaneously, as may be the case with many	Telemedicine services can be provided to patients, but distant providers are still subject to the regulatory documentation requirement as if they are part of the facility providing direct care.

Table 16.3C. Regulations pertaining to charting patient encounters in the medical record (*Continued*)

Regulatory Body	Regulation	Interpretive Guideline	Comments
	to, the requirements in paragraphs (a)(1) through (a)(7) of this section with regard to the distant-site telemedicine entity's physicians and practitioners providing telemedicine services.	teleradiology services. "Simultaneously" means that the clinical services (for example, assessment of the patient with a clinical plan for treatment, including any medical orders needed) are provided to the patient in "real-time" by the telemedicine physician or practitioner, similar to the actions of an on-site physician or practitioner. "Non-simultaneously" means that, while the telemedicine physician or practitioner still provides clinical services to the patient upon a formal request from the patient's attending physician, such services may involve after-the-fact interpretation of diagnostic tests to provide an assessment of the patient's condition and do not necessarily require the telemedicine practitioner to directly assess the patient in "real-time."	
https://www.cms.gov/regulations-and-guidance/guidance/manuals/downloads/som107ap_a_hospitals.pdf			
Example state medical record regulations (Utah)	R432-100-35. Medical Records. (1) The licensee shall establish a medical records department or service that is responsible for the administration, custody, and maintenance of medical records. (a) The hospital administrator shall establish administrative direction of the medical records department and in accordance with the organizational structure and policies of the hospital. (b) The licensee shall retain the technical services of either a registered health information administrator or a registered health information technician through employment or consultation. If retained by consultation, the individual shall visit at least quarterly and document visits through written reports to the hospital administrator. (2) The licensee shall provide secure storage, controlled access, prompt retrieval, and equipment and facilities to review medical records. (a) The license shall ensure medical records are available for use or review by: (i) members of the medical and professional staff; (ii) authorized hospital personnel and agents; (iii) people authorized by the patient through a consent form; and (iv) department representatives to determine compliance with licensing rules. (b) Medical records may be stored in multiple locations if the record can be retrieved or accessed in a reasonable time period. (c) If computer terminals are utilized for patient charting, the licensee shall have policies governing access and identification codes, security, and information retention. (d) The licensee shall index a hospital medical record according to diagnosis, procedure, demographic information, and physician or licensed health practitioner and ensure the index is current within six months following discharge of the patient. (e) Original medical records are the property of the licensee and shall not be removed from the control of the licensee or the licensee's agent as defined by policy, except by court order or subpoena.		Every State has regulations for medical providers and facilities that need to be considered. When Federal and State regulations are in conflict the most stringent of the two apply.

Table 16.3D. Regulations pertaining to charting patient encounters in the medical record (*Continued*)

Regulatory Body	Regulation	Interpretive Guideline	Comments
	(f) The licensee shall manage medical records for individuals who have received or requested admission to an alcohol or drug program in accordance with the Code of Federal Regulations, Title 42, Part 2, Confidentiality of Substance Use Disorder Patient Records. (3) The licensee shall ensure that any medical record entries are legible, complete, authenticated, and dated by the person responsible for ordering the service, providing, or evaluating the service, or making the entry. The author shall review prepared transcriptions of dictated reports, evaluations, and consultations before authentication. (a) The authentication may include written signatures, computer key, or other methods approved by the governing body and medical staff to identify the name and discipline of the person making the entry. (b) Use of computer key or other methods to identify the author of a medical record entry may not be assignable or delegated to another person. (c) The licensee shall maintain a current list of individuals approved to use the methods of authentication. Hospital policy shall identify sanctions for the unauthorized or improper use of computer codes. (d) Qualified personnel shall accept and transcribe verbal orders for the care and treatment of the patient and authenticate them within 30 days of the patient's discharge. (4) The licensee shall ensure medical records are organized according to hospital policy. (a) medical records are reviewed at least quarterly for completeness, accuracy, and adherence to hospital policy; (b) records of discharged patients are collected, assembled, reviewed for completeness, and authenticated within 30 days of the patient's discharge; (c) medical records are retained for at least seven years and medical records of minors are kept until the age of 18 plus four years, but in no case less than seven years. (d) the licensee may destroy medical records after retaining them for the minimum period of time, and before destroying medical records, the licensee shall notify the public by publishing a notice in a newspaper of statewide distribution a minimum of once per week for three consecutive weeks to allow a former patient to access their records; (e) the licensee shall permanently retain a master patient or person index that shall include: (i) the patient name; (ii) the medical record number; (iii) the date of birth; (iv) the admission and discharge dates; and (v) the name of each attending physician. (f) if a licensee ceases operation, the licensee shall provide secure, safe storage and prompt retrieval of any medical records, patient indexes, and discharges for the period specified in Subsection R432-100-34(4)(c); and (g) the licensee may arrange for storage of medical records with another hospital, or an approved medical record storage facility, or may return patient medical records to the attending physician if the physician is still in the community. (5) The licensee shall establish and maintain a complete medical record for each patient admitted, or who receives hospital services. Emergency and outpatient medical records shall contain documentation of the service provided and other pertinent information in accordance with hospital policy. (6) The licensee shall ensure that each medical record contains: (a) patient identification and demographic information to include at least the patient's name, address, date of birth, sex, and emergency contact information;		

Table 16.3E. Regulations pertaining to charting patient encounters in the medical record (*Continued*)

Regulatory Body	Regulation	Interpretive Guideline	Comments
	(b) initial or admitting medical history, physical, and other examinations or evaluations. (c) admitting, secondary, and primary diagnoses; (d) results of consultative evaluations and findings by individuals involved in the care of the patient; (e) documentation of complications, hospital-acquired infections, and unfavorable reactions to medications, treatments, and anesthesia; (f) properly executed informed consent documents for any procedures and treatments ordered for, and received by, the patient; (g) documentation that the facility requested of each admitted person whether the person has initiated an advanced directive as defined in the Title 75, Chapter 2a, Advance Health Care Directive Act; (h) practitioner orders, nursing notes, reports of treatment, medication records, laboratory and radiological reports, vital signs, and other information that documents the patient condition and status; and (i) a discharge summary including outcome of hospitalization, disposition of case with an autopsy report when indicated, or provisions for follow-up.		
https://adminrules.utah.gov/public/rule/R432-100/Current%20Rules?searchText=hospital			
Part 424—Conditions for Medicare Payment	424.535 Revocation of enrollment in the Medicare program. (a) Reasons for revocation. CMS may revoke a currently enrolled provider or supplier's Medicare billing privileges and any corresponding provider agreement or supplier agreement for the following reasons:	(1) *Noncompliance.* The provider or supplier is determined to not be in compliance with the enrollment requirements described in this subpart P or in the enrollment application applicable for its provider or supplier type, and has not submitted a plan of corrective action as outlined in part 488 of this chapter. The provider or supplier may also be determined not to be in compliance if it has failed to pay any user fees as assessed under part 488 of this chapter. (i) CMS may request additional documentation from the provider or supplier to determine compliance if adverse information is received or otherwise found concerning the provider or supplier. (ii) Requested additional documentation must be submitted within 60 calendar days of request. (2) Provider or supplier conduct. The provider or supplier, or any owner, managing employee, authorized or elegated official, medical director, supervising physician, or other health care personnel of the provider or supplier is— (i) Excluded from the Medicare, Medicaid, and any other Federal health care program, as defined in § 1001.2 of this chapter, in accordance with section 1128, 1128A, 1156, 1842, 1862, 1867 or 1892 of the Act. (ii) Is debarred, suspended, or otherwise excluded from participating in any other	Revocation of participation in the Medicare program can occur if the participant fails to provide "True" information or "Access" to review the medical record.

Certification: Compliance with the CMS Conditions of Participation   **339**

Table 16.3F. Regulations pertaining to charting patient encounters in the medical record (*Continued*)

Regulatory Body	Regulation	Interpretive Guideline	Comments
		Federal procurement or nonprocurement program or activity in accordance with the FASA implementing regulations and the Department of Health and Human Services nonprocurement common rule at 45 CFR part 76. (3) Felonies. (i) The provider, supplier, or any owner or managing employee of the provider or supplier was, within the preceding 10 years, convicted (as that term is defined in 42 CFR 1001.2) of a Federal or State felony offense that CMS determines is detrimental to the best interests of the Medicare program and its beneficiaries. (ii) Offenses include, but are not limited in scope or severity to— (A) Felony crimes against persons, such as murder, rape, assault, and other similar crimes for which the individual was convicted, including guilty pleas and adjudicated pretrial diversions. (B) Financial crimes, such as extortion, embezzlement, income tax evasion, insurance fraud and other similar crimes for which the individual was convicted, including guilty pleas and adjudicated pretrial diversions. (C) Any felony that placed the Medicare program or its beneficiaries at immediate risk, such as a malpractice suit that results in a conviction of criminal neglect or misconduct. (D) Any felonies that would result in mandatory exclusion under section 1128(a) of the Act. (iii) Revocations based on felony convictions are for a period to be determined by the Secretary, but not less than 10 years from the date of conviction if the individual has been convicted on one previous occasion for one or more offenses. (4) False or misleading information. The provider or supplier is certified as "true" but provided misleading or false information on the enrollment application to be enrolled or maintain enrollment in the Medicare program. (Offenders may be subject to either fines or imprisonment, or both, in accordance with current law and regulations.) (10) Failure to document or provide CMS access to documentation. (i) The provider or supplier did not comply with the documentation or CMS access requirements specified in §424.516 (f) of this subpart.	

https://www.govinfo.gov/content/pkg/CFR-2019-title42-vol3/pdf/CFR-2019-title42-vol3-part424.pdf

Summary: None of the regulations reviewed above have specifically defined formats for documenting in the medical record. There are some required time frames for the medical record documentation that need to be considered when creating policies and procedures for documentation.

Case Study

The CMS *Conditions of Participation* require that a licensed physician must see and review the care of the residents of a nursing facility at least once every 30 days for the first 90 days after admission, and at least once every 60 days thereafter. Once the physician has completed the initial comprehensive visit in the nursing facility, the physician may then delegate alternate visits to an advanced practice provider such as a physician assistant (PA) or nurse practitioner (NP).

During a site visit survey of a skilled nursing facility (SNF), the surveyors found that the medical director, a physician, has taken a six-month leave of absence, delegating responsibility for the care of the SNF residents to another physician. During this time, the covering physician delegated all the new resident evaluations to the medical director's nurse practitioner to formally admit them to the facility and to review and approve their medications, treatments, and care planning. The covering physician is only seeing residents who were admitted prior to the medical director's leave of absence to monitor and approve the residents' ongoing treatment and care. The surveyors find that this practice does not comply with the *Conditions of Participation* and the facility was cited for this deficiency.

Case Study Questions

1. What is the noncompliance issue in this case, and why did the surveyors cite this facility?
2. What steps should the skilled nursing facility have taken to avoid this citation?
3. How should the skilled nursing facility prevent issues such as this from occurring in the future?

Review Questions

1. Compare and contrast accreditation, licensure, and certification, and construct a case in which a healthcare organization would need to be in compliance with each of these.

2. Which type of healthcare organization review is performed to fulfill legal or licensure requirements?
    a. Voluntary review
    b. Complimentary review
    c. Vocational review
    d. Compulsory review

3. This organization has been responsible for accrediting healthcare organizations since the mid-1950s and determines whether the healthcare organization is continually monitoring and improving the quality of care it provides.
    a. Commission on Accreditation of Rehabilitation Facilities
    b. American Osteopathic Association
    c. National Committee for Quality Assurance
    d. The Joint Commission

4. Your facility is expecting a Joint Commission survey in the next year. You have several new employees who have never experienced this survey process. These employees would like a better understanding of their role in the survey to ease their anxiety about it. Create an outline of the survey process detailing the typical steps so that your employees will know what to expect.

5. State the pros and cons of a healthcare organization's decision to seek voluntary accreditation.

References

42 CFR 482: Conditions of participation for hospitals. 1986 (June 16). https://www.ecfr.gov/current/title-42/chapter-IV/subchapter-G/part-482.

AAAHC (Accreditation Association for Ambulatory Health Care). 2024. "About Us." https://www.aaahc.org/about-us/.

CMS (Centers for Medicare and Medicaid Services). n.d. "SFF Scoring Methodology." Accessed January 19, 2024. https://www.cms.gov/Medicare/Provider-Enrollment-and-Certification/CertificationandComplianc/Downloads/SFFSCORINGMETHODOLOGY.pdf.

CMS (Centers for Medicare and Medicaid Services). 2023. "Conditions for coverage & participation: Hospitals." https://www.cms.gov/medicare/health-safety-standards/conditions-coverage-participation/hospitals.

CARF (CARF International). 2023a. "About CARF." https://carf.org/about/.

CARF (CARF International). 2023b. "Our Standards." https://carf.org/accreditation/our-standards/.

CARF (CARF International). 2023c. "Steps to Accreditation." https://carf.org/accreditation/steps-accreditation/.

DNV. 2024. "Hospital Accreditation." https://www.dnv.us/services/hospital-accreditation-218999.

Joint Commission. 2024a. "Who We Are." https://www.jointcommission.org/who-we-are/#:~:text=The%20mission%20of%20The%20Joint,the%20highest%20quality%20and%20value.

Joint Commission. 2024b. *Hospital Accreditation Standards*. Oakbrook Terrace, IL: Joint Commission Resources.

Joint Commission. 2024c. "Glossary." In *Hospital Accreditation Standards*. Oakbrook Terrace, IL: Joint Commission Resources.

Joint Commission. 2023d. "Find Accredited Organizations." https://www.jointcommission.org/who-we-are/who-we-work-with/find-accredited-organizations/#numberOfResults=25.

NCQA (National Committee for Quality Assurance). 2023. "About NCQA." http://www.ncqa.org/about-ncqa.

Resources

Best-Boss, A. 2018. "How to Survive a Joint Commission Visit." https://www.hospitalrecruiting.com/blog/3572/how-to-a-survive-joint-commission-visit/.

Implementing Effective Information Management Tools for Performance Improvement

17

Learning Objectives

- Explain the reasons why contemporary information technologies are important to quality improvement in healthcare
- Use the information management tools commonly used in the performance improvement process
- Examine current developments in healthcare information technologies that will enhance performance improvement activities in the future
- Describe how information resources management professionals can help performance improvement teams pursue their improvement activities

Key Terms

Artificial intelligence (AI)
Business intelligence (BI)
Data collection
Data governance (DG)

Data repository
Information management standards
Information warehouse

Performance improvement (PI) in healthcare is an information-intensive activity. Because PI models are based on the continuous monitoring and assessment of performance measures, effective management of the data and information collected is crucial to the success of the PI program. Developing effective data and information management systems requires a clear picture of the ramifications of data and information management for PI activities.

The American Recovery and Reinvestment Act (ARRA) included provisions for health information technology in the Health Information Technology for Economic and Clinical Health (HITECH) Act, which required healthcare organizations and providers to make significant investments in information systems that have "meaningful use" (HHS 2017). The objective was to focus the attention of healthcare organizations and providers on the attributes of healthcare information systems that would make the greatest positive impact on the care provided to patients, residents, and clients. These impacts were primarily of a technological nature, but it is important to recognize that most attributes of healthcare information systems have a significant impact on quality as well. Because of this advancement in technology, organizations and providers continue to have a greater volume of and access to their clinical and administrative data. This increase in readily available data has given organizations and providers the ability to make data-driven decisions to improve quality of care.

As technology continues to advance, more efficient and robust tools to assist organizations in performance improvement activities are likely to develop. Management of information resources for PI purposes must facilitate the transformation from data to information and from information to knowledge. **Data collection**, the process by which facts are gathered, falls into one of three categories in healthcare organizations:

- *Patient-specific*: Pertains to the care services provided to each patient
- *Aggregated*: Summarizes the experiences of many patients regarding a set of aspects of their care
- *Comparative*: Uses aggregated data to describe the experiences of unique types of patients with one or more aspects of their care

However, these data are only meaningful in context. They must be formatted, filtered, and manipulated to be transformed into information and knowledge that can be acted on for decision-making in PI programs. This chapter will discuss the following topics related to the effective information management for PI: information governance, comparative performance data, and information resources management professionals.

Data Governance

Data governance (DG) is "the overall administration, through clearly defined procedures and plans, that assures the availability, integrity, security, and usability of the structured and unstructured data available to an organization "(Buttner et al. 2021, 1). Healthcare organizations must embrace data governance standards because of the large volumes of data and information being collected, analyzed, manipulated, stored, and reported on quality of care and patient safety issues. Without a basic framework for data governance, organizations will not have the knowledge necessary to use and protect their information as an asset. This framework should "consist of the policies, procedures, standards, ownership, decision rights, roles and responsibilities, and accountability related to the data" (Buttner et al. 2021, 2). Figure 17.1 lists the AHIMA's data governance guiding principles.

Figure 17.1. Data governance program guiding principles

Data is a strategic asset that has value and risk.
Data-related decisions should be made at the lowest level possible.
Not all data will be treated equally; data will be valued and governed [or] managed based on business impact, stakeholder needs, and application policy [or] regulation (e.g., protected health information (PHI).
Data definitions, standards, processes, and policies will be developed and maintained with an organization-wide approach.
Data stewards define the business terms and definitions, approve data values, data relationships, business rules, data quality standards, and monitor data quality and data asset value, while IT maintains the systems that capture and manage data through their life cycle.
Individuals who create or acquire data are accountable for the quality of that data and must record it in accordance with its definition.
Data quality and integrity will be addressed by the individuals who create the data and who are closest to the data, understand its meaning and business implications to the specifications of the data stewards, with support from the central DG program.

Source: (Buttner et al. 2021, 2).

Business Intelligence

As technology advances, healthcare organizations use **business intelligence (BI)** applications (such as application-program interface [API] and extract-transfer-load [ETL]) as a means to turn their data into information. BI is the end product or goal of knowledge management as part of the organization's data governance adoption model analytics competency. BI processes are used in healthcare organizations to make use of massive amounts of data being collected and stored in their information systems. BI technologies are used to acquire healthcare data that is then manipulated or cleaned. After this cleaning and transformation, trends are identified using predictive analytics, and finally, new knowledge about healthcare issues, problems, and opportunities are discovered (Stedman and Burns 2024). This process has been referred to as the business intelligence life cycle (see figure 17.2).

Figure 17.2. Business intelligence life cycle

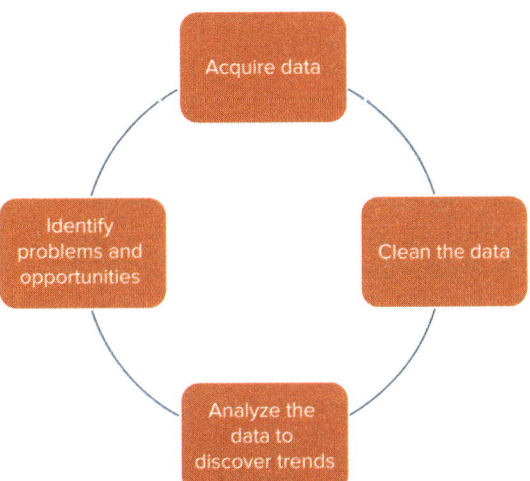

Source: Adapted from Stedman and Burns, 2024.

We have seen that common organization-wide performance improvement process steps are: identify performance measures, measure performance, analyze and compare to internal or external data, identify improvement opportunities, and perform ongoing monitoring. Data from this organization-wide performance improvement process are presented to organization leaders in the form of dashboards or other standardized reports that are reviewed regularly for trends. Figure 17.3 is an example of a PI report used by a hospital to track its important measures on a quarterly basis.

This review of organization-wide PI processes often leads to more questions about the healthcare organization, which then lead to PI team activities. The leaders ask a question about the data and then a PI team is formed to investigate this question. In some circumstances, an existing PI team has questions that need more detailed data to assist them in their improvement processes. BI technologies can be deployed in these instances too.

The first step for the PI team is to gather additional data and information on the issue. This begins the BI cycle using the extract, transform, load (ETL) framework (Manickam and Indra 2022):

- The *extract* step involves pulling the data from multiple sources, such as electronic health records, data repository, or other health information systems.
- The *transform* step involves cleaning the data—duplicates are removed, quality checks may be used to comply with requirements, and data may be normalized or filtered to improve data integrity.
- The *load* step disseminates the data into a data warehouse for use by PI teams.

At this point, the PI team has enough information to make decisions to improve healthcare processes because of the actionable data discovered through the BI process.

Another BI tool with wide-ranging impacts to healthcare is **artificial intelligence (AI)**. This tool, along with machine learning, has the potential to amplify the BI capabilities of healthcare organizations. AI allows organizations to find patterns in their vast amount of data that would take individuals years to analyze. By using this data, organizations are able to make predictions and identify patterns or correlations to assist in operations. Because AI works with machine learning, these tools continue to learn and improve over time (Bharadiya 2023). The full potential impact and application of these tools in healthcare is yet to be determined. The Coalition for Health AI has recommended development of a laboratory environment to evaluate AI in a safe manner to provide "a shared definition of value and components such as registries of tools, templates of legal agreements, as well as sandbox environments for testing tools" (CHAI 2023, 16). Such an environment will assist healthcare organizations in developing best practices and a code of conduct for AI use. Healthcare organizations are creating policies and procedures around the use and application of these AI tools and determining their safe and reliable integration to their processes. At this time, the use and application of AI continues to evolve, and many organizations are still investigating the best use of this technology while continuing to provide excellent patient care. The issues of risk, safety, privacy, and security are at the forefront of a thoughtful approach for healthcare administrators and quality managers to further develop their organizational use of AI.

Data Repositories

In the late 1990s, some healthcare organizations began to develop data repositories to facilitate PI activities and long-range strategic planning. A **data repository** is an open-structure database that is not dedicated to the software of a particular vendor or data supplier, in which data from diverse sources are stored so that an integrated, multidisciplinary view of the data can be achieved. Organizations that have deployed this technology are copying every instance of every datum collected in the course of providing healthcare services to customers. In addition, they are collecting the secondary data acquired in the course of using the technologies to support care, such as those collected to provide audit trails and to support other administrative aspects of running information systems. Which users entered data, which access terminal was used, and the date and time of entry are key examples of this type of administrative data. These repositories are common in healthcare information systems implementations and provide healthcare professionals involved in PI activities with timely data and information that can be used continuously to monitor the quality of many different aspects of the care they provide.

Figure 17.3A. Example of a routine PI report for a community hospital

General Statistics

Statistics	Jan–March 2023	April–June 2023	July–Sept 2023	Oct–Dec 2023	2023 Average	2023 Average
Admissions	625	711	802	775	728.25	747.25
Discharges	789	690	766	759	751.00	789.25
Patient days	1,657	1,671	1,623	1,611	1,640.50	1,910.00
Lost work hours	0*	33*	22*	17*	18*	17*
Observation patients	146	125	137	144	138.00	153.25
Inpatient mortality rate	1.32%	1.35%	1.03%	0.81%	1.13%	1.11%
Deliveries	234	221	232	245	233.00	268.25
Emergency department visits	5,523	5,683	5,890	5,789	5,721.25	6,232.50
Inpatient/outpatient operative encounters	687	664	665	676	673.00	728.75
Outpatient operative encounters	546	524	530	568	542.00	585.25

Patient Care

Measure	Benchmark	Jan–March 2023	April–June 2023	July–Sept 2023	Oct–Dec 2023	2023 Average	2023 Average
Discrepancies: Preop/postop/pathological (op report indicates specimen removed)	100% (I)	37%	47%	86%	85%	64%	40%
Procedure appropriateness: Criteria met	100% (I)	100%	100%	100%	100%	100%	100%
Patient preparation for procedure: Adequate	100% (I)	86%	79%	87%	89%	85%	83%
Procedure performance and patient monitoring: Intraoperative incidents	0% (I)	0.13%	0.0%	0.38%	0.29%	0.20%	0.21%
Procedure performance and patient monitoring: Unplanned returns to OR (M)	0% (M)	0.13%	0.13%	0.38%	1.1%	0.44%	0.27%
Postprocedure care: Complications of postprocedure care	0% (I)	0.26%	0.40%	0.25%	0.43%	0.34%	0.03%
Postprocedure patient education completed	100% (I)	51%	67%	75%	74%	67%	67%

Figure 17.3B. Example of a routine PI report for a community hospital (Continued)

Patient Care (continued)						
Medication Use						
Prescribing or ordering: Orders changed as result of MD clarification	NI	NI	89%	95.4%	93.8%	92.7%	89%
Preparing and dispensing: Dispensing errors	0% (I)	0%	≤1%	0%	0%	≤0.25%	≤1%
Preparing and dispensing: Medication delivery time—preop antibiotics within 2 hours of surgery (hips, knees, appendectomies, hysterectomies)	≤2 hours (N)	89%	93%	93%	91%	92%	87%
Administering: DUE—appropriateness of dosage	90% (I)	73%	67%	73.8%	81.0%	73.7%	89.0%
Monitoring the effects on patients: Adverse reactions	0.1% (I)	0.04%	0.09%	1.0%	0.22%	0.34%	0.36%
Monitoring the effects on patients: Drug–drug interactions	NI	23	2	4	1	7.5	16.0
Monitoring the effects on patients: Drug–food interactions	NI	7	23	44	62	34.0	20.0
Adverse effects during anesthesia	NI	NI	NI	NI	NI	NI	NI
Use of Restraints						
Documented evidence of less restrictive measures used	NI	3	3	11	6	6	NI
Use of Blood and Blood Components						
Ordering: Blood usage appropriate	100% (I)	100%	100%	100%	100%	100%	100%
Distributing, handling, and dispensing	NI	NI	NI	NI	NI	NI	NI
Administering: Blood slips completed and on chart	100% (I)	88.2%	81%	82.6%	86.4%	84.6%	85.7%
Administration: Cross-match:transfusion ratio	≤2:1 (I)	1.8:1	1.6:1	2.2:1	1.8:1	1.9:1	2.0:1
Monitoring blood and blood component effects on patients: Potential transfusion reactions	NI	0.0%	0.0%	0.0%	0.0%	0.0%	0.0%
Monitoring blood and blood component effects on patients: Confirmed transfusion reactions	0% (I)	0.0%	0.0%	0.0%	0.0%	0.0%	0.0%

Figure 17.3C. Example of a routine PI report for a community hospital (*Continued*)

Continuum of Care

Measure	Benchmark	Jan–March 2023	April–June 2023	July–Sept 2023	Oct–Dec 2023	2023 Average	2023 Average
Utilization management: Patients admitted as inpatients not meeting appropriateness criteria on initial review	100% (I)	NI	NI	NI	NI	NI	NI
Utilization management: Continuing stay criteria met	100% (I)	NI	NI	NI	NI	NI	NI
Utilization management: Patients remaining inpatients after discharge criteria met	100% (I)	NI	NI	NI	NI	NI	NI

Important Processes and Outcomes

Measure	Benchmark	Jan–March 2023	April–June 2023	July–Sept 2023	Oct–Dec 2023	2023 Average	2023 Average
Autopsy results: Number performed/number met criteria	—	NI	NI	NI	NI	NI	NI
Critical occurrences		0	1	0	0	0.25	0
C-section rate (O)	12% (M); 17% (N)	15.3%	12.8%	11.8%	12.4%	13.1%	12.1%
VBAC rate (O)	50% (M); 36% (N)	37.5%	38%	38%	34%	37%	50%
Primary C-section rate (O)	6.5% (O)	9.7%	7.8%	5.7%	6.1%	7.3%	7.9%
Percentage of total C-section (O)	50% (O)	56.9%	55.8%	42.5%	43.6%	49.7%	59.2%
Repeat C-section rate (O)	65% (O)	62.5%	62.1%	62.2%	65.9%	63.2%	50.0%
X-ray discrepancies resulting in change of care (O)	1.0% (O)	0.7%	0.42%	0.36%	0.4%	0.5%	NI
Unplanned return to emergency department within 72 hours (M)	0.6% (O)	0.53%	0.5%	0.7%	0.7%	0.6%	0.6%
Patients in emergency department more than 6 hours (M)	12% (I)	14.7%	10%	13.1%	8.8%	11.7%	12.0%
Unplanned return to special care unit (M)	0.0% (I)	1.9%	2.3%	1.8%	2.5%	2.1%	NI
Unplanned admits from outpatient surgery (M)	2.0% (I)	2.3%	1.9%	2.4%	6.9%	3.4%	1.8%
Cancelled surgeries (M)	1.4% (I)	1.0%	1.0%	1.9%	1.6%	1.4%	1.3%
Cancelled endoscopies (M)	1.1% (I)	1.2%	1.9%	1%	1.4%	1.4%	1.1%

Figure 17.3D. Example of a routine PI report for a community hospital (Continued)

Quality Control Activities

Measure	Benchmark	Jan–March 2023	April–June 2023	July–Sept 2023	Oct–Dec 2023	2023 Average	2023 Average
Clinical lab: Number of QC functions completed/number required	100% (I)	0.0%	1.54%	0.78%	2.0%	1.1%	1.2%
Diagnostic radiology: Number of QC functions completed/number required	100% (I)	NI	NI	NI	NI	NI	NI
Dietary: Number of QC functions completed/number required	100% (I)	NI	NI	NI	NI	NI	NI
Equipment used to administer medication: Number of QC functions completed/number required	100% (I)	NI	NI	NI	NI	NI	NI
Pharmacy equipment used to prepare medication: Number of QC functions completed/number required	100% (I)	NI	NI	NI	NI	NI	NI
Equipment malfunctions	0% (I)	NI	1	0	6	2	3

Patient Rights

Measure	Benchmark	Jan–March 2023	April–June 2023	July–Sept 2023	Oct–Dec 2023	2023 Average	2023 Average
Overall patient satisfaction	68% (I)	67.2%	63.8%	68.3%	73.8%	68.3%	63.0%
Advance directives: Patients asked whether they have an advance directive	100% (I)	67.7%	68.6%	66.7%	82.6%	71.4%	NI
Advance directives: Patients provided information about advance directives	100% (I)	100%	100%	100%	100%	100%	NI

Human Resources

Measure	Benchmark	Jan–March 2023	April–June 2023	July–Sept 2023	Oct–Dec 2023	2023 Average	2023 Average
Employee satisfaction: Overall annual employee satisfaction rate	NI	NI	NI	NI	NI	NI	NI
Annual turnover rate	NI	8.6%	9.7%	5.6%	8.6%	8.1%	41.0%
Complete new hire orientation	100% (I)	100%	100%	100%	100%	100%	100%

Figure 17.3E. Example of a routine PI report for a community hospital (*Continued*)

Information Management

Measure	Benchmark	Jan–March 2023	April–June 2023	July–Sept 2023	Oct–Dec 2023	2023 Average	2023 Average
Data quality monitoring: Documentation appropriateness	90% (I)	95.3%	97.1%	95.4%	97.8%	96.4%	NI
Medical record delinquency: Overall	50% (J)	8.7%	8.4%	8.8%	11.1%	9.3%	11.1%
Medical record delinquency: History and physicals	≤2% (I)	1.0%	0.3%	0.3%	0.12%	0.43%	0.6%
Medical record delinquency: Operative reports	≤2% (I)	3.0%	4.1%	3.6%	4.8%	3.9%	2.9%
Verbal orders countersigned	100% (I)	68.0%	NI	81.3%	95.6%	81.6%	NI
Medical records dated (all entries)	90% (I)	48%	NI	53%	NI	51%	NI

Surveillance, Prevention, and Infection Control

Measure	Benchmark	Jan–March 2023	April–June 2023	July–Sept 2023	Oct–Dec 2023	2023 Average	2023 Average
Nosocomial surgical site infection rate	2.5% (I)	0.8%	1.2%	0.6%	2.2%	1.2%	1.2%
Postop nosocomial pneumonia rate	1.0% (I)	0.0%	0.3%	0.3%	0.6%	0.3%	0.13%

New Programs

Measure	Benchmark	Jan–March 2023	April–June 2023	July–Sept 2023	Oct–Dec 2023	2023 Average	2023 Average
Measures of new program effectiveness	NI	NI	NI	NI	NI	NI	NI

Benchmarking Key: N = national; J = Joint Commission; I = internal; O = ORYX; M = Maryland Quality Indicator Project; NI = no information

*Number of incidents per 200,000 hours worked

Information Warehouses

An **information warehouse** allows organizations to store reports, presentations, profiles, and graphics interpreted and developed from stores of data for reuse in subsequent organizational activities. For example, a report developed by a PI team on the occurrence of methicillin-resistant *Staphylococcus aureus* infection in a neonatal intensive care unit subsequently could be used by the perinatal morbidity and mortality committee in a monthly review of infant morbidity. A marketing report on the need for services pertinent to women and children in an organization's locale could be used by a PI team that wants to delineate the important aspects of customer satisfaction with women's and children's services. Employees with access can query any materials available in a warehouse. These can be downloaded or printed for use by PI team members.

Web-Based PI Team Collaboration Technologies

Everyone in the organization who is concerned with quality issues must be kept apprised of the current status of PI activities. A PI team working on one issue in a specific work unit of the organization may discover important information that could be used by another PI team working on a different issue in another work unit. Without good communication of PI activities throughout the organization, the second team might capture information that has already been captured or analyze collected data that have already been analyzed, thereby wasting time and money.

Communication among PI teams may be accomplished through a variety of tools, which are commonly web-based applications that allow real-time interaction between PI team members. Some of the capabilities of these applications allow video conferencing or messaging that provides team members a way to share information and collaborate in a live environment. In today's healthcare environment, team members may not be located in the same facility, city, state, or even country, so face-to-face meetings are not always feasible. Therefore, virtual meetings, which allow team members to participate in the PI process regardless of their physical location, are commonplace. Likewise, these and similar technologies allow the results from PI team and organization-wide quality and patient safety issues to be communicated to employees and other stakeholders.

Check Your Understanding 17.1

1. With an increased use of technology, including electronic health records, healthcare organizations are collecting unprecedented amounts of electronic data. Explain how an information governance program provides the framework not only for the effective use of the data, but also to protect it as an organizational asset.

2. Community Hospital has just been merged into the Northern Hospital Organization (NHO). The leadership of the larger organization is interested in the work the Community Hospital PI team has been doing. It is not feasible for all the PI team members and NHO administrators to travel to one location. Based on this scenario, create a plan for how this communication can occur without travel.

Comparative Performance Data

As discussed earlier in this text, benchmarking can make an important contribution to the improvement of performance in healthcare organizations. Also known as comparative performance measurement, benchmarking is so important that the Centers for Medicare and Medicaid Services (CMS) and accrediting organizations require participating organizations to perform national benchmarking activities through reported quality measures and patient satisfaction surveys. In turn, the organizations have access to data from these measures. The organization then can compare its performance with the performance of similar organizations. The comparison can ensure that the organization is performing up to industry standards or when necessary, help identify opportunities for improvement.

As an example, the Joint Commission categorizes its performance measures into *accountability* and *nonaccountability* measures. Healthcare organizations must create *accountability measures* that meet the following criteria to ensure quality patient outcomes (Joint Commission 2024a):

- Research: Strong scientific evidence exists demonstrating that compliance with a given process of care improves health outcomes (either directly or by reducing risk of adverse outcomes).
- Proximity: The process being measured is closely connected to the outcome it impacts; there are relatively few clinical processes that occur after the one that is measured and before the improved outcome occurs.
- Accuracy: The measure accurately assesses whether the evidence-based process has actually been provided. That is, the measure should be capable of judging whether the process has been delivered with sufficient effectiveness to make improved outcomes likely.
- Adverse effects: The measure construct is designed to minimize or eliminate unintended adverse effects.

Nonaccountability measures are more suitable for secondary uses, such as exploration or learning within individual healthcare organizations, and are good advice in terms of appropriate patient care. Currently, only accountability measures will be evaluated statistically for reporting on hospital performance and used in rating an organization against national experience or against other similar organizations (Joint Commission 2024a).In addition to the activities of the Joint Commission and CMS, many other agencies and organizations contribute benchmark frameworks for use in PI activities (see figure 17.4).

Figure 17.4A. Sample of US quality measurement organizations

Healthcare reimbursement has been tied to quality of care through initiatives like value-based purchasing and accountable care organizations. Quality measurement organizations have gained a more national prominence.

Many organizations develop, endorse, implement, and promote performance measures. Trying to decipher and understand the interplay of organizations involved with quality measures can be challenging.

Following is a list of some of the country's quality improvement and measurement efforts.

Healthcare Quality Organizations

Agency for Healthcare Research and Quality (AHRQ)

https://www.ahrq.gov/cpi/about/otherwebsites/qualityindicators.ahrq.gov/qualityindicators.html

Quality Indicators (QIs) are used to highlight potential quality concerns, identify areas that need further study and investigation, and track changes over time. Currently, the AHRQ Quality Indicators are only for use with administrative data in acute care hospitals, and are not available for other types of settings (e.g., long-term care, outpatient, ambulatory, hospice, individual practice, emergency department, or diagnostic centers) or populations (e.g., mental health or substance abuse, emergency preparedness, patient falls, rehabilitation, readmission, surgery, heparin therapy, c. difficile, or nursing quality).

Centers for Medicare and Medicaid Services (CMS)

https://www.cms.gov/medicare/quality/measures

CMS has developed quality measures for most levels of healthcare. These quality measures are tools that help measure or quantify healthcare processes, outcomes, patient perceptions, and organizational structure and/or systems that are associated with the ability to provide high-quality health care and/or that relate to one or more quality goals for health care. These goals include: effective, safe, efficient, patient-centered, equitable, and timely care.

Institute for Healthcare Improvement (IHI)

http://www.ihi.org

IHI brings awareness of safety and quality to millions, catalyzes learning and the systematic improvement of care, develops solutions to previously intractable challenges, and mobilizes health systems, communities, regions, and nations to reduce harm and deaths.

Figure 17.4B. Sample of US quality measurement organizations (*Continued*)

The Joint Commission

http://www.jointcommission.org

The Joint Commission identifies, tests, and specifies standardized performance measures. It engages in performance measurement research and development activities. The Commission presides over a growing national comparative performance measurement database that can inform internal healthcare organization quality improvement activities, external accountability, and pay-for-performance programs and advance research.

Leapfrog Group

http://www.leapfroggroup.org

The Leapfrog Group is a nonprofit watchdog organization that serves as a voice for healthcare consumers and purchasers, using their collective influence to foster positive change in US healthcare. Leapfrog is the nation's premier advocate of transparency in healthcare—collecting, analyzing and disseminating data to inform value-based purchasing and improved decision-making.

National Committee for Quality Assurance (NCQA)

https://www.ncqa.org/about-ncqa/

NCQA uses measurement, transparency, and accountability to highlight top performers and drive improvement. Their work began by measuring and then accrediting health plans, and has grown to measure the quality of medical providers and practices. Most of their employees work on HEDIS and Accreditation, Certification and Recognition programs, and government and private sector clients hire them through contracts and grants to help them measure and improve quality.

National Quality Forum (NQF)

https://www.qualityforum.org/About_NQF/

NQF is a nonprofit, nonpartisan, membership-based organization that works to improve healthcare outcomes, safety, equity, and affordability. Their unique role is to bring all voices to the table to forge multistakeholder consensus on quality measurement and improvement standards and practices that achieve measurable health improvements for all.

Quality Improvement Organizations (QIOs)

https://www.cms.gov/medicare/quality/quality-improvement-organizations

The QIO Program, one of the largest federal programs dedicated to improving health quality for Medicare beneficiaries, is an integral part of the US Department of Health and Human Services (HHS) National Quality Strategy for providing better care and better health at lower cost. By law, the mission of the QIO Program is to improve the effectiveness, efficiency, economy, and quality of services delivered to Medicare beneficiaries. Based on this statutory charge, and CMS's program experience, CMS identifies the core functions of the QIO Program as:

- Improving quality of care for beneficiaries
- Protecting the integrity of the Medicare Trust Fund by ensuring that Medicare pays only for services and goods that are reasonable and necessary and that are provided in the most appropriate setting
- Protecting beneficiaries by expeditiously addressing individual complaints, such as beneficiary complaints; provider-based notice appeals; violations of the Emergency Medical Treatment and Labor Act (EMTALA); and other related responsibilities as articulated in QIO-related law

AHIMA Resources on Quality Measurement

https://ahima.org/advocacy/advocacy-agenda/
AHIMA's Advocacy and Public Policy website tracks a variety of data quality management and data content issues, including quality measurement initiatives. The site offers an overview of standards and activities, resource links, and analysis.

Check Your Understanding 17.2

1. Which of the following organizations' unique role is to bring all voices to the table to forge multistakeholder consensus on quality measurement and improvement standards and practices that achieve measurable health improvements for all?
   a. Centers for Medicare and Medicaid Services
   b. Leapfrog
   c. National Quality Forum
   d. Premier

2. A local skilled nursing facility has been working to improve the quality of care they provide to their residents. They have engaged in several PI initiatives recently, and the facility's internal data shows an improvement in their quality metrics. The facility administrator is pleased with these findings but is also interested in determining how this facility is performing in comparison to other nearby skilled nursing facilities. Recommend what this administrator could do to determine this.

Information Resources Management Professionals

Regardless of the configuration of a healthcare organization's technical infrastructure, the staff involved in PI activities should recognize important resources already developed within the organization, such as health information services managers, information systems managers, knowledge-based librarians, as well as privacy and security officers. These information management professionals possess a wealth of professional expertise that can be extremely useful in PI activities.

Information resources management professionals can assist quality improvement programs in a variety of ways. First, they can help train PI teams to utilize appropriate sources for finding data or other information regarding an improvement opportunity. They can assist the team in evaluating the quality of data extracted from internal sources and the reliability of information retrieved from external sources. When new technology is needed to support specific PI activities, these professionals can assist in the development of system requirements, cost-benefit analysis, and requests for proposal.

Much of the data and information used in PI processes are protected health information (PHI). It is important to note the privacy responsibilities that the Health Insurance Portability and Accountability Act (HIPAA) places on this type of information. There may also be data-gathering situations in which PHI from patient, resident, or client health records is specifically matched with other data from marketing or satisfaction surveys that would require the special protection of HIPAA to be exercised. The organization privacy officer(s) may need to be consulted by PI teams to ensure that PHI is used, stored, and disclosed appropriately to meet the requirements of federal and state laws and regulations. The privacy officer(s) may also be of assistance in treating PI data as appropriate to their status as research versus quality improvement information.

Joint Commission Information Management Standards

Effective information management for PI entails an understanding of the Joint Commission's **information management standards**. The information management standards are listed in a chapter of the Joint Commission's *Hospital Accreditation Standards* that outlines the Joint Commission's requirements regarding the data and information used for various purposes in hospital organizations (Joint Commission 2024b). The information management chapter of the accreditation standards was developed during the mid-1990s to focus healthcare organizations on the importance of information systems issues in the provision of high-quality patient care. Any healthcare organization that uses accreditation as a component of its PI program must ensure that it meets these standards. Even healthcare organizations that do not seek Joint Commission accreditation as a component of their PI programs would be wise to consider the standards in developing PI systems and procedures.

The Joint Commission information management standards focus on information systems issues, not on information systems. Solutions to these issues must be developed and consciously implemented in healthcare organizations so that information systems can contribute properly to high-quality patient care. Information management standards address areas in which information resources management contributes to high-quality and improved patient care. These standards require the Joint Commission-accredited healthcare organization to plan for and organize their information resources and ensure that the confidentiality, privacy, security, and integrity of the information are maintained.

The record of care standards state that the patient record should be detailed enough so the patient can be identified and to support the care provided to include diagnosis, treatments, care results, and staff communication. In addition, care providers should document patient progress in the patient record and use this information to make care decisions. There are also specific standards regarding the use of data and information in the PI function. These standards instruct the healthcare organization to collect and analyze appropriate data to monitor and improve processes within their organization. Figure 17.5 lists the Joint Commission information management standards.

Figure 17.5. Joint Commission information resource standards

Information Management Standards	Record of Care, Treatment, and Services Standards	Performance Improvement Standards
• IM.01.01.01 The hospital plans for managing information. • IM.01.01.03 The hospital plans for continuity of its information management processes. • IM.02.01.01 The hospital protects the privacy of health information. • IM.02.01.03 The hospital maintains the security and integrity of health information. • IM.02.02.01 The hospital effectively manages the collection of health information. • IM.02.02.03 The hospital retrieves, disseminates, and transmits health information in useful formats. • IM.03.01.01 Knowledge-based information resources are available, current, and authoritative.	• RC.01.01.01 The hospital maintains complete and accurate medical records for each individual patient. • RC.01.02.01 Entries in the medical record are authenticated. • RC.01.03.01 Documentation in the medical record is entered in a timely manner. • RC.01.04.01 The hospital audits its medical records. • RC.01.05.01 The hospital retains its medical records. • RC.02.01.01 The medical record contains information that reflects the patient's care, treatment, and services. • RC.02.01.03 The patient's medical record contains documentation on any operative or other high-risk procedures and the use of moderate or deep sedation or anesthesia. • RC.02.03.07 Qualified staff receive and record verbal orders. • RC.02.04.01 The hospital documents the patient's discharge information.	• PI.01.01.01 The hospital collects data to monitor its performance. • PI.02.01.01 The hospital has a performance improvement plan. • PI.03.01.01 The hospital compiles and analyzes data. • PI.04.01.01 The hospital improves performance.

Source: Joint Commission 2024c. Reprinted with permission.

Check Your Understanding 17.3

1. A PI team has been established at a local hospital. Becky is the hospital privacy officer and is tasked with responding to questions about privacy issues within the organization. She is contacted by the PI team leader, Mike, who is aware that there may be instances when he or other team members should consult with Becky, but is unsure what circumstances warrant this contact. Becky should inform Mike that he or his team members would need to contact her for consultation in which of the following circumstances?
   a. To ensure that PHI is used, stored, and disclosed properly
   b. To ensure that the selection of PI team members met organizational guidelines
   c. To determine which organizations should be used for benchmarking purposes
   d. To determine if patients are experiencing high levels of satisfaction with their care

2. As part of his role at the local hospital, Jake is reviewing Joint Commission standards to ensure that the organization is meeting the accreditation requirements. As part of the review, Jake is looking at a specific set of standards primarily focused on documentation. Some of the standard requirements include care provided, procedures that were done on the patient, and the progress of the patient. Based on this scenario, which set of Joint Commission standards is Jake reviewing?
   a. Information management standards
   b. Record of care standards
   c. Performance improvement standards
   d. Information resource standards

Case Study

During the last accreditation survey, a hospital had findings related to quality and timeliness of documentation. The facility is due for another survey very soon. To ensure that the hospital is in compliance with the Joint Commission documentation standards, you need to conduct a quality audit. This audit should carefully assess documentation compliance for history and physicals (H&Ps) and operative reports (Ops). A history and physical report must be available in the patient's health record before any surgical procedure can begin. The H&P can be completed up to 30 days prior to the procedure as long as the surgeon updates any information prior to starting the procedure. The Op must be dictated by the surgeon within 24 hours of the procedure to be compliant. You have assigned one of your staff to collect data from patient records to accomplish this task. The staff member collected data for the month of December for quality and timeliness of documentation. The data collected are presented in figure 17.6.

Case Study Tasks

1. Review the collected data.
2. Assign the appropriate quality code using the key located at the bottom of figure 17.6.
3. Analyze the data:
   a. Which quality code is most common?
   b. Is there one service that seems to be a problem?
   c. What can you conclude from the data about compliance with documentation standards?
4. What measures do you need to implement to correct any documentation compliance issues?

Figure 17.6. Data for timeliness of documentation study

PATIENT	DISCHARGE DATE	SERVICE	QUALITY CODE	Admit Date & Time	Physician Action	Procedure Start Time	Procedure End Time
1	12/23/24	CD		12/23/2024; 12:30	No time noted on H&P update stamp	12/23/2024; 16:20	12/23/2024; 17:50
2	12/04/24	EN		12/04/2024; 07:04	H&P dated June 2024	12/04/2024; 09:15	12/04/2024; 09:45
3	12/10/24	EN		12/10/2024; 06:47	H&P signed, dated & timed on 12/10/2024 at 05:05	12/10/2024; 08:44	12/10/2024; 09:45
4	12/19/24	EN		12/19/2024	Op report dictated 12/22	12/19/2024; 13:02	12/19/2024; 14:26
5	12/09/24	EN		12/07/2024; 06:14	No date/time on H&P	12/07/2024; 07:51	12/07/2024; 09:15
6	12/26/24	GS		12/26/2024	H&P dated 11/24/2024		
7	12/26/24	GS		12/26/2024	Op report not dictated	12/26/2024; 11:21	12/26/2024; 14:08
8	12/26/24	GS		12/26/2024	H&P dated 11/21/2024		
9	12/30/24	GS		12/21/2024	Op report dictated 01/09/19		12/21/2024
10	12/23/24	NE		12/15/2024; 08:26	H&P dictated 12/18/2024	12/15/2024; 11:44	12/15/2024; 15:32
11	12/20/24	NE		12/18/2024; 05:26	H&P dictated 11/03/2024	12/18/2024; 07:25	12/18/2024; 08:45
12	12/11/24	NE		12/11/2024	H&P dictated post-op	12/11/2024; 07:22	12/11/2024; 11:46
13	12/16/24	NE		12/16/2024; 04:56	H&P dictated 12/16; 05:59	12/16/2024; 07:51	12/16/2024; 09:01
14	12/27/24	OB		12/24/2024; 22:15	Op report dictated 12/29/2024	12/25/2024; 16:00	12/25/2024; 16:42
15	01/03/24	OB		12/29/2024; 02:14	Op report dictated 12/29/2024; 1500	12/29/2024; 13:51	12/29/2024; 14:40
16	12/04/24	OR		12/04/2024; 04:30	Op report dictated 12/23/2024	12/04/2024; 05:25	12/04/2024; 06:32
17	12/17/24	OR		12/17/2024; 09:52	H&P dictated 12/15	12/17/2024; 12:47	12/17/2024; 14:03
18	12/18/24	OR		12/15/2024; 05:14	Limited H&P completed 12/15; 07:30	12/15/2024; 07:39	12/15/2024; 12:41
19	12/12/24	OR		12/04/2024; 10:10	Limited H&P signed/dated/timed as 1100 after analysis	12/04/2024; 13:09	12/04/2024; 16:53
20	12/06/24	OR		12/03/2024; 17:10	No H&P dictated	12/03/2024; 23:46	12/04/2024; 01:28
21	12/15/24	OR		12/15/2024; 06:45	Op report dictated 12/16/2024; 1055	12/15/2024; 08:54	12/15/2024; 10:42
22	12/05/24	UR		12/05/2024; 07:00	H&P update dated/timed 12/5; 0900 post analysis	12/05/2024; 08:14	12/05/2024; 09:59

Key
1 = H&P >30 days
2 = No H&P prior to surgery
3 = No update to H&P prior to surgery
4 = No Operative report within 24 hours after surgery

Review Questions

1. Which business intelligence tool allows organizations to find patterns in their vast amount of data to make predictions and identify patterns or correlations to assist in operations?
   a. Data governance
   b. Artificial intelligence
   c. Comparative performance data
   d. Team collaboration technologies

2. Identify ways in which information resources management professionals can assist quality improvement programs.

3. This technology allows organizations to store reports, presentations, profiles, and graphics interpreted and developed from stores of data for reuse in subsequent organizational activities.
   a. Data repository
   b. Information warehouse
   c. Comparative performance data
   d. PI database

4. The Joint Commission's quality measures are designed to produce the greatest impact on patient outcomes when a hospital demonstrates improvement. Argue why these four criteria are necessary when developing an accountability measure.

5. A PI team is investigating a performance improvement issue. How would they use the extract, transform, load BI framework to accomplish their task?

References

Buttner, P., M. Meyer, R. Mikaelian, N. Miller, and B. Ruhnau-Gee. 2021. "Healthcare Data Governance." https://journal.ahima.org/page/practice-brief-healthcare-data-governance-14.

Bharadiya, J. P. 2023. Machine learning and AI in business intelligence: Trends and opportunities. *International Journal of Computer (IJC)* 48(1):123-134.

CHAI (Coalition for Health AI). 2023. "Blueprint for Trustworthy AI Implementation Guidance and Assurance for Healthcare." https://www.coalitionforhealthai.org/papers/blueprint-for-trustworthy-ai_V1.0.pdf.

HHS (US Department of Health and Human Services). 2017. "HITECH Act Enforcement Interim Final Rule." https://www.hhs.gov/hipaa/for-professionals/special-topics/hitech-act-enforcement-interim-final-rule/index.html.

Joint Commission. 2024a. "Measures." https://www.jointcommission.org/measurement/measures/.

Joint Commission. 2024b. "Information Management." In *Hospital Accreditation Standards*. Oakbrook Terrace, IL: Joint Commission Resources.

Joint Commission. 2024c. "Information Management, Performance Improvement, and Record of Care Standards." In *Hospital Accreditation Standards*. Oakbrook Terrace, IL: Joint Commission Resources.

Manickam, V. and M.R. Indra. 2023. Dynamic multi-variant relational scheme-based intelligent ETL framework for healthcare management. *Soft Computing* 27:605–614.

Stedman, C. and E. Burns. 2024. "Business Intelligence." Tech Target Business Analytics. https://www.techtarget.com/searchbusinessanalytics/definition/business-intelligence-BI.

Resources

Gimbel, E. 2024. "Roundtable: Healthcare Organizations Put Generative AI Under the Microscope." https://healthtechmagazine.net/article/2024/02/roundtable-healthcare-organizations-put-generative-ai-under-microscope.

National Library of Medicine. 2018. "PubMed." http://www.ncbi.nlm.nih.gov/sites/entrez.

Managing Healthcare Performance Improvement Projects

18

Learning Objectives

- Practice the function of project management in performance improvement programs
- Apply the specific knowledge and skills required for team leadership
- Analyze project life cycles and the group dynamics of team life cycles
- Use the steps a team leader should follow to successfully implement and complete a project

Key Terms

PERT chart

Gantt chart

Initiating a performance improvement (PI) program requires a project team that will be responsible for formulating and implementing the program. Thus, to perform effectively, PI team members need to develop project management skills.

Project management is defined in a number of ways—from a narrowly focused approach with a small, task-oriented team to a much broader, organization-wide philosophy that is reflected in organizational culture, behavior, and structure. Project management as a discipline is rooted in engineering and is oriented toward quantitative application methods. Over time, project management has embraced organizational behavior as a critical element of the knowledge and skills necessary for successful implementation of a project.

PI projects in modern healthcare organizations range from small efforts involving only a few departments to larger ones that affect the organization in very significant ways. Healthcare professionals are likely to be assigned to project teams and, in some cases, may lead them.

When a PI team is formed, the life cycle of the team and project begins. Generally, the organization leadership first determines the composition of the team. Then team roles are established. The mission of the team should be developed in alignment with the organization's overall mission and vision.

Project Management and Organizational Structure

Organizational culture and structure are critical to the success of project management. Bureaucratic organizations with highly structured hierarchies are less accepting of project management concepts than more dynamic and flexible organizations are. Organizations in which employees regularly interact across organizational boundaries are more likely to be open to project management, and their employees will likely perform better on project teams.

Project Life Cycle

The length of time a project will take over its entire life cycle varies depending on its scope and size. Large building projects may take months or years, but most projects will last from a few weeks to a few months. The life cycle of a project is composed of several phases; the number of phases and their definitions vary depending on who determines the phases and the industry involved. Most projects have between four and six phases.

A Guide to the Project Management Body of Knowledge (PMBOK® Guide), 7th edition, compares several life-cycle phases representative of different industries as well as five process groups within these life-cycle phases (PMI 2021). Some experts in the project management field have chosen to focus on a series of processes from the *PMBOK® Guide* that organize project management into five life-cycle phases that are appropriate for service industries such as healthcare delivery. For the sake of simplicity, these phases are used in this chapter. The five phases are:

- Initiating processes
- Planning processes
- Executing processes
- Monitoring and controlling processes
- Closing processes

Initiating Processes

The initiating processes phase begins with the determination that a gap exists between organization performance and expected outcomes. The leadership then identifies an opportunity for improvement and assesses the feasibility of the project. A team charter is developed during this phase.

Sponsorship

One or more individuals in an organization normally sponsor a project. The personal commitment a sponsor brings to a project coincides with the degree of empowerment a project manager will have. Sponsorship by top leadership, therefore, must be characterized by commitment and clear articulation of expectations.

Team Member Selection

Leadership will select members for the project team and identify any other resources needed to complete the project. Team members should be selected by identifying individuals who possess a variety of skills and expertise. If all project team members are selected from the same department and have similar experience and skills, the team runs the risk of overlooking viable alternative solutions that might be raised by a team with more diverse experience and skills. Organizational leadership usually completes much of the initiation phase, during which preliminary definitions of the project objectives, activities, and expectations are prepared. Once formed, the team refines these processes.

Mission Statement

If a mission statement has not been articulated by leadership, the project team's first priority is to establish one at the beginning of the team's life cycle. A clear mission and vision statement will serve as a guide in the development of objectives and goals.

Project Phases and Processes

Once a project team has been formed, project management steps similar to the cycle of a team-based PI process are followed. There are seven steps in the cycle of PI team processes:

1. Identify an improvement opportunity.
2. Research and define performance expectations.
3. Design and redesign process or education.
4. Implement process or education.
5. Measure performance.
6. Document and communicate findings.
7. Analyze and compare internal and external data.

These steps parallel the phases of a project. As a project progresses through the steps, it moves from one phase to the next. Figure 18.1 lists the processes that occur within each of the five phases of a project.

Figure 18.1. The PI process cycle

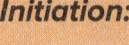

Team Group Dynamics

Just as a project is often defined by its phases, the project team will experience a series of stages and adjustments at various times throughout the life of the project. The project team leader and members will be better prepared to complete the project if they understand the group dynamics of team development. A newly formed team will normally go through all stages of team development, regardless of how well the members know one another.

Models of team development uniformly define four stages of progression: cautious affiliation (forming), competitiveness (storming), harmonious cohesiveness (norming), and collaborative teamwork (performing). Some authors add a fifth stage, adjourning, to this process. See figure 18.2 for an explanation of the four main stages (Levi 2017, 44–46).

Figure 18.2. Four stages of team development

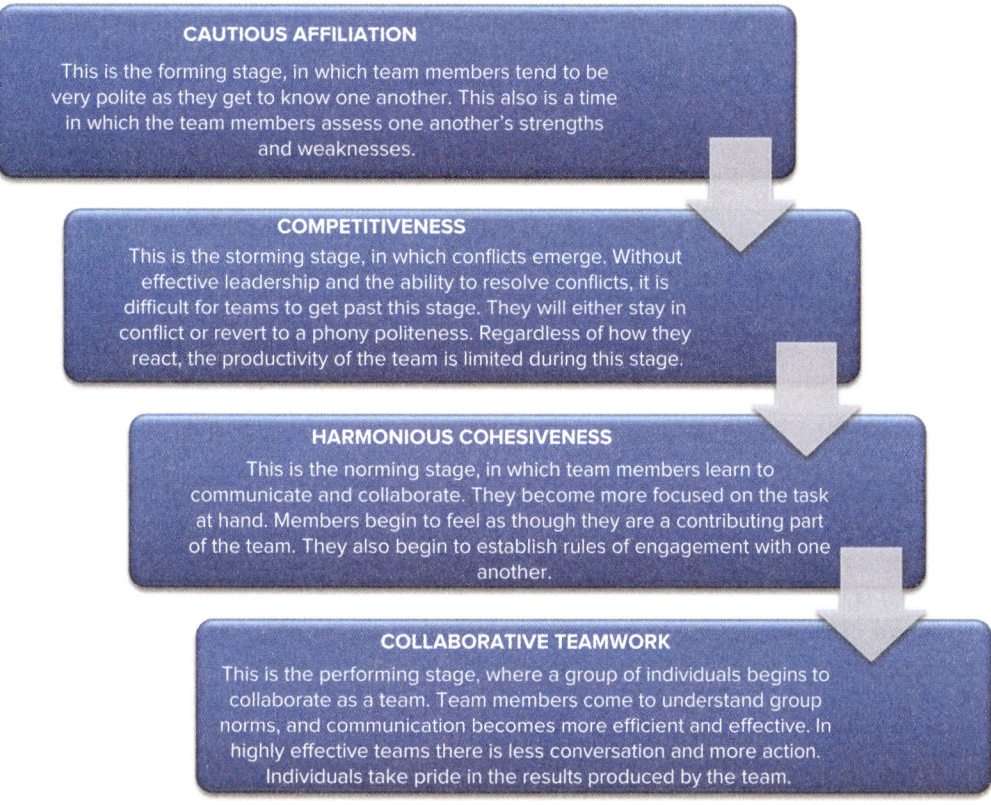

Source: Adapted from Levi 2017.

The team leader needs to be prepared for the natural shift in dynamics of a group as it matures, and they must be able to facilitate team development. Team leaders should allocate time for forming, storming, norming, and performing every time the team meets (Levi 2017, 47–48). This progression of stages is not necessarily linear. Even though a team may mature to norming or performing, events may occur that cause the team to revert to storming.

Allotting a few minutes at the beginning of each meeting to check in can help move the team along toward greater maturity. Checking in can be as simple as asking each team member to tell the team what they are prepared to bring to the meeting that day. If there is a change of even one team member, the team returns to the forming stage and the progression through the four stages begins again.

When the fifth stage, adjourning, is included, it marks the dissolution of a group. If handled appropriately, it provides positive closure for the team members. This is a time to celebrate successes and recognize team member contributions and accomplishments.

Leadership

A successful team leader must possess job task competencies and behavioral competencies (PMI 2021). A technically competent individual may not necessarily be a good project team leader unless this person also possesses behavioral competencies that enable them to understand team dynamics and positively influence team members. Situational leadership is a useful model for understanding and leading project teams (Henkel et al. 2019, 9). A team leader who understands which level of maturity their team has reached can select an appropriate, effective leadership style. The team leader should be more task oriented and directive with newly formed groups, and more relationship oriented and supportive of team members as they mature.

The project team leader is usually an employee from a functional area of the organization who is assigned responsibility for leading the team to completion of a project. This may put the leader in a position that divides attention and loyalty between the project team and the parent organization if the vision, goals, and objectives of the two do not align. A key role for the team leader is to bring these three elements into harmony.

Planning Processes

Organization leadership should make clear to project team members the importance of the project and the expected impact on the organization. However, once objectives for the project are established, the team should feel free to proceed without interference from leadership. Periodic feedback through reports and briefings can be done to keep leadership informed of how the project is progressing.

A critical element of the planning phase is the identification of final system requirements or criteria that set standards for measuring success. Without these standards in place, determining whether a project has succeeded becomes difficult.

Design

The most important contribution that team members can make during the design phase is the development of alternative solutions. If the organizational culture truly embraces PI and problem solving, a team will be able to develop alternative solutions and work through a step-by-step process to decide which alternative provides the optimal solution.

As alternatives are developed and discussed, the cost of implementing a recommended solution should be considered. Costs should be divided into two categories: fixed and operating. Fixed costs are one-time expenses, such as purchasing new software or equipment and other types of start-up costs. Operating costs are incurred to sustain the project on an ongoing basis.

Once the team decides to recommend an optimal solution, it needs to develop a schedule for implementation. This is a critical element of the planning function in project management. Planning must identify tasks, their duration, and who will be responsible for them.

Gantt Charts

An effective tool for planning and tracking the implementation of a project is the **Gantt chart**. A Gantt chart is a graphic tool used to plot tasks; it shows the duration of project tasks and overlapping tasks. This project management methodology is used for planning and tracking patient care processes. For example, a Gantt chart can be used to improve the scheduling process for a busy operating room by tracking schedules for multiple operating rooms and surgeons. Figure 18.3 is an example of a Gantt chart used to show the tasks and schedule for the five phases of a project.

PERT Charts

If a more quantitative approach is required, the program evaluation and review technique (PERT) may be used. This is also called the critical path method (CPM). PERT provides a structure that requires the project team to identify the order and projected duration of activities needed to complete a project. The most helpful element of PERT is that it identifies those critical activities that must be completed on time to enable the entire project to meet its final deadline.

A **PERT chart** depicts a network of activities, represented by arrows, as shown in figure 18.4. The numbers above the arrows represent the time required to complete the activities (hours or days). To construct a PERT chart, the PI team must identify all activities required and determine the order in which activities should proceed. The letters below the arrows represent the activity. Circles or ovals, called events, represent the beginning of an activity.

Figure 18.3. Gantt chart depicting the five phases of a project

Phase / Tasks	Responsible Parties	Week 1	2	3	4	5	6	7	8	9	10	11	12
Initiation		←——→											
First meeting of team leaders	Hospital administrator and county health officer	▼											
Mission statement	Hospital administrator	—											
Team member selection and appointment of team leader	Hospital administrator		—										
Team orientation meeting	County health officer				▼								
Planning					←—————→								
Planning meeting to brainstorm and identify problem(s)	Emergency services				▼								
Assign individual tasks	Emergency services					▼							
FEMA coordination planning	County health officer					—	—	—	—	—			
Admission and medical information management	Health information					—	—	—					
Equipment storage and access	Physical facilities					—	—	—					
Infection management	Infection control					—	—	—					
Identify locations suitable for patients	Physical facilities and nursing					—	—	—					
HVAC issues	Physical facilities					—	—	—					
Media management	Public affairs					—	—	—					
Develop training plan	Emergency services							—	—	—			
Execution									←————→				
Collect team input and write the final plan	All team members								—	—	—		
Training	All team members									—	—	—	—
Monitoring and Controlling					←————————————→								
Monitor project progress and adherence to timeline	Emergency services					—	—	—	—	—	—	—	—
Closure											←——→		
Submit plan for federal funding												▼	
Rehearsal exercise	All team members and hospital staff											▼	
Prepare and submit final report	Emergency services											—→	
Begin ongoing evaluation													▼

Figure 18.4. Example of a PERT chart

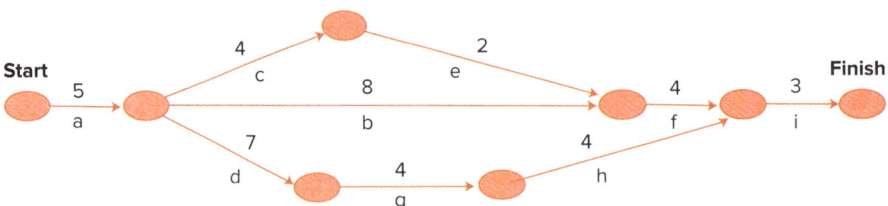

Some activities may be concurrent. These are called parallel activities. By following any path of arrows through the network from start to finish and adding the duration times of each activity, you can determine the total amount of time that series of activities will require. The path with the greatest total duration time is called the critical path and represents the longest amount of time required to complete the total project. The critical path in figure 18.4 is the sequence a → d → g → h → i, which will require 23 days.

Both PERT and Gantt charts require the planner to identify critical tasks, the duration of each task, and the expected completion dates. This scheduling process must consider those tasks that must be performed in a specific order (dependent on the task before and related to the task after) to complete the project at the proposed time, as well as the duration of each critical task. The costs associated with the tasks and the resources needed to complete them must also be considered. Within the critical path, noncritical tasks may be scheduled as resources to accomplish them become available and as their prerequisite tasks are completed.

Executing Processes

Once project planning is completed, execution (also called implementation) begins. This is where installation of equipment or construction begins, and any policy or procedure manuals should be prepared for distribution. Specifications developed in the design (planning) phase should be finalized. Any new systems or processes should be tested for performance.

Individuals involved in implementation and continued operation of a new or reorganized system need training. Thus, the implementation plan should include training and identify who will be trained. The training portion of the implementation plan should identify the content of the training, training objectives, and expected outcomes. If any QI toolbox techniques are to be implemented, they should be part of the training plan.

Execution of a project requires the project manager to coordinate resources, manage stakeholder engagement, and integrate and perform the activities of the project in accordance with the project management plan (PMI 2021). There are, however, some techniques that can help make the execution go as smoothly as possible:

1. *Define the critical success criteria for each phase.* This means identifying and defining the processes, products, and outcomes of each phase of the project plan that need to be accomplished to actually know that a phase is complete and operational. Processes are those actions that people take to make the project actually run. Products are those tangible or intangible outputs that the project produces from the work of its processes and personnel and are defined by the nature of the project undertaken. Outcomes are those elements of change in an organization and its constituent parts that result from undertaking the project.

2. *Organize the work and develop a project schedule that is communicated to leadership and the project team.* Often, project managers will distribute two- and three-year Gantt charts representing the milestones that the project must allegedly meet to be successful in the allotted organizational time frame. However, few individuals are truly able to relate to this kind of presentation on a day-to-day basis. They need to know what they need to accomplish each week and each month to keep the project moving, particularly when the project is large enough to last several years. Project managers who want

to keep their teams focused and motivated need to divide project objectives into smaller windows of time in order so the team members involved understand what is expected and make it happen. Remember that old adage: "How do you eat an elephant? One bite at a time!" Managing the project calendar and schedule ensures that criteria are successfully accomplished on a weekly as well as a project-wide basis.

3. *Make the project calendar public.* It allows everyone on the team to see how their contributions dovetail with everyone else's assignments and how crucial their responsible participation really is.

4. *Manage resource conflicts.* Critical path PERT charts can assist in determining what development or phase of a project needs to be completed before another development or phase. But that is just the first step; sometimes, different phases require the same resources to reach completion. Resources may be such things as the services of personnel with specialized expertise such as electricians or programmers. Or resources may be physical equipment that takes a long process or time period to acquire. Alternatively, resources may be physical spaces or buildings that have to be remodeled before they can be used for the project. Remember, when an organization modifies physical resources, it must also allocate time and money to meet local and state regulatory requirements and acquire permits, adding more time to the process. In any of these cases, management of project timelines is crucial to a project's success.

A number of QI toolbox techniques can be used to measure performance continuously and to evaluate the success or failure of newly implemented processes or systems. Measurement should be undertaken on a weekly and monthly basis against the project calendar. This may be as simple as checking off the success criteria as they are accomplished on a weekly or monthly basis, or it may turn to more sophisticated techniques, such as run charts, as the project actually gears up and begins functioning as it was (or was not) designed to function.

Monitoring and Controlling Processes

Monitoring and controlling are distinct processes, but in project management they work together as a single activity. The monitoring activity is performed to determine the current status of the project, enabling the project to be controlled. The control activity is performed to assess project status in reference to planned activities and their timeline. If the project is off target, a project manager would take action to bring it back on track (PMI 2021). Activities commonly performed in the monitoring and controlling process include regularly measuring and analyzing project performance and ensuring that any variances from the project plan are identified, appropriately vetted, and approved (PMI 2021).

Closing Processes

In closure, stage five of project management, the new system or process is used by the customer. This is the phase in which the project shifts to become an integrated part of organizational operations. During the operational phase, management must continually monitor performance and determine whether the new system or process meets established performance criteria.

As a project shifts from planning to execution to closure, testing performance results against finalized standards must not be ignored. Too often this is where the organization becomes distracted with other issues or new events and does not follow up on the success or failure of the project. This is one reason a project fails.

The project becomes the standard way of doing things in the closure phase. Team members return to their functional roles or move on to newly assigned roles if the project is one that changes their old functional roles. This is the phase in which the lessons learned are cataloged and documented. As the established project continues, it must be evaluated continually to determine whether performance is meeting established criteria and standards. During the process of evaluating results and outcomes, the organization looks for new improvement and innovation opportunities. When a new PI opportunity is identified, a new project is initiated.

Why Projects Fail

The value of PI projects in relation to an organization's outcomes and business performances is undeniable. However, not all PI projects are successful. Antony and Gupta identified the following reasons why process improvement projects fail (Antony and Gupta 2019, 368–372):

- Lack of commitment and support from top management
- Poor communication practices
- Incompetent teams
- Inadequate training and learning
- Faulty selection of process improvement methodology and associated tools and techniques
- Inappropriate rewards and recognition systems and culture
- Scope creep
- Suboptimal team size and composition
- Inconsistent monitoring and control or a lack of expert supervision
- Resistance to change or partial cooperation by employees

Some of the reasons for project failure are self-explanatory. Failing to secure solid business sponsorship has placed the responsibility squarely on an organization's senior leadership. As mentioned previously, executive-level commitment and support of a project are critical to its success. Without the backing of leadership, implementing a new project will be difficult, if not impossible, because of the natural resistance to change that occurs in most organizations.

Developing a viable project process shows that the organization has developed guidelines for standardized and repeatable processes of beginning and completing projects. Project team leaders should not have to start from scratch with each new project. A comprehensive project portfolio consists of a set of files organized into at least six areas that leadership and project team leaders are able to reference. The portfolio should include a file of ideas, charters (or proposed projects), projects in execution, completed projects, suspended projects, and canceled projects. With this collection of information, a project manager can compare their project with past successes and failures and with other activities going on throughout the organization.

It is just as important to plan and organize a team for success, as it is to avoid those things that lead to failure. Careful consideration of the project's team size and composition is needed. Too many members may hinder progress and too few can overburden team members and lead to inaction. Team members should be selected based on their knowledge of the process under consideration and the expertise they bring to the team. Each member of the team should be trained in the organization's PI processes and project management techniques. The communication style and methods should be determined by the team and followed closely so that all members are kept informed.

Getting organized and having a well-conceived plan in place are essential to keeping the project focused so it does not morph into other areas. To find out whether the project is progressing satisfactorily, the team needs to implement a monitoring system that measures success criteria against outcomes. Additionally, the need for an expert in the process is critical to project success.

The last tenet cannot be ignored. It is a natural inclination in humans and organizations to initially resist change. Leadership must be prepared to effectively counter resistance and continue the process of implementation and improvement. Recognizing employees for their contributions to the project can be helpful in getting buy-in to a process change and assist in implementation.

Some organizations are more receptive to change than others. The organization's leadership, project sponsors, and team members must champion the project and be persistent in seeing it through to full implementation.

Check Your Understanding 18.1

1. A local hospital is starting a new PI project to improve the level of customer satisfaction patients experience in the emergency department (ED). The recently hired ED director was chosen as the team leader for the PI project. As the project is moving forward, many team members are uncomfortable about the leader's negative attitude toward the project, which he often shares with team members. Although the project is moving forward and meeting timelines, the team feels that the dynamics of the team are negatively affected. Explain why this leadership style is not conducive to a successful project, even though the project itself seems to be moving forward as planned.

2. The HIM director at Central Valley Community Hospital is preparing to begin a project to improve the satisfaction level of customers of her department's services. She is trying to determine a way to plan and track the project tasks. Which of the following is the best tool for her to use?
   a. Affinity diagram
   b. Gantt chart
   c. PERT chart
   d. Flowchart

QI Toolbox Techniques

Gantt Chart

A Gantt chart is a project management tool used to schedule and track important activities. Gantt charts divide a horizontal scale into days, weeks, or months and a vertical scale into project activities or tasks. Figure 18.3 is an example of a Gantt chart depicting the five phases of a project. The tool provides a graphic method for showing the simultaneous and interdependent tasks for the project.

PERT Chart

The program evaluation and review technique (PERT) is used when a quantitative approach is required to track project progress. This is also called the critical path method (CPM). PERT provides a structure that requires the project team to identify the order and projected duration of activities needed to complete a project. The most helpful element of PERT is that it identifies those critical activities that must be completed on time to enable the entire project to meet its final deadline. A PERT chart depicts a network of activities, represented by arrows, as shown in figure 18.4. The numbers above the arrows represent the time required to complete the activities (hours or days). To construct a PERT chart, the PI team must identify all activities required and determine the order in which activities should proceed. The letters below the arrows represent the activity. Circles or ovals, called events, represent the beginning of an activity.

Real-Life Example

Healthcare accrediting bodies require organizations to have specific plans in place for responding to emergency events. The Centers for Disease Control and Prevention (CDC), Health Resources and Services Administration (HRSA), and the Department of Homeland Security (DHS) work together to ensure that state and local health departments, hospitals, and other health agencies are able to mount a collective response to community-wide emergency events.

Following a recent pandemic event, the local health department and hospital staff determined that their response plan was inefficient and needed improvement. The county health officer approached their local hospital to work together to develop an emergency operations plan for future pandemic events.

This hospital is a 150-bed community hospital, located 35 miles from a large medical center in another county. The hospital has conducted annual disaster drills in compliance with accreditation standards, however, the drills were mass-casualty exercises based on the scenarios of a major fire in an industrial setting, natural disasters, and a transportation accident involving large numbers of injured patients. Previous exercises did not address exposure of large numbers of patients, hospital staff, and emergency response personnel to infectious agents as seen in a pandemic event.

The hospital administrator and the county health officer agree that there is a need to enhance and broaden the scope of disaster planning to include issues that would require triage of patients or strict quarantine of patients exposed to the pandemic virus. The hospital administrator has agreed to appoint a project team that will work with the county health officer to expand the existing disaster plan to include pandemic events.

The county health officer has authorization to spend funds from the DHS to purchase supplies and equipment that the hospital would need in the event of another pandemic. This includes items such as personal protective equipment for hospital personnel assigned to the pandemic response teams. To qualify for the funds, the hospital must coordinate with the county health officer and develop a plan for responding to a pandemic using the DHS framework known as the National Incident Management System. Adoption of this framework is required to be eligible for federal preparedness assistance and funding. For years, the hospital had been using the Incident Command System to orchestrate a response to local disaster situations, but now the response plan needs to be broadened to work with multiple agencies in the region to manage their response to future pandemics.

Because federal funding is involved, the plan must be complete and in place within 12 weeks or the funds will be withdrawn and reallocated to other regions of the country. The hospital is scheduled for an accreditation survey in about nine months, an additional incentive to complete the project in a timely manner.

During the initiation phase of the project, the hospital administrator and the county health officer agree upon the mission to develop an implementation plan for policies and procedures that prepare the hospital to effectively respond to a pandemic event. The combination of individuals selected for the hospital project team is based on ensuring that all the required components of the Incident Command System under unified command are represented. The hospital administrator has decided to appoint the director of emergency services as the hospital project team leader. The team leader will be expected to work closely with the county health officer, along with the leadership of fire, police, emergency medical services, and public works agencies in directing the team's activities. The county health officer will be the overall coordinator of the regional multidisciplinary project team. Under a unified command, agencies will work together through the designated members to analyze intelligence information and establish a common set of objectives and strategies for a single Incident Action Plan. In the case of another pandemic event, it would be likely that the director of emergency services would fill the role of operations section chief for hospital incident activities.

The director of health information services is selected to represent the functions of the public information officer (PIO). This individual is tasked with coordinating the flow of information to the community, news outlets, and other organizations associated with event response. The PIO gathers relevant data and information about the incident to share with all stakeholders.

The infection control nurse's activities become even more important in a pandemic event in collecting data and training staff on procedures that will control further spread of disease from an infected patient. The infection control nurse is selected for the project team to support the operations section chief with technical information and processes for handling the pandemic event.

The director of physical facilities, in support of the operations section chief, is responsible for ensuring that portable triage and isolation tents and other equipment can be located and deployed efficiently in the case of a real event. The director must be able to effectively control heating, ventilation, and air conditioning systems that can be shut down and secured in the event of a pandemic threat to the hospital's internal environment from contaminants present in the external air.

Finally, the director of materials management is selected for the team to represent the Logistics Section, responsible for all support requirements, including communications support, medical support to incident personnel, food for incident personnel, and supplies and ground support.

As part of the initiation phase, the hospital administrator brings the selected members of the project team together for orientation. (See figure 18.3, a Gantt chart depicting the five project phases.) At this point, the planning phase begins. The team will meet to brainstorm and identify problems. In the planning phase, subtasks are assigned to individual team members based on their areas of expertise and responsibility.

As team members bring information and expertise back to the team, the plan begins to take shape, and the team prepares to move into the execution phase. The predominant tasks of the execution phase are writing the final draft of the plan and training staff in preparation for future exercises and the possibility of a pandemic event.

The hospital project team leader will actively monitor the project's progress and ensure that all team members are on target to meet the timeline to ensure that federal funding is secured. If any team members or activities get off track, it is the responsibility of the project manager to take action to bring them back on track.

During the last phase, closure, the team and hospital leadership evaluate the results of the project. The rehearsal exercise will be documented so that lessons learned can be applied to opportunities for continued improvement and demonstrate to accreditation surveyors that an annual exercise that meets the new standards has been conducted.

Case Study

Community Hospital has decided to adopt the principles and behaviors of high reliability organizations. To effectively pilot and then disseminate such a program, it takes robust project management. The following is a list of tasks that need to be completed as part of this initiative.

- Form a multidisciplinary team
- Create a presentation to communicate the details of the PI project
- Determine sources for data collection
- Train staff on new processes
- Develop new process
- Create a project timeline
- Write mission and vision statements
- Collect and analyze data
- Present options to leadership and gain approval
- Assess the environment for unintended consequences of the process change
- Plan a celebratory party for the project team
- Continually analyze data to evaluate the new process for effectiveness
- Initiate the new process

Case Study Questions

1. Using the PI process life cycle, categorize each of the tasks listed into one of the five steps.
2. Develop a Gantt chart that lists the five steps and the corresponding tasks that would be appropriate in that step. Remember to think about activities that are dependent on one another or that may overlap with other activities.

Review Questions

1. This phase in the project life cycle includes clear objectives, importance of the project, and the expected outcome on the organization.
   a. Initiation
   b. Planning
   c. Execution
   d. Closure

2. A PI team in the radiology department determined that the wait time for procedures in their department is too long. This team worked through the steps in the PI process, developed a project and timeline, collected data, and made a recommendation to improve the wait times. The recommendation was to implement a new procedure for the registration process in their department. This project streamlined the registration process and reduced the wait times for patients but failed to collect all of the information necessary to accurately bill and collect payment for services. Administration was not happy because the billing issues they encountered were the first time they had heard about the registration process change. Analyze this scenario, and determine why this project failed.

3. Describe how the function of project management is used in performance improvement programs.

4. You are leading a project to upgrade an existing electronic health record (EHR) system in a busy outpatient clinic. The current system lacks certain functionalities, hindering the clinic's ability to provide efficient patient care. The organization has decided to implement a more advanced EHR system that includes features such as integrated telehealth options and improved data analytics for better decision-making. At this point in the project, you are identifying the key project stakeholders, defining project goals, and securing necessary approvals. Which phase of the project management life cycle is this describing?
   a. Planning
   b. Controlling and monitoring
   c. Initiation
   d. Execution

5. Leading a healthcare project to upgrade an outpatient clinic's EHR system, you are at the point where you are overseeing installation and staff training. Which phase of the project are you currently working in?
   a. Planning
   b. Controlling and monitoring
   c. Initiation
   d. Execution

References

Antony, J. and S. Gupta. 2019. Top ten reasons for process improvement project failures. *International Journal of Lean Six Sigma* 10(1):367-374.

Henkel, T., J. Marion, and D. Bourdeau. (2019). Project manager leadership behavior: Task-oriented versus relationship-oriented. *Journal of Leadership Education* 18(2):1-14.

Levi, D. 2017. *Group Dynamics for Teams*, 5th ed. Los Angeles and Washington, DC: Sage Publishing.

PMI (Project Management Institute). 2021. *A Guide to Project Management Body of Knowledge (PMBOK® Guide)*, 7th ed. Newtown Square, PA: Project Management Institute. https://www.pmi.org/pmbok-guide-standards/foundational/pmbok.

Resources

Kerzner, H. 2022. *Project Management: A Systems Approach to Planning, Scheduling, and Controlling*, 13th ed. New York: John Wiley & Sons.

Olson, B. D. 2020. "Project Management." Chapter 26 in *Health Information Management: Concepts, Principles, and Practice*, 6th ed., edited by P. Oachs and A. Watters. Chicago: AHIMA.

Managing the Human Side of Change

19

Learning Objectives

- Apply change management techniques to implement performance improvements
- Compare and contrast the three phases of change
- Use the key steps in change management

Key Term

Change management

In today's world, there is no such thing as permanent stability. Processes and structures that worked last year may be ineffective this year. Products and services that are considered cutting edge quickly become obsolete. Similarly, healthcare delivery in the US has been in a state of rapid and unpredictable evolution ever since the Medicare and Medicaid programs were implemented in the 1970s and the prospective payment system (PPS) was instituted in the 1980s.

The overarching reason for change in healthcare organizations today is the need to improve the quality of care while controlling the cost of services. Hospitals and other healthcare organizations have performance improvement (PI) programs to meet this need. Systems, processes, and staff competencies undergo a circular cycle of change as improvements are made in the clinical, administrative, and governance areas of the organization.

PI is based on the quantitative analysis of data, processes, and structures, but PI efforts also have a very human side. After all, healthcare is provided by individuals working in extremely complex organizations, not by robots that can be reprogrammed or replaced when change is needed. Failure to consider the human side of PI and the impact of change can derail even the best-conceived improvement efforts.

Healthcare professionals have always understood the importance of what they do. Today, during an era of dramatic and ongoing change, most healthcare professionals strive to improve patient care services and outcomes. In this continued era of rapid change, we see a proliferation of "disruptive technologies and business models that may threaten the status quo but will ultimately raise the quality of care for everyone" (Christensen et al. 2000, 104). Still, most employees find it difficult to alter their work habits, and healthcare professionals are no exception.

The Three Phases of Change

Every change that affects individuals is experienced in three phases. Whether changing their dietary habits or the way they write a patient care plan, all individuals go through a similar process. In his research on human reaction to change, Kurt Lewin called the three phases unfreezing, moving, and freezing, as shown in figure 19.1 (Lewin 1947, 34–35). Lewin observed that during each of these phases, forces in favor of change and forces that resist change work against each other. The analysis of such competing forces in the face of a particular planned change is often called a force-field analysis.

Figure 19.1. Lewin's three phases of change

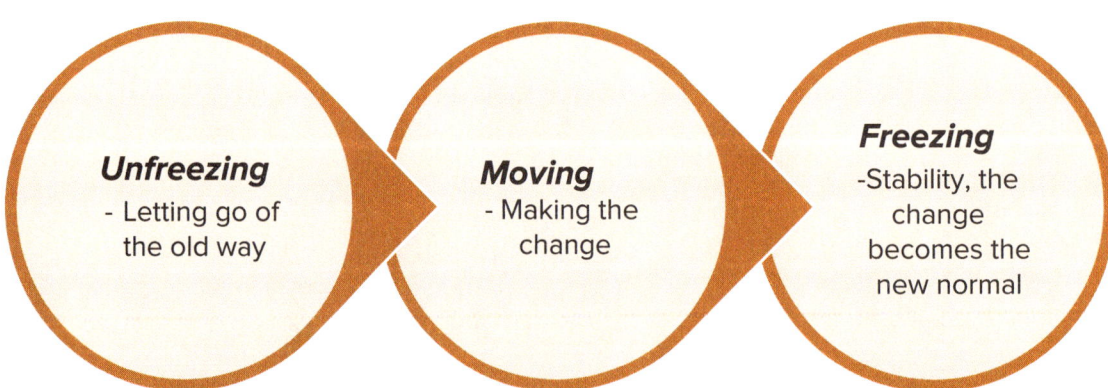

Source: Lewin 1947

These phases also have been referred to as ending, transition, and beginning. The unfreezing/ending phase is characterized by grief and letting go. The moving/transition phase is characterized by confusion and creativity. The freezing/beginning phase is characterized by acceptance and hope for the future.

The three phases of change are not clear-cut steps. Rather, they overlap one another. At any particular point, one of these phases is likely to predominate, while the emotions and concerns associated with the other two phases recede to the background. The movement is gradual as one phase gives way to the next.

Phase 1: Unfreezing/Ending

Grief is a natural human reaction to loss of any kind. Simply defined, grief is the conflicting feelings that come along with the end of something familiar or a change in an accepted pattern of behavior. Employees can experience grief when the way they have been doing their work is changed due to a new process or as their organization experiences significant changes and even realignment. Before individuals can go on to a new beginning, they need to let go of their old identity and/or their old way of doing things. Managers and employees go through these stages at different rates, usually because management is involved in the change process. Taking the time to involve employees in activities such as data collection, data analysis, or decision-making will bring them on board with the change more quickly (Edwards et al. 2020).

Like change, grief occurs in stages. Some propose that the process consists of three stages: shock, despair, and recovery. Still, others posit that the organizational grief process, based on organizational change, includes four stages—equilibrium to immobilization, denial to anger, bargaining to depression, and testing to acceptance (Romadona and Setiawan 2021). Whatever the number and names of the stages, it is clear that a transformation in thinking and perception must occur when employees experience change in the organizations in which they work.

Phase 2: Moving/Transition

Between the ending of the old and the beginning of the new lies a transitional zone. This transitional period is experienced regardless of the desire to change or whether the perception of the change is good or bad. The transitional phase is unsettling and uncomfortable. Individuals often report feeling confusion, anxiety, and unsteadiness in the midst of change. The old way of doing things is gone, but the new way of doing things still feels untried and uncomfortable. The transitional phase is imperative because impactful change cannot happen without it. Ensuring that employees make it through this change by providing clear communication is a must to achieve the desired results (Phillips and Klein 2023, 194).

Left to their own thoughts and feelings and without sufficient information during this phase of organizational change, individuals may decide to escape their discomfort and confusion by leaving the organization. Resistance to change is a common threat to change. However, when the change process is understood, the transitional period can be a time of renewal and creativity. Often, certain individuals within a larger group are optimistic about change. These individuals are more accepting of change and are assets to their organizations (Nwanzu and Babalola 2019).

Phase 3: Freezing/Beginning

During the final phase of change, the beginning of the new way of doing things, the people who make up the organization settle into a more comfortable state. The new processes or staff structures become familiar, and individuals come to understand and accept their new roles. Some may still worry that the new way of doing things may not work or that it may even make things worse. Some may still feel regrets about the ideas or coworkers they had to leave behind. Some may even miss the freedom of the transitional zone and find settling back into a routine rather boring. A beginning also can be a disappointing time when changes seem to have been made for no discernible reason. Eventually the new way of doing things becomes the accepted way. The unfamiliar new task often becomes automatic within the cycle of change.

Change Management

Any organization, and especially a large healthcare organization, thrives when operating with established structures and processes. And when change is necessary, effective management of the phases of change enables an organization to successfully weather the transition. Like PI, change can be thought of as a process to be understood and managed. For the purposes of this chapter, **change management** can be defined as a group of techniques that help individuals understand the process of change and accept PI in work processes. One or more members of the PI team may become the change manager(s) for the project, or a manager in the areas affected by the change may play this role. Many organizations hire consultants to handle the change management process when planned changes will have a significant impact on employees and medical staff.

Eight steps known as "accelerators for change" are shown in figure 19.2. The subsections that follow describe each of these steps.

Figure 19.2. Kotter's eight accelerators for change

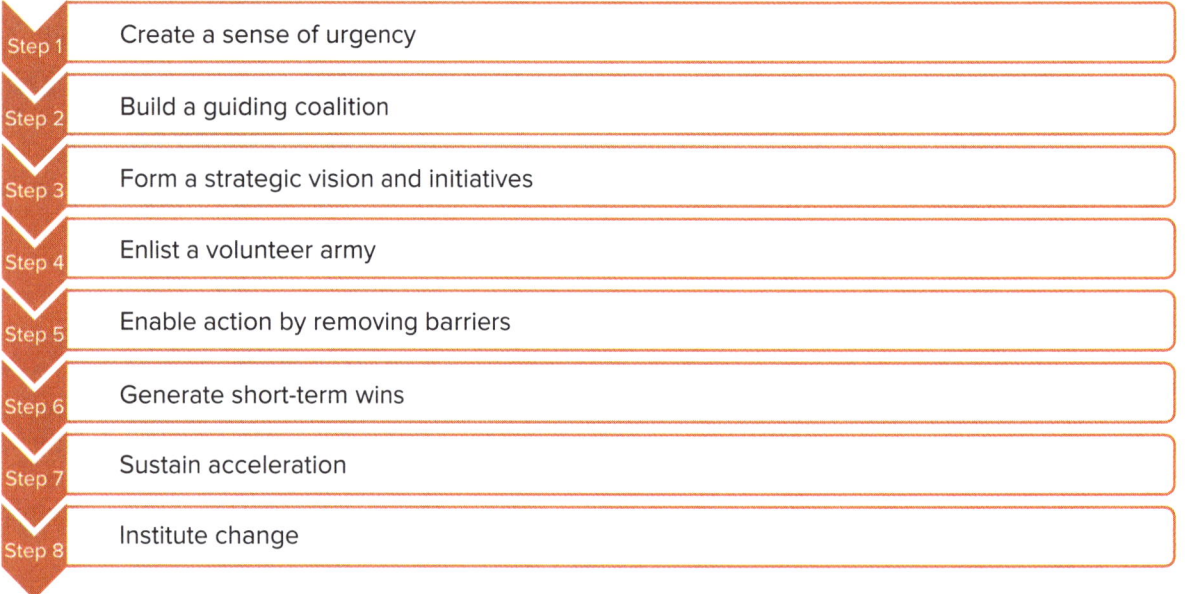

Source: Kotter 2018.

Create a Sense of Urgency

The PI team should describe the proposed improvement in as much detail as possible that will appeal to individuals affected by the change, both logically and emotionally. Using flow charts to map out processes may help the team identify all the areas that will be involved. Changes made in one area may create the need for secondary changes in other areas. The task of the PI team is to explain to affected staff and leaders the benefits of making the proposed change as well as describing the consequences of failing to change (Kotter 2018, 10).

Build a Guiding Coalition

In this step, all members of the PI team must be committed to the change initiative. Without this obvious commitment from the team to making the change, it will be difficult to influence others to change their behavior and processes. Depending on the scope of the change being proposed, the team may need to expand their membership to include individuals from all levels of the organization (management, technical, staff) and both short-term and long-term employees. Including a wide range of individuals allows a broader base of knowledge and experience to help move the organization forward with the change process. The committed PI team that is diverse in membership provides the organization the necessary group to guide the change process (Kotter 2018, 13).

Form a Strategic Vision and Initiatives

To help organizations change it is imperative that the PI team create a clear strategic vision that is simple, flexible, and easily communicated. This vision can help motivate people into action and coordinate activities to move the change process along. The strategic vision should make it clear how the process will be different in the future from what it is now, and why the change is needed. Communication is a key component of this step. The timing and content of communications should be carefully planned as an element of project design. It is crucial that the proposed changes be described in specific detail early in the PI process. If people do not understand the purpose of a change, they will have difficulty accepting it. If they are not sure what the change will entail, they will come to their own conclusions about which processes will end and which will continue. If they are not told how the change will affect them, they may assume the worst (Kotter 2018, 16).

Information about the change project should be communicated consistently and often. Repeating the information in a variety of ways will help people accept the change. Newsletters, special announcements, staff meetings, and other forms of communication can all be used to convey the message. The people affected by the change should be kept up to date as proposed changes are developed, and they should be given an opportunity to provide feedback to the PI team.

Enlist a Volunteer Army

The scale of building an army will be dependent on the change initiative being undertaken. If the change is large (such as the high-reliability initiative discussed later in the Real-Life Example), the organization needs individuals from all levels of the organization to be trained in the new way of working and thinking. These individuals then need to assist in bringing the change to their departments and team members to continue to move the entire organization into this new way of working. However, if the change is on a smaller scale, the volunteer army may be a department or section of a department that needs to change. Regardless of size, at this point in the change process it is important to build excitement around the change so individuals want to change, rather than feel that they have to change. Recognition of your change volunteers is critical to keeping them engaged and to engage new ones (Kotter 2018, 19).

Enable Action by Removing Barriers

Barriers to change can take on many forms. Some common barriers include inefficient processes, organizational silos, and outdated rules or procedures. The change manager or PI team must identify these barriers and then remove them. Managers sometimes make the mistake of criticizing the way things were done in the past as a way of introducing improvements. Creating negative pictures of the past is not effective. Instead, the past should be honored for the positive things accomplished and for the foundations laid for the future. Showing sensitivity to the old process can be helpful in showing employees why the new process or change is needed (Kotter 2018, 22).

Generate Short-Term Wins

A key activity of the change manager or PI team is to keep track of the change process. One reason to do this is to track progress toward the full realization of the change initiative. A second reason is to keep track of short-term wins, lessons learned, processes improved, new behaviors observed, and the like. Each short-term win should be acknowledged by the change manager to reinforce the action for others within the organization. Positive reinforcement of the desired behavior or actions will help generate more of this type of behavior and action in the future by other employees (Kotter 2018, 25).

Sustain Acceleration

At this point in the change management process it is important to stay focused. After some short-term wins or gains toward process change have occurred, the sense of urgency may wane. It is important to stay focused on the goal and to incorporate activities that sustain the sense of urgency for the change. Adding more employees to the change effort brings new energy for the change initiative and a fresh perspective. These new volunteers will bring new ideas for removing the barriers for a successful change (Kotter 2018, 27).

Institute Change

After building new behaviors, attitudes, and processes with steps 1 through 7, the final step requires the organization to look for ways to sustain the change in the future. The new process must become the new norm and replace the old way of doing things. People use ceremonies to mark beginnings as well as endings. The change manager should find a way to help people celebrate their successes in making meaningful changes in the way they perform their work. A ribbon-cutting ceremony at a new facility, an open house for a reorganized department, and a demonstration of new equipment for colleagues outside the department are some examples of celebrations that mark new beginnings. Even the accomplishment of a minor procedural improvement should be acknowledged with a sincere thank-you to all people involved in conceiving, planning, and implementing the change (Kotter 2018, 30).

Real-Life Example

Community Hospital has decided to implement a high-reliability program to improve their quality reporting scores. This program trains individuals across the organization on high-reliability concepts, including mindfulness and zero harm. Implementation of this initiative will be a significant change in the culture of this hospital. The following discussion highlights Kotter's eight-step process of change management that this organization went through as they implemented the high-reliability program.

First, the organization reviewed their quality metrics and compared them to their competitors in the area. Community Hospital had seen a significant drop in their quality scores in patient safety, medication administration, and the Hospital Consumer Assessment of Healthcare Providers and Systems (HCAHPS) scores. This high-reliability initiative is viewed by the organization's leaders as an opportunity for the hospital to improve these metrics. There is a sense of urgency for Community Hospital to improve their quality scores, as this will impact reimbursement and their reputation in the community. Part of this step involves communication with employees to help them understand why this change is needed to improve patient safety and quality of care.

The hospital board of directors appointed the quality and patient safety director as the individual to lead this high-reliability initiative and team. Executive leadership gave their full support to the director to implement this change and provided a budget for the initiative. The director assembled a team of key stakeholders and department managers from the hospital to serve on her team. This team spent time on team-building activities and is committed to implementing the change.

The project team created a vision for implementing the high-reliability initiative. This vision was to "create a culture of zero harm and mindfulness throughout the organization." Strategies for achieving this vision included: understanding the change process and how it affects employees, developing a program to educate all employees throughout the organization about high reliability, and ensuring that this strategy aligns with other quality initiatives and work occurring in the organization.

The first step that Community Hospital took to communicate the high-reliability initiative change was for the executive leadership to share the reasons for the change and steps on how the change will occur through the hospital's employee newsletter. After the newsletter was sent electronically, each department manager met with their employees to discuss the impending changes and how these changes would affect their department functions and job duties. The need and sense of urgency was reiterated by the department managers, and employees were given opportunities to ask questions about the change. The executive leadership, the high-reliability team, and the department managers served as positive role models of the change to model this behavior for employees.

Once the organization's workforce understood the reasons for adopting the high-reliability initiative, more employees began to embrace the idea. Excitement for the program encouraged employees to seek opportunities to be part of the implementation. This shift in thinking about caregiving and safety created a positive energy and facilitated a higher level of buy-in among all employees. The high-reliability team made a concerted effort to recognize those employees who helped to move the initiative forward. This recognition was noticed by employees who were less enthusiastic about the change to high-reliability thinking, which helped change their viewpoint and move them closer to acceptance of the change.

After communicating the high-reliability initiative, the implementation team's next step was to set the plan for change in motion throughout the organization. The team was on the lookout for potential barriers and obstacles as the plan was put into action and they worked to remove these deterrents. The team was cognizant of people or processes that had the potential to undermine the vision for change. As departments embraced the high-reliability culture, they identified opportunities for improvement within their functions and departments. These opportunities for improvement were noted to potentially become smaller team-based PI projects that would incorporate the concepts of high reliability, zero harm, and mindfulness.

Community Hospital set incremental goals to improve the quality scores. The employees were given the tools and support to meet these goals and show improvement in the scores. As short-term metrics were reviewed for quality and patient safety by the team, the scores improved. For each improved metric, the hospital rewarded and recognized all employees who were instrumental in the improvement.

With the success that the high-reliability initiative had at Community Hospital, other initiatives related to quality and patient safety have been recognized. These new initiatives piggybacked on the gains realized by the initial high-reliability project. As the organization has hired new employees and promoted existing employees, those decisions were made based on a fit for the newly developed quality and patient safety culture. Based on their past success, the organization was infused with new projects and ways to improve their quality of care through these further initiatives.

Community Hospital has incorporated criteria in all employee performance appraisals that support the high-reliability initiative. In doing this, the organization reinforced its commitment to improving its quality scores and patient safety, and is rewarding all employees for the change in the organization's culture. This improved performance is recognized in the development of organizational leaders and in the succession process.

 Check Your Understanding 19.1

1. In the context of Kotter's eight accelerators for change, which accelerator specifically focuses on the critical aspect of maintaining the momentum of change initiatives over the long term?
   a. Create a sense of urgency
   b. Enlist a volunteer army
   c. Generate short-term wins
   d. Sustain acceleration

2. Paulo has been working in patient registration for the past two years. Recently, changes have occurred that significantly changed his workflow in the electronic health record. Before the changes were announced, Paul felt that he had a high level of efficiency with the system and was able to provide patients with excellent customer service. Although the changes were difficult to adjust to, Paulo now feels he is back to an acceptable level of proficiency and feels more confident helping patients with their registration. Which phase of change is he now in?
   a. The changing phase, as he is making the changes required of him because of the new workflow.
   b. The unfreezing phase, as he is letting go of the old workflow (the way he used to do his work).
   c. The grief phase because, like any human, he is reacting to the changes associated with the new workflow.
   d. The refreezing phase, as he has become accustomed to the new workflow and his confidence in his abilities has returned.

Case Study

In a large urban hospital, the leadership team has identified a concerning increase in healthcare-associated infections (HAIs) over the past few months. The data reveal a rise in cases, particularly related to a specific unit, despite ongoing efforts to maintain high infection control standards. The hospital's reputation for patient safety is at risk, and there are potential financial implications due to increased healthcare costs.

To address this situation, the leadership recognizes the need for a profound sense of urgency. An in-depth analysis of the infection data indicates a clear trend that demands immediate attention. The rise in HAIs poses a threat to patient well-being and requires swift action to prevent further harm. Several patients have experienced complications associated with the infections, leading to increased lengths of stay and additional medical interventions. Ensuring patient safety becomes a top priority.

The hospital is subject to strict regulatory requirements regarding infection control by state licensing agencies, federal regulators, and their accreditation body. The increasing number of HAIs raises concerns about compliance, and failure to address the issue promptly could result in regulatory penalties. The hospital's reputation for providing high-quality care is at stake. News of rising infection rates may negatively impact public perception, potentially leading to a decrease in patient trust and satisfaction. The financial impact of longer patient stays, increased healthcare costs, and potential legal ramifications necessitates urgent intervention.

Case Study Questions

1. How would you explain the "why" or the need for change based on the current results described in the case?
2. What methods could be used to communicate information about the change within the organization?

Review Questions

1. Community Hospital of the West is experiencing changes occurring throughout the facility. Many of the employees are concerned about how the changes with affect their current position and workflow. Although the employees are aware that changes are occurring in the facility, there has been little communication regarding the changes, and employees are feeling unsettled. Describe the steps the hospital needs to do to better support employees during this transitional phase of change. What are some consequences for the hospital if this type of support is not provided?

2. In his research on human reactions to change, Lewin determined three phases of change. The three phases are_____, _____, and _____.
   a. Unfreezing, thawing, changing
   b. Thawing, refreezing, altering
   c. Unfreezing, moving, freezing
   d. Changing, altering, freezing

3. Darla is the new manager of the pediatric clinic. After a few months in this new role, Darla believes that there is a more efficient way to do several processes in patient registration. As a way of convincing employees that a change needs to occur, she tells them that the past processes are ineffective and should never have been performed in that manner. Assess Darla's technique in introducing the need for change at the clinic and any likely consequences of her approach.

4. When change managers take time to show sensitivity to an old process as a means to help employees understand why a new process or change is needed, they are using which of Kotter's accelerators of change?
   a. Build a guiding coalition
   b. Enlist a volunteer army
   c. Enable action by removing barriers
   d. Institute change

5. In which of Kotter's accelerators of change is it important to build excitement around the change so that individuals want to change, rather than feel they have to change?
   a. Create a sense of urgency
   b. Enlist a volunteer army
   c. Generate short-term wins
   d. Sustain acceleration

References

Christensen, C. M., R. Bohmer, and J. Kenagy. 2000. Will disruptive innovations cure health care? *Harvard Business Review* 5:102–110.

Edwards, K., T. Prætorius, and A. Paarup Nielsen. 2020. A model of cascading change: Orchestrating planned and emergent change to ensure employee participation. *Journal of Change Management* 20(4):342–368.

Kotter, J. 2022. *8 Steps to Accelerate Change in Your Organization*. Cambridge, MA: Kotter Inc. https://www.kotterinc.com/methodology/8-steps/.

Lewin, K. 1947. Frontiers in group dynamics: Concept, method, and reality in social science; social equilibria and social change. *Human Relations* 1(5):5–41, https://journals.sagepub.com/doi/10.1177/001872674700100103.

Nwanzu, C. L. and S. S. Babalola. 2019. Examining psychological capital of optimism, self-efficacy and self-monitoring as predictors of attitude towards organizational change. *International Journal of Engineering Business Management* 11, https://doi.org/10.1177/1847979019827149.

Phillips, J. and J. D. Klein. 2023. Change management: From theory to practice. *TechTrends* 67(1):189–197.

Romadona, M. R. and S. Setiawan. 2021. Researchers' view on R&D organizational change using the grief cycle. *Journal of STI Policy and Management* 6(2):157–171.

Resources

Adelman-Mullally, T., S. Nielsen, and S. Y. Chung. 2023. Planned change in modern hierarchical organizations: A three-step model. *Journal of Professional Nursing* 46:1–6.

Burke, W. W. 2023. *Organization Change: Theory and Practice*, 6th ed. Thousand Oaks, CA: Sage Publishing.

Bushe G. R., and S. Lewis. 2023. Three change strategies in organization development: Data-based, high engagement and generative. *Leadership & Organization Development Journal* 44(2):173–188.

Cameron, E., and M. Green. 2019. *Making Sense of Change Management: A Complete Guide to the Models, Tools and Techniques of Organizational Change*. Philadelphia: Kogan Page.

Understanding the Legal Implications of Performance Improvement

20

Learning Objectives

- Apply legal aspects to performance improvement activities conducted in healthcare organizations
- Explain the significance and relationship of tort law to quality improvement activities
- Relate the concepts of protection and privilege to quality improvement activities
- Distinguish quality improvement activities from research activities

Key Terms

Breach of duty
Causation
Damages
Discoverable
Duty to use due care
Elements of negligence
Generalizable knowledge

Malpractice
Privilege
Privileged information
Protection
Research
Tort

In healthcare organizations, performance improvement (PI) activities are affected by a number of laws, rules, regulations, and accreditation standards. Because PI processes can be complex and at times controversial, understanding the legal context in which these activities are carried out is critical. This chapter addresses the legal implications of PI in relation to the following areas:

- Tort law
- Four basic elements of negligence or malpractice
- Avoidance of risk from a malpractice perspective
- The organized medical staff
- Peer review protection
- Immunity from liability
- Occurrence reports and sentinel events
- Responsibility for disclosing adverse events to the patient or patient's family
- Distinguishing quality improvement from research
- Public health activities

Tort Law

A **tort** is a wrongful act committed against a person or property. A tort is a civil action, as opposed to a criminal act or a breach of contract.

Tort law in the US is primarily based on English law and provides a means for private parties to resolve disputes. Individuals, groups, businesses, corporations, and other nongovernmental organizations can bring many kinds of legal actions, known as lawsuits, under the general heading of tort law in civil courts. In such actions, one party generally seeks monetary payment for harm or damages caused by another party.

In contrast, criminal actions are prosecuted by the government against an individual accused of committing a crime. In criminal actions, the result sought by the government is generally a jail sentence.

In healthcare, the most notable tort is the tort of negligence, also commonly referred to as malpractice. **Malpractice** is the improper or negligent treatment of a patient by a healthcare provider that results in injury, damage, or loss. In malpractice actions, providers or facilities or both are sued for being careless and thereby causing an injury to a patient.

Four Basic Elements of Negligence or Malpractice

Four basic **elements of negligence** must be present and proven to accomplish a successful malpractice action:

1. **Duty to use due care**: A relationship must have been established between the parties in which one party has an obligation, or *duty*, to act as a reasonably prudent person would act toward the other. This duty exists in a provider's relationship with their patients. *Using due care* means acting as a reasonably prudent person (or in this case, a reasonably prudent provider) would act under a given set of circumstances.

2. **Breach of duty**: In a malpractice action, the issue is whether a provider exercised a standard of care that a reasonably prudent provider would have exercised under those circumstances. Failure to exercise due care is a *breach of duty*.

3. **Damages**: The patient must show that actual harm, or *damage*, occurred.
4. **Causation**: There must be a connection between the breach of duty and the damage—evidence that the failure to exercise due care (the breach) *caused* the damage.

The following scenarios illustrate these four elements of negligence.

Hypothetical Situation #1
A physician carelessly administered the wrong drug to a patient, which caused the patient to lapse into a coma. All elements of a malpractice action are met. The physician has a duty to exercise due care in treating a patient, and the physician breached that duty by carelessly administering the wrong drug. As a result of that breach, the patient was harmed, ending up in a coma directly caused by administration of the wrong medication.

Hypothetical Situation #2
A physician carelessly administered the wrong drug to a patient, but the patient was not harmed by this medication error in any way. In such a case, a malpractice action should not succeed because the element of damage is absent, as is causation, since no ill effect was suffered.

Hypothetical Situation #3
State law requires the ratio of nurses to patients in a certain type of nursing unit to be 4 nurses to every 10 patients, and every hospital in the community complies with this standard. In an effort to promote itself as providing the highest quality of care in the community, Hospital X develops a written policy stating that it will provide 5 nurses for every 10 patients. However, shortly after the policy is approved, a significant number of nurses leave Hospital X for other jobs, and the hospital is unable to recruit enough nurses to meet the staffing ratio that it established. During this period, a patient falls and breaks their hip, and the accident is not discovered for 30 minutes. In this case, Hospital X could be found negligent because it failed to comply with the standard set in its own policy, even though no other hospital provides such a high nurse-to-patient ratio.

One of the purposes of PI initiatives is to develop the best possible clinical practices. At a minimum, the organization must meet what is legally referred to as the "community standard of care" or "national standard of care"—the use of practices of care by the provider that are acceptable and expected by other reasonably prudent providers in similar circumstances in the same community. Most PI initiatives strive to exceed this minimum standard and to achieve "best practices," or the highest quality of care that the organization is capable of providing. However, it is important that the organization avoid the trap of setting standards it cannot meet.

There is a natural inclination for providers and facilities to draft policies and statements referring to the "highest" quality of care, or they set standards that they would like to reach rather than those they can realistically reach. From a legal perspective, it is important to provide an acceptable standard of care and to strive to meet the best possible practice but not to overreach when setting standards, drafting policies, or advertising services.

Avoidance of Risk from a Malpractice Perspective

Healthcare professionals need to be concerned with PI because it is the key to ensuring high-quality yet cost-effective care that is desired by payers and consumers. The noble and positive pursuit of best serving patients and clients is the bedrock on which PI initiatives are based. Satisfied customers and the demand for services are the positive rewards for a successful PI program.

In addition to the pursuit of quality, healthcare organizations also want to avoid negative consequences. Failure to meet real or perceived expected performance standards creates risk. In the healthcare setting, this risk is dissatisfied patients, loss of market share, and exposure to legal action in the form of malpractice litigation.

Since the 1970s, technology has improved, costs have skyrocketed, the number of lawyers has grown, and lawsuits have proliferated. This increase in litigation has been particularly dramatic in the healthcare sector. Thus, part of the dedication to PI is driven not only by the benefits of high-quality care but also by the desire to avoid the increased malpractice risk associated with poor quality.

The Organized Medical Staff

The basis for the PI process is the organized medical staff. The medical staff consists of providers who are credentialed and privileged by the healthcare organization to provide patient care services without direction or supervision and within the scope of their license and privileges granted. These providers commonly include physicians, dentists, clinical psychologists, and podiatrists. Additionally, other types of providers may be members of the medical staff or affiliated with the medical staff. They may include certified nurse-midwives, certified registered nurse-anesthetists, nurse practitioners, physician assistants, and pharmacists.

It is important for organizations to have a well-defined recruitment process. At a minimum, the recruitment process generally includes a job posting, job description, and minimum qualifications to be eligible to be considered for the position. These qualifications may include educational and licensure requirements as well as previous experience.

Although employed providers are currently the majority, independent providers still exist. These independent providers most likely will not respond to a job announcement or become employees of a hospital. Instead, they want to remain independent and may want to join a hospital's medical staff because it is close to their private office, because their practice group is associated with the hospital, or because they want to expand their practice by being able to treat patients at a hospital that is convenient for their patients. Because there is not a traditional recruiting process for such independent providers, hospitals need to have a process for identifying these individuals and ensuring that they meet the hospital's credentialing and privileging qualifications for providing services to its patients. Accordingly, legal and operational requirements were developed for organized medical staffs; that is, medical staff bylaws stipulating the rights and responsibilities of medical staff members, and credentialing and privileging processes of medical staff members. Failure to ensure that a medical staff member's qualifications are consistent with their job responsibilities can be a significant legal and compliance problem. This is true for physicians, other healthcare providers, administrators, and staff.

The process for ensuring the qualifications of medical staff members is unique because it is a peer review process, as opposed to a supervisor evaluating an employee. Providers review the credentials of other providers and determine whether they qualify for membership on the medical staff and what services and procedures they are qualified to perform. It has often been said that providers are poor at policing each other. Difficulties with the peer review process are not surprising because peers are required to make decisions about one another that affect their reputations, futures, and livelihoods. It is awkward and difficult for one provider to tell another (who spent years going to medical school and completing an internship and residency program) that they are not qualified to perform a certain procedure. In addition, providers may worry about destroying the reputation of a peer and incurring personal liability for voicing their opinions about another staff member.

Both state and federal legislators have tried to ease the difficulties in peer review by providing protection for peer review materials and meetings and providing immunity from liability for medical staff members in carrying out their peer review responsibilities.

Peer Review Protection

Peer review **protection** means that the discussions, deliberations, records, and proceedings of medical staff committees having responsibility for the evaluation and improvement of quality are kept confidential and are not subject to disclosure outside the medical staff process. This confidentiality protection generally applies to peer review and PI-related information regarding any member of or applicant to the medical staff, meetings of the medical staff, and meetings of standing and ad hoc committees created by the medical staff. The significance of this protection is that information from peer review proceedings, whether oral or written, generally is not discoverable. **Discoverable** means the information is not shielded and can be introduced at trial to support a patient's malpractice action against a provider or facility. Information that has peer review protection is not discoverable, so it is shielded, and cannot be introduced at trial to support a patient's malpractice action.

Most state legislatures have created a peer review protection for public policy purposes. It is accepted that effective PI activities, peer review, and consideration of medical staff applicants must be based on free and candid discussions within the quality improvement process. These state legislatures place a greater importance on effective PI than on an individual plaintiff's ability to obtain information on medical staff discussions that may pertain to a malpractice action.

A protection is often confused with a privilege. A **privilege** applies to discussions and correspondence between persons with a certain type of relationship that has been recognized as needing confidentiality. Examples of such relationships include those between a lawyer and a client, priest and penitent, husband and wife, and doctor and patient. In each of these cases, the person seeking some type of counsel (the client, penitent, spouse, or patient) holds the privilege. Generally, **privileged information** is not admissible at trial unless the holder waives the privilege.

In contrast, documents and discussions generated by peer review and medical staff privileging activities are protected due to their nature. The individual subjects of the documents do not hold the protection and do not have the right or ability to waive the protection. By their very nature, these documents are not admissible as evidence in legal proceedings.

Immunity from Liability

The Health Care Quality Improvement Act (HCQIA) of 1986 (HCQIA 1986) is a federal statute designed to make the peer review process more effective by reducing the fear of legal liability on the part of participants. This statute confers immunity from civil liability for damages under federal and state laws to the following individuals and entities for actions taken by peer review bodies:

- The professional body itself
- Any person acting as a member of or staff to the professional review body
- Any person under a contract or other formal agreement with the professional review body
- Any person who participates in or assists the professional review body with respect to the action

This statute also provides protection from liability for individuals who provide information to professional review bodies during the medical staff appointment and reappointment process, including physicians and staff members of hospitals, medical schools, and insurance companies.

A professional review action is defined as

An action or recommendation of a professional review body which is taken or made in the conduct of professional review activity, which is based on the competence or professional conduct of an individual physician (which conduct affects or could affect adversely the health or welfare of the patient or patients) and which adversely affects (or may affect) adversely the clinical privileges, or membership in a professional society, of the physician.

As with peer review protection, by providing immunity from civil liability for participants in the peer review process, the legislation recognizes the need for candor and the free flow of information for the peer review process to be effective. The HCQIA also created the National Practitioner Data Bank.

Occurrence Reports and Sentinel Events

In addition to credentialing, privileging, and PI initiatives, peer review committees also review specific incidents through the occurrence reporting or sentinel event review process. To foster an environment in which healthcare professionals can honestly and openly review and discuss issues involving the provision of care, including errors and systems that are not working well, the court protects these PI (or peer review) activities from being used as evidence in malpractice cases. However, the peer review protection applies only to the discussions and materials from peer review meetings.

In the event of a malpractice action, the facts of what happened must be disclosed. The patient will have access to their health record, which should include a full description of what happened from the perspective of the clinicians involved. Additionally, providers and staff involved in the incident at issue may be compelled to testify in a deposition and at trial as to their knowledge of what happened. Only the discussions and follow-up judgments in the context of the peer review meetings are protected from discovery.

The law makes a distinction between the facts of what happened, which must be disclosed in court proceedings, and an organization's analysis and response to the incident as an organizational peer review process, which are protected. This distinction is made to foster environments in which problems can be assessed and corrected without fear of having those corrections result in the organization's legal detriment.

Responsibility for Disclosing Adverse Events to the Patient or Patient's Family

Even though it is uncomfortable and may not be in a provider's or hospital's best legal interest, ethical and accreditation standards require that adverse events be disclosed to the patient or the patient's family when the patient is incapacitated or a minor. Adverse events are negative clinical outcomes stemming from a diagnostic test (such as reaction to contrast media), medical treatment (such as medication error), or surgical intervention (such as postoperative wound infection). Adverse events may or may not be the result of clinical error. The treating provider is responsible for disclosure of an adverse event to the patient or the patient's family.

Disclosure should include the following elements:

- A factual explanation of the circumstances surrounding the adverse event
- An explanation of the impact of the adverse event on the patient's treatment, including treatment that may otherwise not have been necessary
- Steps that will be taken to correct or mitigate any injury
- An assurance that the provider and other members of the patient care team will remain available to discuss any concerns that the patient or family may have

Additionally, documentation should be added to the patient's health record that includes the following:

- A factual description of the adverse event (without conjecture as to the cause or attribution of fault)
- A note outlining the substance of the discussion with the patient and family members about the adverse event, including the date, time, and who was present
- A note describing any follow-up discussions with the patient and family members

An occurrence report also should be filed for the adverse event, thereby triggering a review through the organization's PI process. The patient and family have a right to a factual explanation of the circumstances and treatment and the steps that will be taken in regard to the patient. The PI review process, including the occurrence report, discussion of individual fault, and corrective plans implemented to prevent similar errors in the future, is protected and does not need to be disclosed to the patient or the patient's family.

Distinguishing Quality Improvement from Research

Quality improvement initiatives and research studies are similar in that they typically are aimed at improving some element of care or testing the utility of some mode of care or process. However, it is important to distinguish quality improvement from research because they fall under different legal frameworks.

Quality improvement generally involves using data collection and analysis activities as management tools to improve the provision of services to a specific healthcare population. These activities are not intended to have any application beyond the specific organization in which they are conducted. In fact, organizations take measures to keep the results of quality improvement activities confidential so that they do not lose their peer review protection status.

In contrast, **research** is defined by US Department of Health and Human Services regulations as "the systematic investigation, including development, testing, or evaluation, designed to develop or contribute to generalizable knowledge" (CFR 45 164.501). In the context of research, **generalizable knowledge** means that the results of the activity may be applied to populations outside the population being studied. Participants in a research project may or may not benefit directly from the study, but a larger group may benefit from the knowledge obtained in the study. The investigator conducting the research usually intends to publish the results in a scientific or professional journal.

If an activity is research, federal regulations require the researchers to follow a variety of procedures to protect the human subjects involved. Most notably, research involving human subjects must be reviewed and approved by an institutional review board (IRB) before the work may be undertaken. It is the responsibility of the IRB to ensure that subjects are protected from undue risk and from deprivation of personal rights and dignity. Two issues that are the touchstone of ethical research are voluntary participation by the subjects as indicated by informed consent and an appropriate balance that exists between the potential benefits of the research to the subject or to society and the risks assumed by the subject.

Additionally, pursuant to the Health Insurance Portability and Accountability Act of 1996 (HIPAA), patients must authorize the use or disclosure of their protected health information for research purposes. Healthcare organizations require that prior to conducting research with human subjects, all researchers must submit an application to the IRB or a privacy board, where it may be possible to obtain a waiver of patient authorization (CFR 45, Parts 160 and 164).

The difference between quality improvement activities and human subjects research has been distinguished as follows:

> While quality improvement and human subjects research are both rigorous processes and at times involve similar methods, quality improvement and human subjects research have distinctly different overall aims. Quality improvement projects use data-driven methods to improve health delivery and quality. These projects examine changes in human behavior and are largely experiential learning processes. Research is a systematic investigation designed to develop or contribute to generalizable knowledge (Bass and Maloy 2020).

Incorrect classification of investigations as quality improvement or research may have significant implications. On the one hand, research initiatives that are misclassified solely as quality improvement may be conducted without appropriate review, thereby violating federal regulations and potentially resulting in harm to patients and others or endangering federal grants-in-aid to a whole host of healthcare activities. On the other hand, if IRBs had to review all quality improvement initiatives, they would be so overburdened with additional work that they would become inefficient. Additionally, important quality improvement initiatives might be unnecessarily delayed or discarded due to the rigorous and time-consuming requirements for IRB review of proposed research (Bass and Maloy 2020).

Public Health Activities

Public health departments are charged with conducting certain activities to protect the health of a population. Examples include disease surveillance, emergency responses, and program evaluations. They may also include activities to prevent and control disease, injury, or disability; provide information to the Food and Drug Administration regarding adverse drug events; track health-related products; enable product recalls; and conduct postmarketing product surveillance. These public health activities are neither quality improvement nor research.

 Check Your Understanding 20.1

1. Breach of duty is when a provider fails to provide a standard of care that a prudent physician (or other healthcare provider) would provide, thus deviating from the expected quality of care a patient should receive. Breach of duty is a basic element of negligence, or malpractice, that ultimately is a tort. Evaluate the relationship between negligence (or a tort) and quality improvement activities.
2. Which of the following is an example of a quality improvement activity as opposed to a research activity?
    a. Analyzing and optimizing workflow to enhance efficiency and reduce wait times
    b. Comparing the outcomes of different healthcare interventions to determine which is most effective in a real-world setting
    c. Conducting a clinical trial to test the efficacy and safety of a new drug or treatment
    d. Investigating the patterns, causes, and effects of health and disease conditions within a specific population

Case Study

You are the health information (HI) manager at a large urban hospital responsible for managing the department. A formal request is received from another hospital for the minutes of the recent Credentialing Committee meeting regarding Dr. Sarah Johnson, a well-established physician at your hospital. This hospital would like information on Dr. Johnson's credentials and competency as she recently applied for privileges at the hospital across town, triggering their standard credentialing process. The request specifically seeks the minutes of the recent Credentialing Committee meeting where Dr. Johnson's credentials and competency were discussed. Address the following questions regarding this request and the HI manager's response.

1. How should the health information manager respond to this request and why?
2. What other options does the requesting hospital have available to them to obtain information regarding Dr. Sarah Johnson?

Review Questions

1. A patient was taken into surgery at a local hospital for treatment of colon cancer. A large section of the colon was removed, and the patient was taken to the medical floor after surgery. Within the first 24 hours postop, the patient developed fever, chills, and abdominal pain. An abdominal CT scan revealed the presence of a foreign body. The relationship between the provider and the patient in this scenario represents which of the four basic elements of negligence or malpractice?
   a. Duty to use due care
   b. Breach of duty
   c. Damages
   d. Causation

2. What is the primary purpose of provider credentialing?
   a. Enhancing patient engagement
   b. Optimizing billing processes
   c. Ensuring the qualifications and competence of healthcare providers
   d. Expediting the discharge-planning process

3. Which of the following applies to discussions and correspondence between persons with a certain type of relationship that has been recognized as needing confidentiality?
   a. Breach of duty
   b. Peer review
   c. Privilege
   d. Causation

4. Which of the following legislative actions confers immunity from civil liability for damages for actions taken by peer review bodies to certain individuals and entities?
   a. HCQIA
   b. HITECH
   c. Civil Rights Act
   d. National Practitioners Data Bank

5. Explain why there is legal protection for occurrence reporting and peer review activities and how this protection facilitates performance improvement activities.

References

CFR 45 160: General Administrative Requirements. 2000.

CFR 45 164: Security and Privacy. 2000.

Bass, P. F. and J. W. Maloy. 2020. How to determine if a project is human subjects research, a quality improvement project, or both. *Ochsner Journal* 20(1):56–61.

Health Care Quality Improvement Act of 1986. Public Law 99-660.

Glossary

Absolute frequency: The number of times a score or value occurs in the data set

Accreditation: The act of granting approval to a healthcare organization on the basis of whether the organization has met a set of voluntary standards developed by an accreditation agency

Accreditation standards: An accrediting agency's published rules, which serve as the basis for comparative assessment during the review or survey process

Accountable care organization (ACO):   A network of doctors and hospitals that share responsibility for providing care to patients.

Action plan: A set of initiatives that are to be undertaken to achieve a performance improvement goal

Adverse drug event (ADE):   Patient injuries resulting from a medical intervention related to a medication, including harm from an adverse reaction or medication error

Adverse drug reaction (ADR):   "Any response that is noxious, unintended, and undesired and that occurs at doses normally used in man for prophylaxis, diagnosis, or therapy" (WHO 1970)

Affinity diagram: A graphic tool used to organize and prioritize ideas after a brainstorming session

Affordable Care Act of 2010 (ACA):   Legislation that focuses on providing or improving access to healthcare services for millions of US citizens, including new restrictions on the ability of payers to limit coverage on the basis of preexisting conditions, an end to lifetime limits on coverage, and a requirement for payers to spend premium dollars on healthcare costs and not administrative costs

Agenda: A list of the tasks to be accomplished during a meeting

All-hazards approach: Disaster and emergency management method that "supports a general response capability that is sufficiently nimble to address a range of emergencies of different duration, scale, and cause" (Joint Commission 2024, EM 4).

Artificial intelligence (AI):   A technology that uses machine learning, and also has the ability to adapt and has cognitive-type abilities similar to those of human intelligence. AI continues to learn, adapt and change its behavior and output based on this learning. This tool has the ability to quickly assimilate large amounts of data that would have been a time-consuming and tedious task for a human.

Bar graph: A graphic data display tool used to show discrete categories of information

Benchmark: A standard of performance or best practice, for a particular process or outcome

Benchmarking: The systematic comparison of the products, services, and outcomes of one organization with those of a similar organization (external benchmarking), or the comparison of one unit to another unit within the same organization (internal benchmarking).

Blood-borne pathogen: An infectious disease, such as HIV or hepatitis B or C, that is transported through contact with infected body fluids such as blood, semen, and vomitus

Brainstorming: An idea generation technique in which a team leader solicits creative input from team members

Brand name: The name given to the drug by the manufacturer so that is recognizable and distinct

Breach of duty: One of four elements of negligence; in a malpractice action, the issue is whether a physician exercised a standard of care that a reasonably prudent physician would have exercised under those circumstances

Business intelligence (BI): The end product or goal of knowledge management as part of the organization's information governance adoption model analytics competency

Causation: One of the four elements of negligence; in a malpractice action, there must be a connection between the breach of duty and the damage—evidence that the failure to exercise due care, or breach, *caused* the damage

Cause-and-effect diagram: An investigational technique that facilitates the identification of the various factors (that is, manpower, material, methods, and machinery) that contribute to a problem; also called a fishbone diagram

Case management: The principal process by which organizations optimize the continuum of care for their patients

Certification: Process that grants approval for a healthcare organization to provide services to a specific group of beneficiaries

Change management: A group of techniques that help individuals understand the process of change and accept PI in work processes

Check sheet: A data collection tool used to identify patterns in sample observations

Clinical guidelines: The descriptions of medical interventions for specific diagnoses in which treatment regimens and the patient's progress are evaluated on the basis of nationally accepted standards of care for each diagnosis

Clinical Laboratory Improvement Amendments (CLIA): The federal regulations outlining the quality assurance activities required of laboratories that provide clinical services

Clinical practice standards: The established criteria against which the decisions and actions of healthcare practitioners and other representatives of healthcare organizations are assessed in accordance with state and federal laws, regulations, and guidelines; the codes of ethics published by professional associations or societies; the criteria for accreditation published by accreditation agencies; or the usual and common practice of similar clinicians or organizations in a geographical region

Clinical privileges: Permission given by a healthcare organization to practice in a specific area of specialty within that organization

Community-acquired infection: An infection that was present in a patient before he or she was admitted to a healthcare facility

Community needs assessment: A comprehensive evaluation of community health by which health maintenance organizations (HMOs) become acquainted with a community; identify the community as a client; and assess that client by collecting and analyzing information about community healthcare needs, targets for interventions, and its interest in change

Compliance: The process of meeting a prescribed set of standards or regulations to maintain active accreditation, licensure, or certification status

Compulsory reviews: Assessments performed to fulfill legal or licensure requirements

Conditions of Participation: A set of regulations published by the Centers for Medicare and Medicaid Services (CMS) to outline requirements of approved programs providing healthcare services to beneficiaries of Medicare and Medicaid programs

Continuous data: Data that may have an infinite number of possible values in measurements that can be expressed in decimal values

Continuous monitoring: The regular and frequent assessment of healthcare processes and their outcomes and related costs

Continuum of care: The totality of healthcare services provided to a patient and their family in all settings, from the least to the most extensive. The emphasis is on treating individual patients at the level of care required by their course of treatment

Control chart: A chart that can be used to measure key processes over time in that it focuses attention on any variation in the process and helps the PI team determine whether that variation is normal or a result of special circumstances.

Core processes: The processes involved in care, treatment, and services are *assessing* patient needs; *planning* care, treatment, and services; *providing* the care, treatment, and services that the patient needs; and *coordinating* care, treatment, and services. The greatest responsibility for care lies within these processes.

Cost: The amount of financial resources consumed in the provision of healthcare services

CRAF method: Format for recording meeting minutes that includes four categories of recordable information: Conclusions of group discussion; Recommendations made by the committee or team; Actions that the committee, team, or individual members decide to take; and Follow-up activity

Credentialing process: Obtaining, verifying, and assessing qualifications of a licensed healthcare practitioner

Credentials: The recognition by healthcare organizations of previous professional practice responsibilities and experiences commonly accorded to licensed independent practitioners

Critical pathway: A multidisciplinary outline of anticipated care within an appropriate time frame to aid a patient in moving progressively through a clinical experience that ends in a positive outcome

Cross-functional: A term used to describe an entity or activity that involves more than one healthcare department, service area, or discipline

Customers: The recipients of a product or service as a result of an organizational process

Damages: One of the four elements of negligence; in malpractice terms, the patient must show that actual harm, or *damage*, occurred

Dashboard: The regular presentation of monitoring data for boards of directors

Data analysis: The task of transforming, summarizing, or modeling data to allow the user to make meaningful conclusions. Data analysis may be characterized as turning data into information that may be used for operational decision making" (White 2021, 2).

Data collection: The process by which facts are gathered

Data governance: "The overall administration, through clearly defined procedures and plans, that assures the availability, integrity, security, and usability of the structured and unstructured data available to an organization" (Buttner et al. 2021, 1)."

Data repository: An open-structure database that is not dedicated to the software of a particular vendor or data supplier, in which data from diverse sources are stored so that an integrated, multidisciplinary view of the data can be achieved

Decision matrix: A tool that is helpful in setting priorities. It assists in evaluating and prioritizing a list of potential improvement opportunities (ASQ 2023).

Deemed status: The term used for the assumption by the Centers for Medicare and Medicaid Services (CMS) that an organization meets the Medicare and Medicaid *Conditions of Participation* as a result of prior accreditation by an organization with deeming authority

Direct observation: A data collection method in which the researchers conduct the observation themselves, spending time in the environment they are observing and recording these observations

Discoverable: Information that is not shielded and can be introduced at trial to support a patient's malpractice action against a physician or hospital

Discrete data: Numerical values that represent whole numbers

Diversion: The removal of a medication from its usual stream of preparation, dispensing, and administration by personnel involved in

Document review: An in-depth study in which accreditation surveyors examine an organization's policies and procedures, administrative rules and regulations, administrative records, human resources records, and the case records of patients

Drug pedigree: A record of the chain of custody of a drug as it moves through the supply chain from manufacturer to pharmacy (FDA 2024).

Due process: Provides for fair treatment through a hearing procedure that is generally outlined in the healthcare organization's medical staff bylaw

Duty to use due care: One of the four elements of negligence; a relationship must have been established between the parties in which one party has an obligation, or *duty*, to act as a reasonably prudent person would act toward the other

Electronic presentations: Software that has significantly streamlined storytelling because it provides standard formatting and key symbols to display the PI tools. Types of electronic presentation might include a poster created as a single slide or a full electronic presentation with multiple slides.

Emergency: A situation created by a natural disaster or a man-made event that can impede a healthcare organization's ability to care for patients (Joint Commission 2024, EM 1)

Emergency operations plan (EOP): "An organization's written document that describes the process it would implement for managing the consequences for emergencies, including natural and human-made disasters, that could disrupt the organization's ability to provide care, treatment, and services" (Joint Commission 2024, GL 13)

Elements of negligence: Four conditions—duty to use due care, breach of duty, damages, and causation—that must be proved in a malpractice case

Evidence-based medicine: The care processes or treatment interventions that researchers performing large, population-based studies have found to achieve the best outcomes in various types of medical practice

Exit conference: A meeting that closes a site visit during which the surveyors representing an accrediting organization summarize their findings and explain any deficiencies that have been identified. The leadership of the organization is allowed an opportunity to discuss the surveyors' perspectives or provide additional information related to any deficiencies the surveyors intend to cite in their final reports

Expectations: Characteristics that customers want to be evident in a healthcare product, service, or outcome

External customers: Individuals from outside the organization who receive products or services from within the organization

Facility quality indicator profile: A report based on the data gathered using the Minimum Data Set for Long-Term Care that indicates what proportion of the facility's residents have deficits in each area of assessment during the reporting period and, specifically, which residents have which deficits

Failure mode and effects analysis (FMEA): A prospective (proactive) tool useful in analyzing potential problems when introducing new systems or equipment or when looking anew at an existing process

Flow charts: Analytical tools used to illustrate the sequence of activities in a complex process

Formulary: A list of drugs approved for use in a healthcare organization. The selection of items to be included in a formulary is based on objective evaluations of their relative therapeutic merits, safety, and cost

Functional: A term used to describe an entity or activity that involves a single healthcare department, service area, or discipline

Funneling: The process of moving questions from a broad theme to a narrow theme in an unstructured interview

Gantt chart: A data display tool used to schedule a process and track its progress over time

Generalizable knowledge: In research, the results of the activity that may be applied to populations outside the population being studied

Generic: The name that represents the chemical makeup of the drug

Goal: The level of attainment or result that you wish to accomplish.

Ground rules: Basic expectations for team members and include a discussion of attendance, time management, participation, communication, decision making, documentation, room arrangements, and cleanup

Hazard vulnerability analysis (HVA): An assessment that helps an organization identify potential hazards, threats, and adverse events and their impact on the care, treatment, and services that must be sustained during an emergency

Healthcare-associated infection (HAI): An infection occurring in a patient in a hospital or healthcare setting in whom the infection was not present or incubating at the time of admission, or it is the remainder of an infection acquired during a previous admission

High reliability organizations (HROs): Organizations that know that unexpected change can sometimes be prevented or at least anticipated and even prepared for through a preoccupation with failure and sensitivity to operations and weak signals of trouble

Histogram: A bar graph used to display data proportionally

Icons: Graphic symbols used to represent a critical event in a process flow chart

Increased transparency: The integration of electronic health records (EHRs), healthcare organizations and facilities had the capability to access, analyze, and share data more efficiently. As organizations were increasingly tasked with tracking and reporting their performance on quality metrics, this information began to be available to consumers, resulting in increased transparency.

Indicator: A performance measure that enables healthcare organizations to monitor a process to determine whether it is meeting requirements

Information management standards: One chapter of the Joint Commission's *Hospital Accreditation Standards* that promulgates the Joint Commission's requirements regarding the data and information used for various purposes in hospital organizations

Information warehouse: Repository that allows organizations to store reports, presentations, profiles, and graphics interpreted and developed from stores of data for reuse in subsequent organizational activities

Institutional review board: A committee within a healthcare organization that preapproves the use of any data-gathering tool. Institutional review board approval is mandated by federal regulations on the use of human subjects in biomedical and health services research. Although policies and procedures vary across organizations, PI teams using such data-gathering methodologies should recognize their responsibility to obtain IRB approval to maintain the highest research standards respecting their human subjects even when the IRB committee may deem the investigation or study to be exempt.

Intensity of service: The type of services or care the patient requires

Internal customers: Individuals within the organization who receive products or services from an organizational unit or department

Interview: A series of open-ended questions delivered to the selected respondents whose answers must be analyzed to identify common themes and perceptions

Kaizen event: Another term for a rapid improvement event that involves relatively simple fixes that improve work processes without going through the whole PI process and without the need to involve other departments. Specifically, Kaizen is a Japanese term meaning continuous improvement (Lean Enterprise Institute 2024).

Leadership group: Body composed of the senior governing, administrative, and management groups of a healthcare organization that are responsible for setting the mission and overall strategic direction of the organization

Lean: A quality improvement technique often seen in the manufacturing sector and has been implemented in many other industries with great success

Lean Six Sigma: A combination of the two methodologies, Lean and Six Sigma. Lean Six Sigma incorporates the attributes of Lean by focusing on the elimination of waste and removal of unnecessary steps in a process in order to increase the speed at which a process is done

Licensed provider: Any individual permitted by law to provide healthcare services without direction or supervision, within the scope of the individual's license as conferred by state regulatory agencies and consistent with individually granted clinical privileges

Licenses: Conferred by state regulatory agencies that allow an individual to provide healthcare services within a specific scope of service and geographical location.

Licensure: A state's act of granting a healthcare organization or an individual healthcare practitioner permission to provide services of a defined scope in a limited geographical area

Likert scale: A measure that records level of agreement or disagreement along a progression of categories

Line chart: A data display tool used to plot information on the progress of a process over time

Malpractice: The improper or negligent treatment of a patient, as by a physician, resulting in injury, damage, or loss

Mean (M): The average value in a range of values, calculated by summing the values and dividing the total by the number of values in the range

Median: The observed values are placed in ascending or descending order; the value that is in the very middle of the set is taken as the median.

Medication administration record (MAR): The record used to document each dose of medication administered to a patient

Medication error: A mistake that involves an accidental drug overdose, administration of an incorrect substance, accidental consumption of a drug, or misuse of a drug or biological during a medical or surgical procedure

Minimum Data Set (MDS) for long-term care: The data set that the Centers for Medicare and Medicaid Services (CMS) requires long-term care facilities to collect on all residents who are federal program beneficiaries.

Minutes: The written record of key events in a formal meeting

Mission statement: A written statement that sets forth the core purpose of an organization or performance improvement team. It is simply an expression of what already exists. The generation of a mission statement usually precedes the formation of the organization's overall goals. It identifies the PI team, what it does, and whom it serves

Multiple drug-resistant organisms (MDROs): Bacteria of any kind that has become resistant to many different antibiotics

National Incident Management System (NIMS): A system that provides guidelines for common functions and terminology to support clear communication and effective collaboration in an emergency situation

National Patient Safety Goals (NPSGs): Healthcare targets established by the Joint Commission to help accredited organizations address specific areas of concern in relation to patient safety

National Practitioner Data Bank (NPDB): A federally sponsored national database that maintains reports on medical malpractice settlements, clinical privilege actions, and professional society membership actions against licensed healthcare providers

Near misses: Occurrences that do not necessarily affect an outcome, but would carry significant chance of being a serious adverse event if they were to recur

Nominal data: Values assigned to name-specific categories; also called categorical data

Nominal group technique: A quality improvement technique that gives each member of the team an opportunity to select the most important ideas from the affinity diagram and allows groups to narrow the focus of discussion or to make decisions without becoming involved in extended, circular discussions.

Normal distribution: Almost all measures, when graphed, take on a bell-shaped or "normal" appearance as the number of observations increases. At the center or vertex of the normal distribution is the calculated mean of what is called a normal distribution. Approximately 68 percent of the observations occur in the interval under the curve from $-1\ SD$ from the mean to $+1\ SD$ from the mean.

Occurrence report: A structured data collection tool that risk managers use to gather information about potentially compensable events; also called an incident report

Opening conference: A meeting conducted at the beginning of the accreditation site visit during which the surveyors outline the schedule of activities and list any individuals whom they would like to interview

Operational definition: Terminology that reduces ambiguity and can improve data collection

Opportunity for improvement: A healthcare structure, product, service, process, or outcome that does not meet its customers' expectations and, therefore, could be improved

Ordinal data: Express the comparative evaluation of various characteristics or entities and relative assignment of each, to a class according to a set of criteria; also called ranked data

Outcome: The results of care, treatment, and services in terms of the patient's expectations, needs, and quality of life, which may be positive and appropriate or negative and diminishing

Outcome measure: Indicates the result of the performance (or nonperformance) of a function or process

Pareto chart: A bar graph used to determine priorities in problem solving

Patient advocacy: The function performed by patient representatives (sometimes call ombudsman) who respond personally to complaints from patients, and/or their families

Patient-centered care: Care that involves the patient and the patient's family in care decisions; a respect for the patient's values, preferences, and expressed needs; and an emphasis on the provider's cultural competence

Peer review: Review by like professionals, or peers, established according to an organization's medical staff bylaws, organizational policy and procedure, or the requirements of state law

Performance improvement: The continuous and adaptation of a healthcare organization's functions and processes to increase the likelihood of achieving the desired outcomes

Performance improvement council: The leadership group that oversees performance improvement activities in some healthcare organizations

Performance improvement team: Members of the healthcare organization who have formed a functional or cross-functional group to examine a performance issue and make recommendations with respect to its improvement—to examine the process.

Performance measure: "A gauge used to assess the performance of a process or function of any organization" (CMS 2023)

Performance measurement: The indicator of a healthcare organization's performance in relation to a specified process or outcome

Pharmacy and therapeutics (P and T) committee: The multidisciplinary committee that oversees and monitors the drugs and therapeutics available for use, the administration of medications and therapeutics, and the positive and negative outcomes of medications and therapeutics used in a healthcare organization

Pie chart: A data display tool used to show the relationship of individual parts to the whole

Pivot table: A Microsoft Excel tool used "to summarize data according to categories. Pivot tables also provide flexibility for the end user or analyst to organize and filter data in various ways before finalizing the analysis" (Adebayo 2017, 13)

Plan, do, check, act (PDCA): Cycle wherein parties follow four steps: *Plan* the change, *Do* or test the change, *Check* or analyze the test, *Act* on the results of the test (American Society for Quality 2018)

Plan, do, study, act (PDSA): Cycle wherein parties follow four steps: *Plan* the change; *Do* or test the change; *Study* the change; *Act* based on the findings

Potentially compensable events (PCEs): Occurrences that result in injury to persons in the healthcare organization or property loss

Predictive analytics: Process that takes the products of statistical analysis and utilizes them in a way that provides organizations the ability to predict future events

Privilege: Condition that applies to discussions and correspondence between persons with a certain type of relationship that has been recognized as needing confidentiality

Privileged information: Documents or discussions not admissible at trial unless the holder waives the privilege

Process: The interrelated activities of healthcare organizations—including governance, managerial support, and clinical services—that affect patient outcomes across departments and disciplines within an integrated environment

Process measure: A measure that focuses on a process that leads to a certain outcome, meaning that a scientific basis exists for believing that the process, when executed well, will increase the probability of achieving a desired outcome

Process redesign: The steps in which focused data are collected and analyzed, the process is changed to incorporate the knowledge gained from the data collected, the new process is implemented, and the staff is educated about the new process

Program evaluation and review technique (PERT) chart: Display tool that depicts a network of activities, represented by arrows, and the time required to complete the activities

Prospective payment systems: Providers receive a fixed, predetermined payment for the services they provide

Protection: Condition that signifies the discussions, deliberations, records, and proceedings of medical staff committees having responsibility for the evaluation and improvement of quality are kept confidential and are not subject to disclosure outside the medical staff process

QI toolbox techniques: This textbook calls these quality improvement tools collected from traditional quality improvement practice and theory

Quality: The degree or grade of excellence of goods or services. In healthcare, this means meeting expectations for outcomes of care. Performance improvement is the continuous adaptation of a healthcare organization's functions and processes to increase the likelihood of achieving the desired outcomes

Quality assurance (QA): Audit activities designed to measure the quality of services, products, or processes followed by remedial action to improve care delivery

Quality improvement organizations (QIOs): Nongovernmental agencies contracted by the Centers for Medicare and Medicaid Services (CMS) to monitor the care provided by independent healthcare practitioners

Quarterly report: Document based on the recorded meeting minutes and should include information about PI activities, such as summaries of data collection, conclusions, and recommendations

Rapid improvement team: A group of staff assembled to construct relatively simple fixes that improve work processes without going through the whole PI process and without the need to involve other departments

Ratio: A calculation found by dividing one quantity by another and listed as a percentage when reported

Relative frequency: The percentage of time a characteristic appears within a data set

Report cards: A means of presenting data on an organization's performance with respect to a preestablished set of criteria relevant to the organization's segment

Research: "The systematic investigation, including development, testing, or evaluation, designed to develop or contribute to generalizable knowledge" (CFR 45 164.501)

Retrospective payment system: A type of fee-for-service payment in which providers are paid for the services they provided to a patient in the past

Risk: An exposure to the chance of injury or financial loss and its associated liability

Risk manager: An individual responsible for managing organizations' risk exposure and improve processes so that the threat of injury and its associated liability is minimized

Root-cause analysis (RCA): A process in which a sentinel event is evaluated from all aspects (human, procedural, machinery, and material) to identify how each contributed to the occurrence of the event and to develop new systems that will prevent recurrence

Safety data sheets (SDSs): Documents that give detailed information about a material, including any associated hazards

Sampling: The recording of a smaller subset of observations of the characteristic or parameter, making certain, however, that a sufficient number of observations have been made to predict the overall configuration of the data

Scatter diagram: A diagram used to show the relationship or association between two variables, also called a scatter plot (White 2021, 54).

Sentinel events: Instances that usually involve significant injury to or the death of a patient or an employee through avoidable causes

Severity of illness: Refers to how sick the patient is, or what level of care the patient requires, such as intensive care or general medical care

Six Sigma: Methodology that uses statistics for measuring variation in a process with the intent of producing error-free result

Site visit: An in-person review conducted by an accreditation survey team

Skewing: When there are many very high or very low values in the observations that distort the calculated mean and may shift the distribution one direction or the other

Specific, Measurable, Achievable, Relevant, Time-related (SMART) goals: A technique used to effectively define a goal in terms of specific, measurable, achievable, relevant, and time-related criteria.

Social determinants of health (SDOH): The health of individuals was more complex than just providing services and was often directly correlated to their social determinants. These determinants include education, neighborhood, economic stability, healthcare access, and social and community context.

Standard deviation (*SD*): A complex analysis technique used in developing control charts for the display of some PI data

Standard precautions: The use of infection prevention and control measures to protect against possible exposure to infectious agents

Standards of care: An established set of clinical decisions and actions taken by clinicians and other representatives of healthcare organizations in accordance with state and federal laws, regulations, and guidelines

Storyboard: A physical display presentation on a cardboard trifold, which may be created using printouts of documents and graphs created on a computer

Storytelling: A report format that explains the PI purpose, process undertaken, analysis, and results of team activities in an easily understood manner by anyone interested (Ishikawa 1990, 254–255)

Strategic plan: A document in which the leadership of a healthcare organization identifies the organizations overall mission, vision, and goals to help set the long-term direction of the organization as a business entity

Structure: The foundation of caregiving, which includes buildings, equipment, technology, professional staff, and appropriate policies

Survey team: A group of individuals sent by an accrediting agency to review a healthcare organization for accreditation purposes

Survey tool: A research instrument used to gather data and information from respondents in a uniform matter through the administration of a predefined and structured set of questions and possible responses

SWOT analysis: Strategic planning process in which leaders complete an assessment of the organization's *S*trengths, *W*eaknesses, *O*pportunities, and *T*hreats

Systems: The foundations of caregiving, which include buildings (environmental services), equipment (technical services), professional staff (human resources), and appropriate policies (administrative systems)

Systems thinking: An objective way of looking at work-related ideas and processes with the goal of allowing people to uncover ineffective patterns of behavior and thinking and then finding ways to make lasting improvements

Team charter: A document that explains the issues the team was initiated to address, describes the team's goal or vision, and lists the initial members of the team and their respective departments

Team facilitator: A performance improvement (PI) team role primarily responsible for ensuring that an effective PI process occurs by serving as advisor and consultant to the PI team; remaining a neutral, nonvoting member; suggesting alternative PI methods and procedures to keep the team on target and moving forward; managing group dynamics, resolving conflict, and modeling compromise; acting as coach and motivator for the team; assisting in consensus building when necessary; and recognizing team and individual achievements

Team leader: A performance improvement (PI) team role responsible for championing the effectiveness of PI activities in meeting customers' needs and for the *content* of a team's work

Team member: A performance improvement team role responsible for participating in team decision making and plan development; identifying opportunities for improvement; gathering, prioritizing, and analyzing data; and sharing knowledge, information, and data that pertain to the process under study

Team recorder: A performance improvement team role responsible for maintaining the records of a team's work during meetings, including any documentation required by the organization

Timekeeper: A performance improvement (PI) team role responsible for notifying the team during meetings of time remaining on each agenda item in an effort to keep the team moving forward on its PI project

Tort: A wrongful act committed against a person or a piece of property. A tort is a civil action as opposed to a criminal act or a breach of contract

Total quality management (TQM): Management theory that mobilizes individuals directly involved in a work process to examine and improve the process with the goal of achieving a better product or outcome

Tracer methodology: A process surveyors use during the on-site survey to analyze an organization's systems with particular attention to identified priority focus areas, by following individual patients through the organization's healthcare process in the sequence experienced by its patients

Transfusion reaction: Signs, symptoms, or conditions suffered by a patient as the result of the administration of an incompatible transfusion

Triggers: Alerts to a possible or actual adverse event or patient safety issue in a healthcare organization

Utilization review (UR): The process of determining whether the medical care provided to a specific patient is necessary according to pre-established objective screening criteria at time frames specified in the organization's utilization management plan

Value-based purchasing: A payment model that holds healthcare providers accountable for both the cost and quality of care they provide (Healthcare.gov 2023).

Values statement: Describes the values and standards governing the operation of the organization and its relationship with customers, suppliers, employees, the local community, and other stakeholders

Vision statement: Describes what the organization or performance improvement (PI) team initiative will look like in the future, or it describes some milestone the organization or PI team will reach in the future

Voluntary reviews: Examinations of an organization's structures and processes conducted at the request of a healthcare facility seeking accreditation from a reviewing agency

Check Your Understanding Answer Key

CHAPTER 1

1.1

1.

ACS' The Minimum Standard	Modern practices	
That physicians and surgeons privileged to practice in the hospital be organized as a definite group or staff.	This practice exists today, providers must apply for privileges at each healthcare organization they wish to practice at. This includes mid-level providers today such as nurse practitioners and physician assistants.	
That membership upon the staff be restricted to physicians and surgeons who are (a) full graduates of medicine in good standing and legally licensed to practice in their respective states or provinces; (b) competent in their respective fields; and (c) worthy in character and in matters of professional ethics.	Prior to granting privileges to any provider of care at a healthcare organization, verification of education, license status, and any board specializations must occur. In addition, references would be checked. All new applicants and reappointments must be verified in the National Practitioners Data Bank to ensure that there has not been or is not currently any malpractice judgements made about the applicant.	
That the staff initiate and, with the approval of the governing board of the hospital, adopt rules, regulations, and policies governing the professional work of the hospital.	This is still the same practice today.	
That accurate and complete records be written for all patients and filed in an accessible manner in the hospital.	This standard is still required today.	
That diagnostic and therapeutic facilities under competent supervision be available for the study.	These services still must be provided in the hospital, and standards regarding them exist.	

2. Flexner documented the unacceptable variation in curricula that existed across the schools. He also noted that applicants to medical schools frequently lacked knowledge of the basic sciences. Flexner reported how the absence of appropriate hospital-based training limited the clinical skills of medical school graduates. Perhaps most importantly, he documented the huge number of graduates produced by the colleges each year, most with unacceptable levels of medical expertise.

   Several reform initiatives grew out of Flexner's report and the recommendations made by the AMA's Committee on Medical Education. One reform required medical college applicants to hold a baccalaureate degree. Another required that the medical curriculum be founded in the basic sciences.

Reforms also required that medical students receive practical, hospital-based training. Flexner recommended the closing of most medical schools in the country. Most of these recommendations were instituted over the decade after the release of Flexner's report, but only about half of the medical colleges actually closed. By 1920, most of the colleges met rigorous academic standards and were approved by the AAMC.

1.2

1. In 1965, the US Congress passed Public Law 89-97, an amendment to the Social Security Act of 1935. Title XVIII of Public Law 89-97 established health insurance for adults age 65 and older and individuals with disabilities. This program soon became known as Medicare. Title XIX of Public Law 89-97 provided grants to states for establishing medical assistance programs for low-income individuals and families. The Title XIX program became known as Medicaid. The objective of the programs was to ensure access to healthcare for people who could not afford to pay for it themselves. The impact of this legislation on the healthcare industry was significant; hospitals were now guaranteed payment for the care they delivered, and patients were guaranteed care. Consumers were now more likely to seek the care that they needed, and in some ways began to expect quality healthcare as their right rather than a privilege, which is still reflected today in the healthcare debate.

2. **c.** To foster trust and accountability: Transparency in healthcare aims to foster trust between patients and healthcare providers by providing clear and accessible information about healthcare services, costs, and outcomes.

1.3

1. **c.** Physical environment: Physical environment is a critical social determinant of health as it encompasses factors such as housing, neighborhood safety, access to healthy food, and opportunities for education and employment. These conditions can significantly influence an individual's overall health and well-being, contributing to health disparities within the community.

2. **c.** Quality improvement organizations: Contracted healthcare examiners—once called peer review organizations (PROs) and now called quality improvement organizations (QIOs)—retrospectively examine the care provided to Medicare and Medicaid beneficiaries and compare it with comparable providers' performance in different regions of the country.

CHAPTER 2

2.1

1. Most PI models applied in healthcare today share one structural characteristic: they are cyclical in nature. The cyclical model is based on the assumptions that PI activities will take place continually and that services, processes, and outcomes can always be improved.

2. Answers will vary but might include:

   Plan:
   - **Objective:** Reduce patient wait times in the emergency department by 20 percent.
   - **Identify Issues:** Conduct a thorough analysis of the current process to identify bottlenecks and inefficiencies contributing to extended wait times.
   - **Set Targets:** Establish a specific and measurable goal for improvement.

   Do:
   - **Implement Changes:** Introduce changes based on the analysis, such as optimizing staff schedules, improving triage processes, and streamlining communication between departments.
   - **Train Staff:** Ensure that all staff members are trained on the new processes and are aware of their roles in reducing wait times.

   Check:
   - **Collect Data:** Monitor and collect data on patient wait times before and after the implementation of changes.

- **Assess Results:** Compare the data against the established targets to determine the effectiveness of the changes.
- **Gather Feedback:** Obtain feedback from patients, staff, and other stakeholders to identify any unforeseen issues or areas for further improvement.

Act:
- **Adjust:** If the results indicate that the wait times have not met the target, analyze the data to identify areas that need further improvement.
- **Modify Strategies:** Adjust the implemented changes or introduce new strategies based on the feedback and analysis.
- **Standardize:** Once an effective solution is identified, standardize the improved process and update protocols to ensure sustainability.

2.2

1. A critical element of systems thinking is viewing an organization as an open system of interdependencies and connectedness rather than a collection of individual parts and professional enclaves. This approach sees interrelatedness as a whole and looks for patterns rather than snapshots of organizational activities and processes. The shift in healthcare to focus on patient outcomes requires all healthcare workers to work together and understand how their work impacts other healthcare workers before and after them in the flow of care for the patient.

2. **a.** Data mining: Systems analysis can be applied at the team, organizational, and environmental levels. It involves four groups of analysis tools, modeling and simulation, enterprise management, financial engineering and risk management, and knowledge discovery. Data mining is an example of knowledge discovery and can be used to predict future patient populations.

2.3

1. **c.** Employees are preoccupied, rushed, and overloaded: High reliability organizations (HROs) have learned that mistakes and errors occur because of employees' mindlessness and distraction, which occur when employees are hurried or overloaded.

2. **b.** Lean: Deploying Lean in healthcare requires the organization to perform root-cause analysis to determine the causes of the waste of supplies. The Lean methodology requires the organization to determine why the outpatient surgery units would have so many supplies on hand that are expired.

CHAPTER 3

3.1

1. **b.** Relevant: A SMART goal defines the goal in terms of specific, measurable, achievable, relevant, and time-related criteria.

2. **a.** Benchmarking: Benchmarking is the systematic comparison of the products, services, and outcomes of one organization with those of a similar organization. Benchmarking comparisons also can be made using regional and national standards if the data collection processes are similar. In this case, the HIM Director is performing an internal corporate benchmark comparison.

3.2

1. **d.** Brainstorming: Brainstorming is an idea-generation technique in which a team leader solicits creative input from team members. The purpose of a brainstorming session is to generate as many ideas as possible in a short amount of time. Sue was soliciting input from her coding team as to why they have seen a drop in productivity.

2. **c.** Affinity diagram: Affinity diagrams are used to organize and prioritize ideas after the initial brainstorming session. This type of diagram is useful when the team generates a large amount of information. Team members agree on the primary categories or groupings from the brainstorming session, and then secondary ideas are listed under each primary category.

3. **a.** Nominal group technique: The nominal group technique gives each member of the team an opportunity to select the most important ideas from the affinity diagram. This technique allows groups to narrow the focus of discussion and to make decisions without getting involved in extended, circular discussions during which the more vocal members dominate.

CHAPTER 4

4.1

1. **b.** Functional team: A functional team involves staff from a single department or service area; in this scenario the team consists of members from the HIM department who perform the release of information function.

2. **a.** Team charter: Team charters explain the issues the team was initiated to address, describe the team's goal and vision, and list the initial members of the team and their respective departments. Team charters are helpful because they keep the team's objective in focus.

3. **a.** A rapid improvement event team should be created to resolve this issue quickly. Team members should include emergency department staff (nurses, physicians, support staff); quality improvement specialists; and possibly patient representatives for valuable insights. The goal of this team might be to "Reduce patient waiting times in the emergency department by 30 percent within the next two months."

4.2

1. **d.** Team vision: A vision statement describes what the organization or PI team initiative will look like or be in the future, or it describes some milestone the organization or PI team will reach in the future.

2. **c.** Ground rules: Establishing ground rules for meetings helps a team maintain a level of discipline. Ground rules include a discussion of attendance, time management, participation, communication, decision making, documentation, room arrangements, and cleanup. The ground rules will not be the same for every team, because each team should decide how it wants to proceed.

CHAPTER 5

5.1

1. **a.** Check sheet: A check sheet is used to gather data based on sample observations to detect patterns. When preparing to collect data, a team should consider the four W questions: *Who* will collect the data? *What* data will be collected? *Where* will the data be collected? *When* will the data be collected?

2. **c.** Likert scale: A Likert scale allows respondents to state the degree to which they agree or disagree with a statement. It typically ranges from 1 to 5. This type of scale allows the PI team to determine how respondents feel about issues.

5.2

1. **c.** 95 percent: Approximately 95 percent of the observations occur in the interval under the curve from –2 *SD* from the mean to +2 *SD* from the mean.

   Two standard deviations from the mean

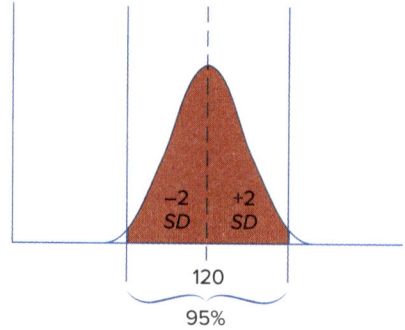

2. **d.** Consistency: The extent which healthcare data are reliable and the same across the entire patient encounter is known as data consistency.

5.3

1. **d.** Line chart: A line chart is a simple plotted chart of data that shows the progress of a process over time. By analyzing the chart, the PI team can identify trends, shifts, or changes in a process over time. The chart tracks the time frame on the horizontal axis and the measurement (the number of occurrences or the actual measure of a parameter) on the vertical axis.
2. **b.** Pareto chart: A Pareto chart is a type of bar graph that uses data to determine priorities in problem solving. The Pareto principle states that 80 percent of costs or problems are caused by 20 percent of the patients or staff.

CHAPTER 6

6.1

1. **b.** Minutes: It is important that the PI committee or team keep track of its progress and activities. Documentation of these activities is often recorded in the form of minutes. Minutes are the written record of key events in a formal meeting.
2. **c.** Quarterly: In addition to documenting meeting activities, the committee or team must provide quarterly reports to the organization's Performance Improvement and Patient Safety Council. The frequency of reporting is usually based on the committee or team meeting schedule. At a minimum, quarterly reports should be submitted to the council. The quarterly report is based on the documented meeting minutes and should include information about PI activities, such as summaries of data collection, conclusions, and recommendations.

6.2

1. **c.** To offer a transparent evaluation of healthcare quality and outcomes: Report cards provide a summary of performance and outcomes related to healthcare services, facilities, and/or providers. These report cards consist of a document or system designed to offer a transparent and easily understandable evaluation of various aspects of healthcare delivery. The goal is to help patients, providers, and other stakeholders make informed decisions about healthcare quality and choose the most appropriate care options.
2. Methods of storytelling include oral presentations, poster presentations, and other types of electronic presentations. A poster presentation is created electronically as a single slide using presentation software such as Microsoft PowerPoint or Prezi. Electronic presentation software has significantly streamlined storytelling because such software provides standard formatting and key symbols to display the PI tools. Both of these presentation techniques are used to summarize the PI team's activities. The decision to create a single-slide presentation versus a full electronic presentation with multiple slides depends on the setting or situation in which the team's results are being presented. For example, if the results are presented in a training session, a multiple-slide presentation may be the best option. If the results are being presented as a snapshot in a common area of the facility, a single-slide presentation may be better.

CHAPTER 7

7.1

1. **a.** External customer: Customers can be placed in one of two categories: internal customers or external customers. Within the healthcare organization setting, internal customers are individuals within the organization or department who receive products or services from an organizational unit or department. In this scenario, the HIM department is an external customer of the admitting registration process because HIM is not part of the registration department.

2. In this scenario, HIM department customer expectations of the patient registration department might include:
   - Accurately identify the patient in the electronic health record at the time of registration.
   - Collect accurate health insurance information for the patient.

3. **a.** To assess patient satisfaction and gather feedback on various aspects of the hospital experience: The Hospital Consumer Assessment of Healthcare Providers and Systems (HCAHPS) survey was initiated to provide a consistent format and process for gathering patient satisfaction and perspectives on hospital care. The HCAHPS survey includes three broad goals: collect consistent data on patients' perspectives of their care that allow for comparison between hospitals; publicly report survey data to incentivize hospitals to improve their quality of care; and enhance accountability for care provided. This process removed the variations of patient satisfaction surveys across the US in an effort to standardize the data collection. This standardization allows organizations and consumers to compare their results more easily.

7.2

1. **b.** Reliability: One aspect of quality that customers may emphasize in their evaluations of healthcare performance is reliability, which refers to the level at which an organization can provide an offered product or service when requested and as advertised. The fact that Community Hospital is meeting this expectation as advertised 96 percent of the time means that in this area, they are reliable.

2. **d.** Survey tool: A survey tool is defined as a research instrument used to gather data and information from respondents in a uniform matter.

7.3

1. **b.** Unstructured interview: Interviews may be unstructured or structured. In an unstructured interview, the sequence of questions is not planned in advance. Instead, the interview is conducted in a friendly, conversational manner. This type of interview is helpful when the interviewer is trying to uncover preliminary problems that may need in-depth analysis and investigation.

2. **a** How likely are to use cafeteria during your shift. Survey items should be arranged from general to specific in an effort to engage the respondent in the survey process. General questions that are easily answered are an effective way to begin the survey. The question of how often an employee uses the cafeteria is appropriate to begin a survey on the satisfaction of the cafeteria. If the employee does not use the cafeteria, it will difficult for them to assess the quality of services. The other three questions address could provide important information on the cafeteria services, but may be emotionally charged and affect all other responses to the survey.

CHAPTER 8

8.1

1. **c.** Heart failure 30-day mortality rate: The VBP program supports the CMS three-part aim: better care for individuals, better health for populations, and lower costs. Hospitals are no longer paid solely on the volume of services they provide but also on the quality of care and how well the hospital adheres to best-practice standards. This VBP program includes four domains: safety, clinical outcomes, efficiency and cost reduction, and person and community engagement. Heart failure 30-day mortality rate is a measure in the clinical outcomes category.

2. **d** Hospital readmission reduction program. The hospital readmission reduction program (HRRP) lowers payments to inpatient prospective payment system hospitals with too many readmissions. This program is designed to improve care coordination and postdischarge planning. CMS calculates an excess readmission ratio (ERR) for hospitals, which is the ratio of predicted-to-expected readmissions. This ERR is determined for each of the following conditions and procedures: Acute myocardial infarction; Chronic obstructive pulmonary disease; Heart failure, Pneumonia; Coronary artery bypass

graft surgery; and Elective primary total hip arthroplasty or total knee arthroplasty. Any readmissions to any acute-care hospital for any condition is factored into the readmission rate.

8.2

1. **a.** Preadmission care planning: Preadmission care planning is initiated when a provider contacts a healthcare organization to schedule an episode of care service for the patient. The patient's projected needs are reviewed, admission criteria are established, and any required preauthorizations are completed. The case manager may also contact the patient directly to obtain further information.

2. **d.** Discharge planning: As the patient's requirements for care decrease and the patient moves toward discharge, the case manager undertakes final discharge planning. In this step, the patient's continued care after discharge is planned. In this case, the patient will be discharged to a rehabilitation center.

8.3

1. **c.** Severity of illness: Severity of illness refers to how sick the patient is or what level of care the patient requires, such as intensive care or general medical care.

2. **c.** Gantt chart: A Gantt chart is a project management tool used to schedule important activities. Gantt charts divide a horizontal scale into days, weeks, or months and a vertical scale into project activities or tasks.

CHAPTER 9

9.1

1. **d.** Assessing the patient's needs: The cornerstone of good patient care is the initial assessment, which determines the patient's appropriateness for admission to the facility and the level of care to be rendered. Specific admission criteria based on defined services help determine which patients will benefit most from services the facility offers during the assessment and reassessment period.

2. **d.** Care pathway: Providing the care, treatment, and services that the patient needs requires care interventions based on the plan of care. Often these plans are based on an established protocol or guideline in a care pathway.

9.2

1. **d.** Transfusion reaction: The cause of every transfusion reaction (the signs, symptoms, or conditions suffered by a patient as a result of the administration of an incompatible transfusion) must be investigated. Most deaths resulting from hemolytic transfusion reactions were primarily attributable to incomplete patient-identification processes for blood verification.

2. **c.** Poor documentation: A key quality and performance concern is the adequate and reliable documentation of care. Poor documentation leads to the largest number of risk management and legal situations in the industry. Accreditation and licensing agencies have standards on the documentation of patient care and expect that a sample of clinical documentation will be regularly reviewed as part of an organization's PI activities. The expectation is that all records have been authenticated and contain the necessary reports and that they appropriately document the condition and treatment of the patient.

9.3

1. Telehealth removes the barriers of distance in the provision of care by using readily accessible technology to provide treatment and medical guidance. For those living in remote locations, telehealth allows convenient care to occur. Practitioners in rural areas are able to utilize this technology to connect with larger facilities or specialists who can assist them in managing difficult cases that the rural provider may not often encounter. Because of the limited number of specialists in rural areas, telehealth provides a mechanism for patients and providers to access these specialists without the barrier of distance.

2. The universal protocol for surgery includes three steps: conduct a pre-procedure verification process, mark the procedure site, and perform a time-out. Each of these steps would have helped to prevent

Diane's wrong-site surgery. The pre-procedure verification process involves verification of the correct procedure, patient, and operative site; marking the procedure site with a marker by having the patient assist the clinical staff in identifying the correct operative site; and finally, conducting a time-out before the start of the procedure can ensure that all staff present in the operative suite know what procedure is to be performed, whether this is the correct patient, and which body part to operate on.

CHAPTER 10

10.1

1. **c.** Standard precautions: Standard precautions can be defined as the use of infection prevention and control measures to protect against possible exposure to infectious agents. The concept behind these general precautions is that every individual encountered in the healthcare setting should be treated as if they may have an active blood-borne pathogen disease.

2. **a.** Healthcare-associated infection: A healthcare-associated infection (HAI) is an infection occurring in a patient in a hospital or healthcare setting in whom the infection was not present or incubating at the time of admission, or it is the remainder of an infection acquired during a previous admission. In this scenario, the pneumonia developed postoperatively and would be a healthcare-associated infection.

CHAPTER 11

11.1

1. Some of the potential risks for Katie include the following:
   - A medical error during her treatment from the variety of tests and procedures she had during her stay
   - A medical mistake made by one of her many healthcare providers
   - A fall from bed due to her sedated state
   - Theft or loss of her personal belongings that would have been removed before treatment and surgery
   - Unresponsiveness to treatment as expected and a negative outcome, even if the correct care and treatment were provided; this is especially possible because of the comorbidities she had prior to treatment

2. In 1999, the Institute of Medicine (IOM) published a report on medical errors in healthcare titled *To Err Is Human: Building a Safer Health System*, which sent shock waves through the American healthcare industry. The report was eye opening for both the public and healthcare organizations revealing that "at least 44,000 [people], and perhaps as many as 98,000 [people], die in hospitals each year as a result of medical errors" that could have been prevented. Not only did the report increase awareness of medical errors, but it also began a movement toward an increased focus on quality and safety issues for all stakeholders including both government and the private sector.

11.2

1. The risk manager's principal tool for capturing the facts about PCEs is the occurrence report, sometimes called the incident report. Effective occurrence reports are structured and are valuable for the risk manager as they allow the collection of data, information, and facts in a relatively simple format. Because they facilitate collection of necessary data, information, and facts, these can be tracked in an electronic system. The content of the occurrence report can help to facilitate a root-cause analysis and even recommendations for policy changes.

2. **d.** Near miss: The situation presented was a near miss as it did not affect the outcome, but if the wrong drug would have been administered before the error was caught, it had the chance of being a serious adverse event. Near misses include occurrences that do not necessarily affect an outcome, but if they were to recur they would carry a significant chance of being a serious adverse event. Near misses fall under the definition of a sentinel event but are not reviewable by the Joint Commission

under its current sentinel event policy. Near misses are a valuable tool for evaluation of processes and procedures, especially in high-risk or high-volume areas of facilities.

11.3

1. **b.** Cause-and-effect diagram: In this case the toolbox technique used by the administrator and director of nursing was the cause-and-effect diagram. The toolbox technique used most often in RCA is the cause-and-effect diagram, also called a fishbone diagram. A cause-and-effect diagram is an investigational technique that facilitates the identification of the various factors or causes that contribute to a problem. This technique structures the root-cause inquiry and ensures that investigators examine the situation from all perspectives.

2. **c.** Reducing patient safety incidents and improving quality of care: Root-cause analysis helps healthcare professionals investigate the root or fundamental causes of incidents that may compromise patient safety. By understanding the root causes, healthcare organizations can implement targeted interventions and improvements to prevent similar incidents from happening again. The ultimate goal of RCA in healthcare is to enhance the quality of care provided to patients by addressing systemic issues and improving processes.

CHAPTER 12

12.1

1. **a.** Adverse drug event: In this case, Holly did everything right while administering the pain medication to Dylan; however, Dylan is having an adverse reaction to the medication. Adverse drug events (ADEs) are patient injuries resulting from a medical intervention related to a medication, including harm from an adverse reaction or medication error.

2. Examples will vary depending on which abbreviations the student chooses to use. The Joint Commission's "Do Not Use" abbreviation list for medication orders is shown in Figure 12.2. It can also be found online at https://www.jointcommission.org/resources/news-and-multimedia/fact-sheets/facts-about-do-not-use-list/.

   When medication orders are received there is a chance of error in communication. To avoid the risk of a medication error and better ensure patient safety, abbreviations that can be mistaken for another meaning are not safe to use.

CHAPTER 13

13.1

1. **a.** Hazard vulnerability: Rick's role as the director of environmental services includes being tasked with determining all types of threats to the hospital. To do this, Rick must conduct a hazard vulnerability analysis. An annual hazard vulnerability analysis (HVA) is conducted to identify potential hazards, threats, and adverse events and assess their impact on the care, treatment, and services that must be sustained during an emergency.

2. Paul has been trained on the proper method used to train healthcare staff for fire responses. This is the response based on the acronym RACE. **R** = Rescue anyone in immediate danger of the fire; **A** = Activate alarms; **C** = Confine fires (close doors and windows); and **E** = Extinguish fires using PASS and prepare to evacuate patients. Paul would first want to rescue anyone that is in immediate danger. Because the room is vacant, and the rooms next to it are vacant, Paul moves to the "A" activate alarm and activates the nearby fire alarm. Paul then confines the fire as best he can (using PASS) and begins to extinguish the fire while waiting for a response from hospital staff.

3. **b.** Medical equipment management, life safety management, and safety management: The seven written safety standards or plans for the environment of care cover the following areas: safety management, security management, hazardous materials and waste management, life safety management, medical equipment management, utilities management, smoking policy management.

13.2

1. To determine if employees have retained and understood the material presented to them, postprogram assessments are commonly used to evaluate employee knowledge of care environment and safety area issues. These assessments are given to employees after they have completed the required training.

2. In this scenario, a hospital employee is injured as they are performing their work duties, making this an occupational injury. The information collection and evaluation system (ICES) consists of many documents, facts, reports, and performance monitoring. One type of information collected and evaluated is employee injuries. The Joint Commission requires monitoring, investigation, and reporting of the following items: patient or visitor injuries; incidents of property damage; occupational injuries or illnesses; security incidents; hazardous materials and waste spills and exposures; fire prevention problems, deficiencies, and failures; equipment problems, deficiencies, and failures; and, utility systems problems, deficiencies, and failures. This incident would need to be reported and investigated.

CHAPTER 14

14.1

1. **b.** Establishing a culture of teamwork and collaboration among diverse staff members: In a hospital setting, fostering a culture of teamwork and collaboration is crucial for several reasons. Teamwork enhances communication among healthcare professionals, leading to improved patient care and outcomes. Collaboration promotes a supportive work environment, where different skills and expertise can be leveraged to address complex medical challenges. This approach contributes to the overall success of the organization by creating a cohesive and efficient healthcare team, ultimately benefiting both staff satisfaction and patient well-being.

2. **d.** Clinical privileges: In this case, Landmark Hospital is using physician assistants (PAs) to provide a higher level of care they need, but there is a limit to their scope of practice. Each provider who practices under the auspices of a healthcare organization must do so in accordance with delineated clinical privileges based on the practitioner's training, experience, and proven clinical competence.

CHAPTER 15

15.1

1.

Board of Directors	Chief Executive Officer (CEO)
Ultimate responsibility for quality and safety of patient care	Has the responsibility to implement board directives
Establishes policies and directs the monitoring and assessing of all services to ensure standards of care and service are acceptable	Acts as a board representative in managing the operations of the hospital
Operates under a set of bylaws and provides a framework to support quality patient care, treatment, and services	Partial or full voting member of the board
Designates the CEO	Responsibility to ensure that the board of directors is knowledgeable about its governing duties
Responsible for proper functioning of the organization	
Both the Board of Directors and the CEO work together to: identify the needs of their community, set and pursue the goals of the organization, plan, budget, conduct PI, and ensure patient satisfaction.	

2. **d.** Strategic plan: The organizational leaders are responsible for planning (strategic plan) and creating the environment within the organization in which the mission, vision, and organizational goals can be achieved. Leaders are responsible for ensuring that a process is in place to measure, assess, and improve the hospital's governance, management, clinical, and support functions.

15.2

1. **c.** Data security and compliance. When selecting a new electronic health record (EHR) system for a hospital, data security and compliance are critical factors. Healthcare organizations handle sensitive patient information that must be protected to ensure patient privacy and comply with regulations such as the Health Insurance Portability and Accountability Act (HIPAA). The decision matrix should prioritize the EHR systems that meet the highest standards for data security and compliance, as this directly impacts the integrity and confidentiality of patient records. This consideration ensures that the selected EHR system aligns with legal requirements and best practices in safeguarding patient information.

2. **b.** Trended performance measures vary significantly and unfavorably from the standards, benchmarks, or statistical process controls : As part of the PI process, data regarding performance measures is aggregated and analyzed to look for trends in the data. Trends in the data are reviewed when trended performance measures significantly and undesirably vary from those of other organizations, requiring a more detailed review; when they significantly and undesirably vary from recognized standards, benchmarks, or statistical process controls; or when the occurrence of an event is questionable or too infrequent to make judgments about patterns in care or to analyze statistical significance.

15.3

1. Executive summary—The executive summary section of the PI review summarizes the main points of the annual report. This section highlights the results of key PI initiatives undertaken by the organization in the previous year.

    Overview—This section highlights the organization's philosophy and strategy related to all quality and PI activities. It includes how these PI activities relate to the organization's mission, vision, values, and strategic plan, and how organization leaders use this information to prioritize operations for the future.

    PI structures—The leaders and staff responsible for the organization's quality and PI activities are described here. How PI teams are developed and guided toward improvement activities are outlined, as well as how this information is communicated throughout the organization and leaders. The process for ongoing monitoring and the identification of critical data collection activities are provided.

    Improvement opportunities—Trends from aggregate data analysis, interventions, corrective actions or improvements, or changes in policies and procedures, may be highlighted in the improvement opportunities section using graphic representation and PI presentation of findings rather than detailed reports. Data should show evidence of continued and sustained improvement. System improvements may be broken into four areas: patient-focused improvements, organizational improvements, ongoing measurements, and quality data reporting.

    PI team activities—The PI team activities part of the report should highlight the work of PI teams sanctioned by the organization's PI council and should provide information on their effectiveness.

    Other PI Review Topics—Other topics that may be addressed in the organization's PI plan review may include areas of focused change or improvement.

2. Possible answers might be:
    - Has the team's work resulted in measurable and sustained improvements?
    - What process changes and training occurred to support and sustain the improvement(s)?
    - Has the organization's staff assigned to PI team projects been effectively trained to work on PI teams?
    - Is staff willing and able to take on the important roles in team activities?
    - Does staff participate and interact well at team meetings to work through PI processes?
    - Can they document important team milestones with appropriate tools?

- Have they implemented the organization's PI model appropriately?
- Have they learned to listen and question effectively in interpersonal communication?
- Can they effectively communicate the team's process and outcomes to the rest of the organization?

15.4

1. The tool that should be recommended is a dashboard. Kevin and his PI team are presenting too much data to the board, and it is overwhelming and difficult to use for decision-making. The best tool would be a dashboard, which provides a concise and clear overview of key monitoring data. This report provides valuable information that is in an easily readable format and can be used as a guide by the board for making management decisions.

2. In healthcare settings, findings from peer review activities are aggregated and reported to the executive committee of the medical staff, as well as to clinicians' professional files for consideration in the recredentialing process. The peer review process is a critical part of ensuring that providers are meeting the expectations for patient care and treatment. This process is also important because provides insight into potential PI improvement opportunities. Because the findings are reported to the executive committee, the documentation of the findings also gives needed evidence that PI activities are occurring in the facility.

CHAPTER 16

16.1

1. The *Conditions of Participation* for healthcare facilities cover issues related to medical necessity, level of care, and quality of care. CMS contracts with nongovernmental agencies across the country to monitor the care provided by independent healthcare practitioners. These agencies, called quality improvement organizations (QIOs), retrospectively review patient records to ensure that the care provided by practitioners meets the federal standards for medical necessity, level of care, and quality of care.

2. **a.** AAAHC: The Accreditation Association for Ambulatory Health Care (AAAHC) surveys and accredits ambulatory care facilities, with a primary focus on ambulatory surgery centers. In addition, AAAHC also accredits multispecialty and single-specialty group practices, dental group practices, community and student health services, independent practice associations, employer-based and retail clinics, and endoscopy, diagnostic imaging, and radiation oncology centers (AAAHC 2024).

16.2

1. **b.** Deemed status: CMS accepts accreditation by organizations with deeming authority in granting what it calls **deemed status**. When granting deemed status, CMS assumes that the organization meets the *Conditions of Participation* if it is currently accredited by one of these organizations. In addition, CMS may conduct a validation survey of accredited facilities to ensure compliance with the *Conditions of Participation*. Many state licensing agencies routinely survey organizations to qualify them for deemed status.

2. **d.** Tracer methodology: The on-site survey for the Joint Commission utilizes a tracer methodology that permits assessment of operational systems and processes in relation to the actual experiences of selected patients currently under the organization's care. Tracer methodology analyzes an organization's systems, with particular attention to identified priority focus areas, by following individual patients through the organization's healthcare process in the sequence experienced by its patients.

16.3

1. **c.** A department of health surveyor will visit the nursing home: After a complaint by a resident, family member, or employee, a state department of health surveyor may visit a facility at any time to perform a special investigation. This investigation is to ensure that proper care is being received by the resident in question and others at the facility.

2. a. How the correction will be continually enforced and an ongoing monitoring plan. With the determination of the scope and level of the deficiencies, the survey agency may recommend enforcement remedies that range from directed plans of correction, to civil penalties, up to the termination of the provider agreements. In most cases, a plan of correction is the first step, with the facility or organization required to submit a plan that covers four distinct elements:

- How the correction will be accomplished
- Title or position of the individual who will be responsible for correction implementation
- How the correction will be continually enforced, along with a monitoring plan to prevent the reoccurrence of the deficiency
- The date the correction will be in place or accomplished.

In the scenario the correction plan included all of the required elements except how the correction will be continually enforced, along with a monitoring plan to prevent the reoccurrence of the deficiency.

CHAPTER 17

17.1

1. Healthcare organizations must make information governance a priority to view the data and information accumulated in their facilities as an asset. For it to be an asset, it must be managed, protected, and utilized within a framework. Just because organizations are collecting data does not mean that they are handling the data appropriately. Information governance provides the basis to ensure that all aspects of data management are provided for and that the data are used in the most meaningful ways.

2. Communication between teams or groups is necessary to keep all members up to date on PI activities occurring within an organization. In this scenario, the larger organization is interested in the current PI activities of Community Hospital. Although communication is critical within organizations to keep all relevant stakeholders informed, it is also necessary to insure quality patient care. Technology has advanced to where meetings can be effectively held through web-based technologies that allow participants to communicate and share information when travel is not necessary or possible. The plan would include: setting up an appointment time for the meeting; sending information to each team member, how to access the web-based technology, and an agenda for the meeting; and facilitating the meeting using the technology.

17.2

1. **c.** National Quality Forum: The National Quality Forum (NQF) is a nonprofit, nonpartisan, membership-based organization that works to improve healthcare outcomes, safety, equity, and affordability. Their unique role is to bring all voices to the table to forge multistakeholder consensus on quality measurement and improvement standards and practices that achieve measurable health improvements for all.

2. The facility administrator should do comparative performance measurement known as benchmarking. Comparative performance measurement (benchmarking), such as a nursing home comparison in this case, allows facilities to determine how the facility does in comparison to similar facilities. Facilities report their performance and in turn, have access to data from these measures. The comparison can ensure that the organization is performing up to industry standards or help the organization identify opportunities for improvement when necessary.

17.3

1. **a.** To ensure that PHI is used, stored, and disclosed properly: In this instance, Mike and his team would need to contact Becky (the privacy officer) when they have questions about managing PHI for various PI projects they may be doing. Organizational privacy officers may need to be consulted by PI teams to ensure that PHI is used, stored, and disclosed appropriately to meet the requirements of

federal and state laws and regulations. The privacy officers may also be of assistance in treating PI data as appropriate to their status as research versus quality improvement information.

2. **b.** Record of care standards: Based on the scenario, it can be deduced that Jake is reviewing the record of care standards. These standards should be detailed enough so the patient can be identified, and should also support the care provided to include diagnosis, treatments, care results, and communication between staff. Care providers should also document patient progress in the patient record. This information is used to make care decisions.

CHAPTER 18

18.1

1. Although the project itself seems to be moving along as planned, a good project team leader must provide more than the ability to manage the technical aspects of the project. A successful team leader must possess job task competencies and behavioral competencies. A technically competent individual may not necessarily be a good project team leader unless they also possesses behavioral competencies that enable them to understand team dynamics and positively influence team members. In this case, the leader has the technical skills but is missing the behavioral skills needed for the project.

2. **b.** Gantt chart: The HIM director is looking for a tool to help her plot the tasks of her project. The best tool for her to use would be a Gantt chart, which is an effective tool for planning and tracking the implementation of a project. It is a graphic tool used to plot tasks that shows the duration of project tasks and overlapping tasks. This tool is the best choice because it fits the project scope and meets the director's needs.

CHAPTER 19

19.1

1. **d.** Sustain acceleration: At this point in the change management process it is important to stay focused on the goal and to incorporate activities that sustain the sense of urgency for the change.

2. **d.** The refreezing phase, as he has become accustomed to the new workflow and his confidence in his abilities has returned: Paulo has experienced the unfreezing and moving phases, and probably has experienced some grief along with that, but now has moved into the refreezing phase. He is experiencing stability in the new workflow and the new processes have begun to feel normal. He is once again able to help patients effectively, and his confidence has returned.

CHAPTER 20

20.1

1. Healthcare organizations must be concerned with the quality of their patient care. Performance improvement is critical to ensuring the high-quality yet cost-effective care expected by payers and consumers. This is the basis of PI activities' noble and positive pursuit of best serving patients and clients, which is the bedrock on which PI initiatives are based. Satisfied customers and the demand for services are the positive rewards for a successful PI program. In addition to the pursuit of quality, healthcare organizations also want to avoid negative consequences. **Malpractice** is the improper or negligent treatment of a patient by a healthcare provider that results in injury, damage, or loss. Failure to meet real or perceived or expected performance standards creates risk and can even expose the healthcare organization to legal action through malpractice litigation.

2. **a.** Analyzing and optimizing workflow to enhance efficiency and reduce wait times: Research activities and quality improvement (QI) activities in healthcare facilities serve distinct purposes, although they both contribute to the overall advancement of healthcare. Quality improvement generally involves using data collection and analysis activities as management tools to improve the provision of services

to a specific healthcare population. These activities are not intended to have any application beyond the specific organization in which they are conducted. Analyzing and optimizing workflows to enhance efficiency and reduce wait times is a performance improvement activity; the other three options are research activities.

Index

A
Absolute frequency, 76, 80, 93
"Acceptable to Use" orders, 210, 211
Accidental release measures, 231
Accountable care organization (ACO), 13, 131, 154
Accreditation
    Accreditation Association for Ambulatory Health Care, 322
    acute care and other facilities, 324–329
    CARF, 331–332
    case study, 340
    CMS Conditions of Participation, 322
    Commission on Accreditation of Rehabilitation Facilities and, 321
    compliance with CMS Conditions of Participation, 332
    compulsory reviews, 320
    definition, 320
    DNV, 321
    Joint Commission, 320–321, 324–329
    National Committee for Quality Assurance, 322
    policies and procedures, 323
    psychiatric and rehabilitation care facilities, 331–332
    public disclosure, 329
    real-life example, 333–339
    regulations pertaining to charting by exception, 334–339
    site visit, 324
    standards, 320–322
    state licensure, 322
    survey process, 323–324
    voluntary reviews, 320
Accreditation Association for Ambulatory Health Care (AAAHC), 322
Action plan, 56, 66
Activities of daily living, 159
Activity-pursuit patterns, 159
Adverse drug events (ADEs), 206–207
Adverse drug reaction (ADR), 207, 213
Affinity diagrams, 47
Affordable Care Act (ACA), 13
    health of community as focus with, 131
Agenda, 57, 61, 64–65
Aggregated data, 344
All hazards approach, 233–234
Ambulatory payment classification (APC), 12
Ambulatory surgical center quality reporting (ASCQR) program, 134

American Health Information Management Association (AHIMA), 8
American Medical Association (AMA), history of, 6
American Public Health Association (APHA), 164
American Recovery and Reinvestment Act of 2009 (ARRA), 17, 344
Application-program interface (API), 345
Artificial intelligence (AI), 82–83, 346
Association for Professionals in Infection Control and Epidemiology (APIC), 164
Association of American Medical Colleges (AAMC), 6
Assurance, 113
Avian influenza, 164

B
Bar graph, 73–74, 84, 89–90
Benchmark
    definition, 28
    external *vs.* internal, 29
    in performance measures, 28
    Six Sigma with, 33
Benchmarking
    definition, 44
    identifying, 44
Bird flu, 164
Blood-borne pathogen, 167–169
Blood products, evaluations of use, 155
Board of directors
    dashboard report, 313
    defined, specific accountabilities, 312
    performance improvement activities, 311–312
Boas, Ernst P., 8
Brainstorming, 44, 47
Brand name, 211
Breach of duty, 388
Bubonic plague, 164
Bush, George W., 186
Business intelligence (BI), 345–351
Business intelligence life cycle, 345

C
Calderone, Mary Steichen, 9
Callen, Maude E., 8
Canadian Medical Association (CMA), 10
Care planning at time of admission, 136

Case management, 135–138, 142–143
Causation, 389
Cause-and-effect diagram, 199–200
Centers for Disease Control and Prevention (CDC)
  infectious disease, 164, 165, 167
  laboratory services regulated by, 155
Centers for Medicare and Medicaid Services (CMS)
  compliance with, 332
  Conditions of Participation, 320, 322–325, 330, 332
  deemed status, 323
  long-term care facilities, 330–331
  pay-for-performance, 131
  policies and procedures, 323
  Quality Indicator Survey for, 331
Certification, 320
  case study, 340
  compliance, 320
  compulsory reviews, 320
  Conditions of Participation, 320, 322–325, 330, 332
  definition, 320
  long-term care facilities, 330–331
  policies and procedures, 323
  real-life example, 333–339
  standards, 320–322
  voluntary reviews, 320
Change
  Kotter's eight accelerators for, 380
  three phases of change, 378–379
Change management
  build guiding coalition, 380–381
  case study, 384
  create sense of urgency, 380
  definition, 380
  enable action by removing barriers, 381
  enlist volunteer army, 381
  form strategic vision and initiatives, 381
  generate short-term wins, 381
  institute change, 382
  real-life example, 382–383
  sustain acceleration, 382
Check sheet, 72–73, 84–85, 87
Chemical labeling provision, 227
Chief clinical officer (CCO), 272
Chikungunya, 164
Cholera, 164
Clinical guidelines, 158
Clinical Laboratory Improvement Amendments (CLIA), 155
Clinical practice standards, 156
Clinical privileges, 265, 269–271
Clinton, Bill, 186
Closing processes, project life cycle, 369
Cognitive loss and dementia, 159
Commission on Accreditation of Rehabilitation Facilities (CARF), 321
  document review, 332
  psychiatric and rehabilitation care facilities, 331–332
Communication
  CRAF method, 97
  minutes, 96–98
  quarterly reports, 96, 98
  report cards, 101
  storytelling, 96, 99–101
Community-acquired infection, 166–168
Community needs assessment, 135–136, 142–143
Comparative data, 344

Compliance, 320
  with Conditions of Participation, 332
Composition/information on ingredients, 227
Compulsory reviews, 320
Conditions of Participation, 320, 322–325
  compliance with, 332
  deemed status, 323
  long-term care facilities, 330
  policies and procedures, 323
Connector icons, 171
Continuous data, 74, 84
Continuous monitoring, 28
Continuum of care
  case study, 144
  definition, 126
  example, 140–141, 148–149
  healthcare in US, 126–131
  optimal spending for optimal health, 128
  QI toolbox techniques, 139–141
  shift to paying for value, 131–135
  steps to success, 135–138
Control chart, 80, 82, 87–88
Core processes in patient care
  assessing patient's needs, 149–150
  coordinating care, treatment, and services, 151, 153
  definition, 148
  planning care, treatment, and services, 150–151
  providing care, treatment, and services, 151
Cost, 15
COVID-19 pandemic, 158, 164, 167, 177
  emergency operations plan, 233
  vaccination, 168
CRAF method, 97–98
Credential and extend privileges, 269–271
Credentialing process, 269, 271, 289
Credentials, 265, 269–271
Critical pathway, 135
Critical to process (CTP), Six Sigma, 34
Critical to quality (CTQ), Six Sigma, 34
Crosby, Philip, 14
Cross-functional PI team, 54–55
Customers
  definition, 108
  expectations, 108–110
  external, 108–109, 112
  internal, 108–109, 112
  types, 108–111
Customer satisfaction
  case study, 121
  data analysis, 114
  data collection, 114
  examples, 119–121
  identification of products and services, 112–113
  identify internal and external customers, 112
  identify opportunities for improvement, 115
  interview design, 118
  monitoring and improving, 111–118
  QI toolbox techniques, 115–118
  quality measures and satisfaction scales, 113–114
  survey design, 115–117

D
Damages
  defined, 389
  immunity from civil liability for, 391

Dashboard, 311
Data analysis
    customer satisfaction, 114
    data quality, 78–79
    performance improvement data, 78–89
    statistical analysis, 79–82
Data collection, 302, 344
    customer satisfaction, 114–118
    monitoring performance through, 27–30
    performance improvement model, 27–30
    tools, 72–77
Data display tools, 84–89
Data governance (DG), 344–345
Data repository, 346
Data sets, management of, 77–78
Decision icons, 170
Decision matrix, 305–306
Deemed status, 323
Dehydration and fluid maintenance, 159
Delirium, 159
Dementia, 159
Deming, W. Edwards, 14, 24
Design phase, project life cycle, 366
Diagnosis-related group (DRG), 12
    standardized payments, 129
Dickinson, Robert Latou, 8
Dimock, Dr. Susan, 7
Direct observation, 114
Discharged not final billed (DNFB) rate case, 50
Discharge planning, 138
Disclosure of adverse events, 392
Discoverable, 391
Discrete or count data, 74
Disease diagnoses, 159
Disposal considerations, 231
Diversion, 214
DNV accreditation, 321
Dock, Lavinia Lloyd, 8
Document review, 332
Domestic violence, 227
Donabedian, Avedis, 14
"Do Not Use" abbreviations, 210
Drug pedigree, 209
Due process, 271
Duty to use due care, 388

E
Ebola, 164
Ecological information, 231
Educational and screening programs, in infection surveillance, 169
Education, performance improvement activities, 314–315
Electronic health record (EHR), 28, 67, 108, 154, 346
Electronic presentations, 99
Elements of negligence, 388–389
Emergency, 233
Emergency department (ED), 186
Emergency management
    annual evaluation, 253–255
    Joint Commission accreditation standards manual, 321
Emergency operations plan (EOP), 233
    emergency management plan, 242–244
    implementation of incident command structure for, 238, 240, 241
    monitor and improvement of, 233–245
    six critical areas of, 234

Empathy, 113
Employee-to-employee harassment, 226
Employee training, 231
Employee turnover rate, performance improvement model, 28–29
End-stage renal disease (ESRD), 134
Environmental tour and facility audit, 249–252
Environment of care
    case study, 257–258
    criteria for annual evaluation, 253–255
    emergency operations plan, 219, 233–245
    hazardous materials and waste management program, 219, 227–233
    improvement, 220–253
    information collection and evaluation system, 255
    Joint Commission accreditation standards manual, 321
    life (fire prevention) safety management plan, 219, 245–247
    medical equipment management program, 219, 247–248
    QI toolbox techniques, 256
    real-life example, 257
    safety management program, 219, 221
    security management program, 219, 221–227
    utilities management program, 219, 248–253
Evidence-based medicine, 158
Excess readmission ratio (ERR), 135
Execution processes, project life cycle, 368–369
Exit conference, 329
Expectations, customers, 108–110
Exposure controls/personal protection, 231
External customers, 108–109, 112
Extract-transfer-load (ETL), 345

F
Facility quality-indicator profile, 160
Failure mode and effects analysis (FMEA), 214–216
Falls, 159
Features, 113
Fire drill tracking summary, 246–247
Firefighting measure, 231
Fire prevention program, 245–247
First-aid measures, 227
Flexner, Abraham, 7
Flow charts, 170–176
Food services department, 119–121
Formulary, 209
Freezing, 379
Full-time equivalent (FTE) staff, 263
Functional PI team, 54
Funneling, 118

G
Gantt chart
    in continuum of care, 137, 139, 142
    five phases of project in, 367
    project life cycle, 366–367
    sample format, 137
Generalizable knowledge, 393
Generic medications, 211
Goal, 42–43
Grief, 379
Ground rules, 61–62
A Guide to the Project Management Body of Knowledge
    (PMBOK Guide), 362

H

Handling and storage, 231
Hanta virus, 164
Harassment, 226
Hazard Communication Standard, 227
Hazard determination provision, 231
Hazard identification, 227
Hazardous materials inventory, 232
Hazardous materials management program, 219, 227–233
Hazard vulnerability analysis (HVA), 234
Hazard vulnerability planning activities, 239
Healthcare
    AHRQ, 353
    authoritarian approach, 130
    community-acquired *vs.* infections associated with, 167–168
    continuum of care for US, 126–131
    DNV, 321
    early quality improvements, 4–10
    evolution of quality in, 14–18
    historical perspectives in PI, 5
    home patient care monitoring, 159–160
    incident command structure for organization, 240, 241
    infection surveillance, 167–169
    modern, 11–14
    organization risk management plan, policies, and procedures, 188
    quality improvement in, 4–10
    quality in, 14–18
    staff roles in patient-centered approach, 129
Healthcare-associated infection (HAI), 164–166, 168
Healthcare Common Procedure Coding System (HCPCS), 12
Healthcare Effectiveness Data and Information Set (HEDIS), 322
Healthcare institutions, 4–6
Health Information Technology for Economic and Clinical Health Act (HITECH), 17, 344
Health Insurance Portability and Accountability Act of 1996 (HIPAA) regulations, 169
Health professions, other, 8
Health value-based purchasing model (HHVBP), 134
High reliability organizations (HROs), 33, 35–36
Histogram, 75, 84–85
Hospital Consumer Assessment of Healthcare Providers and Systems (HCAHPS) survey, 113, 114
Hospital hazard vulnerability assessment tool, 234–237
Hospital organization chart example, 295
Hospital readmission reduction program (HRRP), 135
Human resources. *See* Staff and human resources
Humors, 6
Hurricanes, 233

I

Icons
    connector, 171
    decision, 170
    line connector, 171
    manual input, 171
    predefined process, 170
    process, 170
    QI toolbox techniques, 170–171
    start/end, 171
Immunity from liability, 391
Improvement opportunities, performance improvement program, 309
Improving Medicare Post-Acute Care Transformation Act (IMPACT Act), 17

Incident command structure
    emergency operations plan implementation of, 238, 240, 241
    for healthcare organization, 240, 241
Indicator, 139
Indwelling catheter status, 159
Infection prevention and control, Joint Commission accreditation standards manual, 321
Infection surveillance
    educational and screening programs, 169
    employee health and illness, 168
    facility vaccine program, 168
    food preparation areas, 169
    healthcare-associated *versus* community-acquired infections, 167–168
    healthcare environment, 168–169
Infectious disease
    case study, 177–178
    educational and screening programs, 169
    epidemiologic investigations, 167–169
    managing, 165–178
    QI toolbox techniques, 170–171
    real-life example, 171–177
    sample list of reportable diseases, 166
    standard precautions, 167
Influenza, 164
Information collection and evaluation system (ICES)
    accrediting bodies requirements, 255
    environment of care, 255
Information management, Joint Commission accreditation standards manual, 321
Information management standards, 355
Information management tools
    business intelligence, 345–351
    case study, 357–358
    comparative performance data, 352–355
    data collection, 344
    data governance, 344–345
    data repository, 346
    information resources management professionals, 355
    information warehouse, 352
    Joint Commission standards, 355–357
    routine PI report for community hospital example, 347–351
    web-based collaboration technologies, 352
Information warehouse, 352
Initiating processes, project life cycle, 362–366
Inpatient psychiatric facility quality reporting (IPFQR), 134
Institute for Safe Medication Practices (ISMP), 213
Institute of Medicine (IOM), medical errors report published by, 185–186, 207
Institutional review board, 114
Intensity of service, 139
Internal customers, 108–110, 112
Interviews, 114
    appropriate and inappropriate questions, 266
    customer satisfaction, 118
    design, 118
    point-scoring process for, 267
    recruitment process, 265–267
    stress, 266
    unstructured questions, 266

J

Joint Commission
    accreditation activities, 320–321
    accreditation decisions, 329

accreditation standards manual, 321
acute care and other facilities, 324–329
"Do Not Use" abbreviations, 210
emergency operations plan, 233
hazard vulnerability analysis, 234
information management standards, 355–357
minimum criteria for pharmacist reviews, 211
near misses investigated by, 187
NPSGs with 2024 Hospital and Nursing Care Center, 157
Juran, J. M., 14

K
Kaizen event, 54
Kotter's eight accelerators for change, 380

L
Laboratory services, evaluations of use, 155
Leadership
    Joint Commission accreditation standards manual, 321
    performance improvement activities, 294–296
    project life cycle, 365–366
Leadership group, 30–31
Lean, 33–35
Lean Six Sigma, 35
Leapfrog Group, 207
Legal implications of performance improvement
    background and significance, 388
    case study, 394
    disclosure of adverse events to patients and family, 392
    four elements of negligence or malpractice, 388–389
    immunity from liability, 391
    occurrence reports and sentinel events, 392
    organized medical staff, 390
    peer review protection, 390–391
    public health activities, 394
    research *versus* quality improvement, 393
    risk from malpractice perspective, 389–390
    tort law, 388
Length of stay (LOS), 70, 71
Lewin, Kurt, 378
Lewin's three phases of change, 378–379
Liability, immunity from, 391
Licensed independent practitioner, 269
Licensed provider, 265
Licenses, 265, 269
Licensure, 320
    case study, 340
    definition, 320
    long-term care facilities, 330–331
    multiple standards and regulations, 323
    real-life example, 333–339
    standards, 320–322
    state, 322
Life Safety Code, 245
Life safety, Joint Commission accreditation standards manual, 321
Likert scale, 74
Line chart, 74, 84, 87
Line connector icon, 171
Long-term care
    certification and licensure, 330–331
    Minimum Data Set for, 159

M
Malpractice
    defined, 388
    disclosing adverse events, 392
    four basic elements of negligence, 388–389
    peer review protection, 390–391
    risk avoidance, 389–390
Managed care, 12–13
Manual input icons, 171
Martin, Dr. Edward, 9
Mass shootings, 233
Mean *(M)*, 79–80
Median, 80
Medicaid, 11–12
    continuum of care for US, 127, 129, 131
Medical equipment management program, 219, 247–248
Medical practice, 6–7
Medical staff, Joint Commission accreditation standards manual, 321
Medicare, 11–12. *See also* Centers for Medicare and Medicaid Services
    continuum of care for US, 127–129, 131–132
    value-based purchasing program, 131–132, 134
Medicare Access and CHIP Reauthorization Act of 2015 (MACRA), 17, 18
Medication administration, five rights of, 212
Medication administration record (MAR), 212
Medication error, 195
Medication management
    case study, 217
    Joint Commission accreditation standards manual, 321
    QI toolbox techniques, 215–216
    real-life example, 216
    steps to success, 207–214
Medication management system
    administer medications, 212–213
    building safe and effective, 207–214
    evaluation of, 214
    monitor medication effects on patients, 213
    prepare and dispense medications, 211–212
    safely store medications, 209–210
    select and procure medications, 209
    transcribing medication orders, 210–211
Medication reconciliation, 207
Medication systems and processes, evaluations of, 155
Medication use, 159
Minimum Data Set (MDS), 331
    for long-term care, 159
Minutes, 96–98
    sample minutes from PI meeting, 97–98
Mission statement, 59–60, 65, 66
    project life cycle, 363
Monitoring and controlling processes, project life cycle, 369
Mood and behavior symptoms, 159
Moving, 379
Multidisciplinary accreditation and licensing, 327–328
Multiple drug-resistant organisms (MDROs), 164

N
National Committee for Quality Assurance (NCQA), 322
National Fire Protection Association (NFPA), 245
National Incident Management System (NIMS), 233
National Patient Safety Goals (NPSGs), 15–16, 187, 326
    infectious disease regulations of, 165
    Joint Commission 2024 Hospital and Nursing Care Center, 157
    patient care, 157
National Patient Safety Goals, Joint Commission accreditation standards manual, 321
National Practitioner Data Bank (NPDB), 270

National Toxicology Program (NTP), 231
Natural disasters, 233
Near misses, 187
Newborn intensive care unit (NICU), 217
Nominal data, 73
Nominal group technique, 47–48
Nursing
    Joint Commission accreditation standards
        manual, 321
    practice, 7–8

O
Occupational Safety and Health Administration (OSHA)
    blood-borne pathogen exposure, 169
    Hazard Communication Standard, 227, 231
    infectious disease protection regulations of, 164, 169
Occurrence reports, 187–195, 392
Opening conference, 325, 329, 332
Operating room (OR), 186
Operational definition, 117
Opportunity for improvement, 28
Oral and dental status, 159
Oral and nutritional status, 159
Ordinal data, 74
Organization-wide PI process, 25, 26
Outcome, 15
Outcome measure, 42, 44
Outpatient Quality Reporting (OQR) program, 133

P
Pain, 159
Pareto chart, 85–86
Park, Roswell, 8
PASS, 245
Patient advocacy, 187, 197, 203
Patient care
    blood products use, 155
    care pathways, 156
    case study, 161
    core processes, 148–153
    home healthcare monitoring, 159–160
    improvement example, 160
    integrated care pathway example, 152
    laboratory services use, 155
    long-term care, 159–160
    medication systems and processes, 155
    national standardization of care processes, 158
    NPSGs, 157
    ongoing developments, 157–160
    optimizing, 153–156
    outcomes review, 153–154
    patient-centered care initiatives, 158–159
    policy, procedure, and documentation review, 156
    process cycle, 148–153
    standards of, 156
    use of seclusion, restraints, and protective devices, 154–155
Patient-centered care, 153–154, 158–159
    principles of, 158
    staff roles in, 129
Patient-centered medical homes (PCMHs), 154
Patient rights, 182–185
Patient Safety and Quality Improvement Act of 2005, 186
Patient Safety Council, 96
Patient safety plan, PI, 297–302
Patient-specific data, 344

Pay-for-performance (P4P), 131
Peer review, 314
Peer review protection, 390–391
Perceived quality, 113
Performance assessment, 268
Performance improvement (PI)
    case study, 19
    continuous, 294
    contributions of individuals, 8–9
    healthcare institutions, 4–6
    hospital standardization and accreditation, 9–10
    Joint Commission accreditation standards manual, 321
    managed care, 12–13
    medical practice, 6–7
    Medicare and Medicaid, 11–12
    modern healthcare and, 11–14
    nursing practice, 7–8
    other health professions, 8
    patient safety plan, 297–302
    plan design, 297–305
    quality and, 18
    staff survey questions, 308
Performance improvement activities
    board of director, 311–312
    case study, 102, 316–317
    CRAF method, 97–98
    education, 314–315
    evaluating performance, 307–310
    formal quality management structures, 315
    implementing plan, 306–307
    leading, 294–296
    minutes, 96–98
    plan design, 297–305
    quarterly reports, 96, 98
    real-life example, 101–102
    report cards, 101
    standing committees of medical staff, 314
    storytelling, 96, 99–101
    strategic planning, 296
Performance improvement council, 57
Performance improvement data
    artificial intelligence, 82–83
    case study, 91–92
    data analysis, 78–89
    data collection tools, 72–77
    data display tools, 84–89
    length of stay, 70, 71
    management of data sets, 77–78
    predictive analytics, 83
    QI toolbox techniques, 84–89
    real-life example, 89–90
    statistical analysis, 79–82
    types, 73–76
Performance improvement model
    benchmark, 28, 33
    case study, 37
    continuous monitoring, 28
    as cyclical process, 24–31
    data collection, 27–30
    employee turnover rate, 28–29
    high reliability organizations, 33, 35–37
    leadership group, 30–31
    lean, 33–35
    opportunity for improvement, 28
    PDCA cycle, 24

PDSA cycle, 25
process redesign, 30–31
QI toolbox techniques, 31
real-life example, 36–37
Six Sigma, 33–35
systems analysis tools, 32
systems control tools, 32
systems thinking, 31–33
team-based process, 26, 30–31
Performance improvement program
components of, 308–310
effectiveness and recommendations section, 310
evaluating, 307–310
executive summary section of, 309
improvement opportunities, 309
key questions to evaluate, 310
overview, 309
PI structure, 309
PI team activities, 310
Performance improvement projects
case study, 373
project life cycle, 362–369
project management and organizational structure, 362
real-life example, 371–373
why projects fail, 370–371
Performance improvement team
charters, 57–59
composition of, 54–55
cross-functional, 54–55
functional, 54
ground rules for meetings, 61–62
mission, vision, and values statements, 59–60
people issues, 63–64
problem-solving, listening, and questioning, 62–63
QI toolbox technique, 64–65
roles, 55–57
Performance improvement (PI) team, 30–31
Performance measurement
customers for monitored process in, 45
day surgery registration example, 48–49
definition, 42
DNFB rate case, 50
identifying, 43–45
improvement builds on continuous monitoring for, 43–46
QI toolbox techniques for, 47–48
real-life example, 48–50
steps in, 43–46
Performance measures, 27–28, 43
PERT charts, project life cycle, 366–368
Pharmacy and therapeutics (P and T) committee, 213–214
Physical and chemical characteristics, 231
Physical attacks, 226
Physician quality reporting system (PQRS), 133–134
Pie chart, 74, 86, 90
Pisacano, Nicholas J., 8
Pivot table, 86
Plan design, performance improvement activities, 297–305
Plan, do, check, act (PDCA), 24
Plan, do, study, act (PDSA), 25
Planning phase, project life cycle
design phase, 366
Gantt chart, 366–367
PERT chart, 366–368
Planning processes, project life cycle, 366–368
Pneumonia, 164

Position requisition, 263–265
Postdischarge planning, 138
Posttraining assessment tool, 256
Potentially compensable events (PCEs), 186, 195, 203
PPS-exempt cancer hospital quality reporting (PCHQR), 134
Preadmission care planning, 136
Predefined process icons, 170
Predictive analytics, 83
Pressure ulcer, 159
Pritchett, Henry S., 7
Privilege, 391
Privileged information, 391
Process, 10, 14
Process cycle, project life cycle, 364
Process icons, 170
Process measure, 43–44
Process redesign, 30–31
Progress note, sample, 196
Project life cycle
closing processes, 369
design phase, 366
execution processes, 368–369
Gantt charts, 366
initiating processes, 362–366
leadership, 365–366
mission statement, 363
monitoring and controlling processes, 369
PERT charts, 366–368
phases and processes, 363–364
planning processes, 366–368
process cycle, 364
sponsorship, 363
team development stages, 365
team group dynamics, 364–365
team member selection, 363
Prospective payment system, 12
Protection, 390–391
Provider index summary, 276–286
Provider profile, 273–275, 287–288
Provision of care, treatment, and services
blood products use, 155
care pathways, 156
case study, 161
core processes, 148–153
home healthcare monitoring, 159–160
improvement example, 160
integrated care pathway example, 152
Joint Commission accreditation standards manual, 321
laboratory services use, 155
long-term care, 159–160
medication systems and processes, 155
national standardization of care processes, 158
NPSGs, 157
ongoing developments, 157–160
optimizing, 153–156
outcomes review, 153–154
patient-centered care initiatives, 158–159
policy, procedure, and documentation review, 156
process cycle, 148–156
safety, 157
standards of, 156
use of seclusion, restraints, and protective devices, 154–155

Psychosocial well-being, 159
Public information officer (PIO), 372

Q
QI toolbox techniques, 31
   affinity diagrams, 47
   agenda, 57, 61, 64–65
   brainstorming, 47
   cause-and-effect diagram, 199–200
   continuum of care, 139
   customer satisfaction, 115–118
   environment of care, 256
   failure mode and effects analysis, 214–216
   flow charts, 170–171
   icons, 170–171
   indicator, 139
   infectious disease, 170–171
   medication management, 215–216
   nominal group technique, 47–48
   performance improvement data, 84–89
   performance improvement team, 64–65
   for performance measurement, 47–48
   posttraining assessment tool, 256
   report cards, 101
   risk exposure, 198–201
   root-cause analysis, 200–201
   staff and human resources, 271
Quality
   data, 78–79
   definition of, 4
   in healthcare, 14–18
   measures and satisfaction scales, 113–114
   performance improvement and, 18
Quality assurance (QA), 11, 18
Quality improvement in healthcare
   case study, 19
   contributions of individuals, 8–9
   healthcare institutions, 4–6
   hospital standardization and accreditation, 9–10
   medical practice, 6–7
   nursing practice, 7–8
   other health professions, 8
Quality improvement organizations (QIOs), 322
Quality Indicator Survey (QIS), 331
Quality Payment Program (QPP), 133–134
Quarterly reports, 96, 98

R
RACE, 245
Rapid improvement event, 54
Ratio, 139
Record of care, treatment, and services, Joint Commission accreditation standards manual, 321
Recruitment process, staff and human resources, 263–267
Regulatory information, 231
Relative frequency, 76
Reliability, 112
Report cards, 101
Research, 393
Research studies
   definition, 393
   distinguishing from quality improvement initiatives, 393
Responsiveness, 112
Retention process, staff and human resources, 268–269
Retrospective payment system, 12

Return-to-community referral, 159
Right-to-Know Law, 227
Risk, 185–186
Risk exposure
   case study, 202
   managing, 181–202
   QI toolbox techniques, 198–201
   sample occurrence report, 189–194
   sample progress note, 196
   skilled nursing facility rights, 185
   steps to manage, 186–187
Risk management plan, policies, and procedures, 188
Risk management team, 187
   communication to legal support, 197
   development of insurance strategy, 198
   occurrence reports, 188–195
   patient advocacy function, 197
   practice patterns, trends in risk occurrences, and sentinel events, 195, 197
   structure, process, and knowledge issues, 195
   teaching risk management concepts, 188
Risk manager, 186–188, 195, 197
Root-cause analysis (RCA), 187, 199–201

S
Safety data sheets (SDSs), 227
Safety management program, 219, 221
Sample position requisition, 264
Sampling, 72
Scatter diagram, 88–89
Security management program, 219, 221–227
Security risk assessment, 228–230
Sentinel events, 44, 392
Severe acute respiratory syndrome (SARS), 164
Severity of illness, 139
Site visit, 324, 329–331
Six Sigma, 33–34
   CTP, 34
   CTQ, 34
   lean, 35
Skewing, 80
Skilled nursing facility rights, 185
Skilled nursing facility value-based purchasing program (SNF VBP), 134
Smallpox, 164
SMART goal, 42–43
Smoking policy management, 221
Social determinants of health (SDOH), 17–18
Social Security Act of 1935, 11
Sponsorship, project life cycle, 363
Stability and reactivity, 231
Staff and human resources
   case study, 273–288
   credential and extend privileges, 269–271
   development, 263–271
   Joint Commission accreditation standards manual, 321
   key leadership functions, 262
   new employees, onboarding of, 267
   performance appraisal process, 268
   QI toolbox techniques, 271
   real-life example, 272
   recruitment process, 263–267
   retention process, 268–269
   steps to success, 263–271

Standard deviation *(SD)*, 80–82
Standardization
    patient care processes, 158
    performance improvement with accreditation and, 9–10
Standard precautions, 167
Standards of care, 156
Standing committees of medical staff, 314
Start/end icons, 171
Statistical analysis
    mean, 79–80
    median, 80
    normal distribution, 81–82
    standard deviation, 80–82
Storytelling, 96, 99–101
    benefits of, 100–101
    key elements, 99
    methods of, 99–100
Stranger violence, 227
Strategic plan, 303
    defined, 295–296
    performance improvement activities, 296
    PI opportunities in document of, 303–304
Stress interview, 266
Structure, 8, 14
Survey design, 115–117
Survey process, 323–329
Survey team, 324–325, 329
Survey tools, 114
Suspicious package/substance, 234, 237
Swine flu, 164
SWOT analysis, 296
Systems, 42, 43
Systems analysis tools, 32
Systems control tools, 32–33
Systems thinking, 31–33

T
Team-based process, PI, 26, 30–31
Team charter, 57–59, 65, 66
Team development stages, project life cycle, 365
Team facilitator, 56
Team group dynamics, project life cycle, 364–365
Team leader, 5, 55, 62, 66
Team member, 55–58, 61–66
Team member selection, project life cycle, 363
Team recorder, 56–57
Teamwork
    action plan in, 56, 66
    agenda in, 57, 61, 64–65
    case study, 67
    cross-functional PI team in, 54
    functional PI team in, 54
    ground rules in, 61–62
    mission statement in, 65, 66
    performance improvement council in, 57
    rapid improvement event in, 54
    real-life example, 65–66
    timekeeper in, 57, 61
    values statement in, 59–60
    vision statement in, 59–60, 65, 66
Terrorist activity, 233
Threatening behavior, 226
Timekeeper, 57, 61
To Err is Human: Building a Safer Health System (IOM), 185, 207
Tort law, 388
Total quality management (TQM), 14
Toxicological information, 231
Tracer methodology, 325, 329
Training platform, 269
Transfusion reaction, 155
Transplant safety, Joint Commission accreditation standards manual, 321
Transport information, 231
Triggers, 328
Tuberculosis, 164

U
Unfreezing, 379
Urinary incontinence, 159
US quality measurement organizations guide, 353–354
Utilities management program, 219, 248–253
Utilization review (UR), 128, 136, 142–143

V
Value-based purchasing (VBP) program, 13, 15, 131–132, 134
Values statement, 59–60
Verbal abuse, 226
Verbal or written threats, 226
Vision function, 159
Vision statement, 59–60, 65, 66
Voluntary reviews, 320

W
Waived testing, 321
Waste management program, 219, 227–233
Worker Right-to-Know legislation, 227
Workplace violence, 226–227
Written implementation program, 231

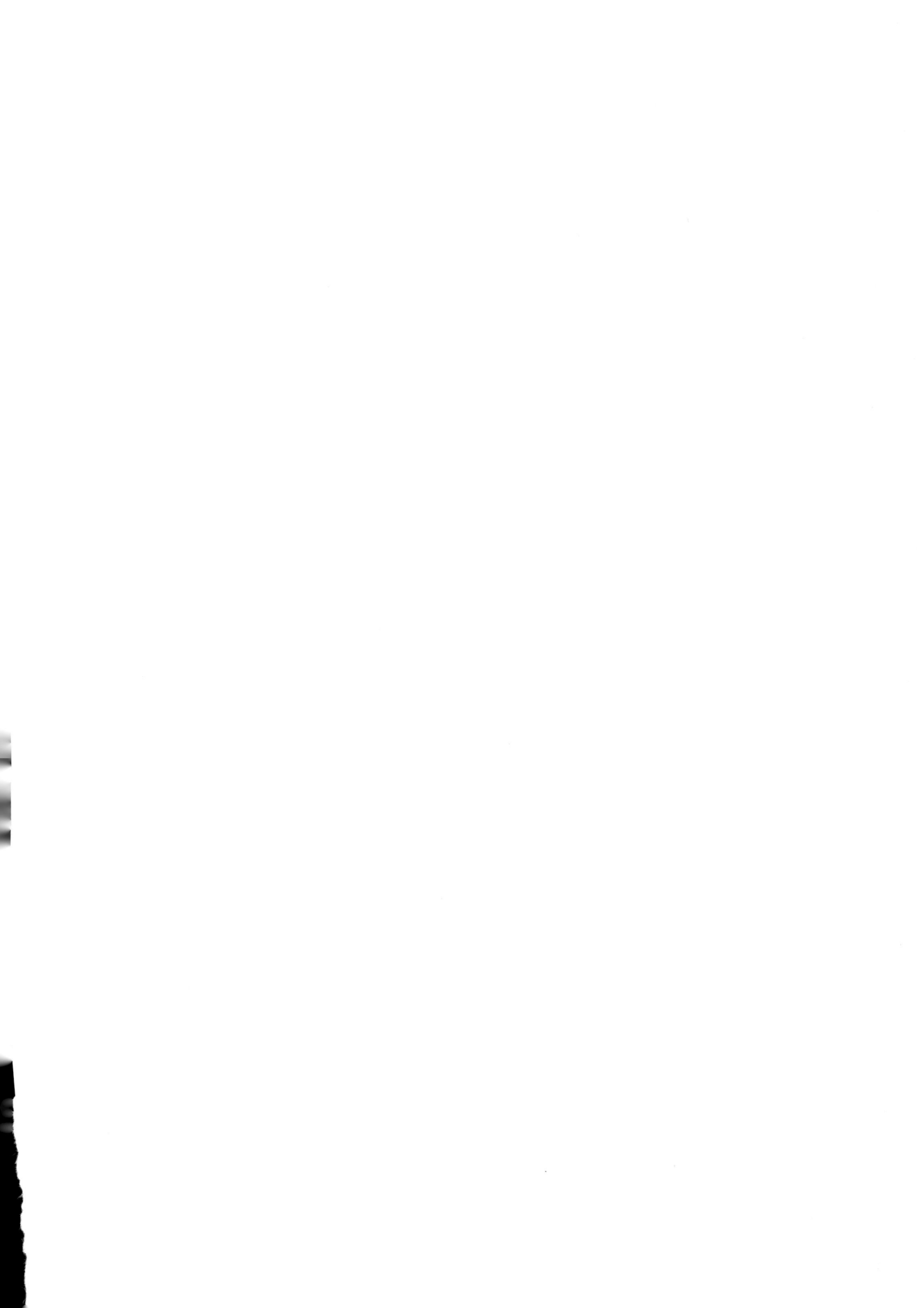